Differential Diagnosis of Common Complaints

ROBERT H. SELLER, M.D.
Professor of Family Medicine and Professor of Medicine
State University of New York at Buffalo
School of Medicine and Biomedical Sciences

Differential Diagnosis of Common Complaints

FOURTH EDITION

W.B. SAUNDERS COMPANY
A Division of Harcourt Brace & Company
Philadelphia London Toronto Montreal Sydney Tokyo

W.B. SAUNDERS COMPANY
A Division of Harcourt Brace & Company

The Curtis Center
Independence Square West
Philadelphia, Pennsylvania 19106

Library of Congress Cataloging-in-Publication Data

Seller, Robert H.
Differential diagnosis of common complaints / Robert H. Seller.—
4th ed.

p. cm.

Includes bibliographical references and index.

ISBN 0-7216-8017-8

1. Diagnosis, Differential. I. Title.
[DNLM: 1. Diagnosis,
Differential. WB 141.5 S467d 2000]

RC71.5.S45 2000 616.07′5—dc21

DNLM/DLC 99-27918

DIFFERENTIAL DIAGNOSIS OF COMMON COMPLAINTS ISBN 0–7216–8017–8

Printed in the United States of America

Last digit is the print number: 9 8 7 6 5 4 3 2 1

To the medical students,
physicians, and other health care providers
of the 21st century

NOTICE

Preface

The purpose of the fourth edition of *Differential Diagnosis of Common Complaints* remains the same as the first—to help physicians accurately and efficiently diagnose common complaints. This book emphasizes a clinical approach to diagnosis rather than one that relies largely on diagnostic studies. Most medical school curricula, texts, and continuing education courses deal with diseases. Patients, however, usually come to their physician complaining of headache, backache, or fatigue—not migraine, spinal stenosis, or depression. To address this reality, this book is organized around common presenting complaints—the patients' symptoms rather than the disease. The 36 symptoms reviewed account for more than 80% of the chief complaints with which physicians are confronted. The physician who has mastered the differential diagnosis of these symptoms will be able to diagnose accurately almost all the problems seen in a typical medical practice.

Each chapter deals with different common complaints, which are discussed alphabetically. The chapters are organized to approximate the problem-solving process that most physicians use to make a diagnosis. Initially, the presenting symptom suggests several diagnostic possibilities. Then this diagnostic list is further defined and reduced by additional, more specific, historic findings; by the patient's physical findings; and then by the results of diagnostic studies. The index lists all complaints, symptoms, and diagnoses in the text.

The fourth edition was revised to include suggestions by colleagues and students who like the book's clinical orientation and practical approach to differential diagnosis. Each chapter has been revised to include new information with emphasis on the latest clinical and diagnostic studies. Since the last edition, five new chapters have been added: Breast Lumps, Forgetfulness, Swelling of the Legs, Vision Problems, and Voiding Disorders and Incontinence. The diagrams and illustrations for the chapter on pain in the upper and lower extremities and skin problems have been extensively revised.

The text does not deal extensively with pathophysiology or therapy except in situations in which this information is particularly useful in the diagnostic process. The most useful diagnostic studies for differential diagnosis are reviewed. The text concentrates on the most likely diagnoses and common illnesses that include many serious illnesses. It also notes when the physician must rule out extremely serious diagnostic possibilities.

The format of each chapter has remained the same:

Introduction. Includes relevant definitions, as well as a list of the most common causes of the symptoms.

Nature of patient. Identifies those conditions that are most prevalent within a particular subgroup (e.g., children, elderly, premenopausal, diabetic, hypertensive, immunocompromised).

Nature of symptoms. Further identifies conditions by amplifying additional characteristics of the symptoms (how, when, where, radiation, acute/chronic, and so on).

Associated symptoms.

Precipitating and aggravating factors.

Ameliorating factors.

Physical findings.

Diagnostic studies.

Less common diagnostic considerations.

Differential diagnosis table. A concise table located at the end of each chapter summarizes the salient differential diagnostic features of the most common clinical entities that cause a particular complaint.

Selected references. Most articles represent an approach to differential diagnosis of problems rather than a review of a specific disease.

Clinicians and students may use this book for general information about the many causes of common chief complaints. They can also use it as a reference text when treating a patient who has a specific symptom (e.g., facial pain, shortness of breath, fever) when the diagnosis is not apparent.

Differential Diagnosis of Common Complaints was written to be useful. I hope you find it so . . . remember the adage, "If you don't think about it, you will never diagnose it."

Robert H. Seller

Acknowledgments

Carolyn Doueck, CGF Health Sciences Libraries, provided invaluable assistance with the literature reviews. I wish to thank my faculty colleagues at the State University of New York at Buffalo School of Medicine for reviewing each chapter.

I also wish to thank two editors at W.B. Saunders Company:

Lisette Bralow (Editor-In-Chief, Medical Books), who as acquisitions editor saw the potential of what became the first edition of this book, and

Raymond Kersey (Senior Editor), who encouraged me to write the subsequent editions.

Contents

Differential Diagnosis of Common Complaints

CHAPTER 1

Abdominal Pain in Adults

The most common causes of abdominal pain are discussed here, with special attention given to the acute abdomen and recurrent abdominal pain. The term *acute abdomen* is medical jargon that refers to any acute condition within the abdomen that requires immediate surgical attention. Acute abdominal pain may be of nonabdominal origin and does not always require surgery. The majority of patients who consult a physician for abdominal pain do not have an acute abdomen, although their chief complaint may be a sudden or acute onset of abdominal pain. In studies involving analysis of large series of patients presenting to emergency rooms with acute abdominal pain, nonspecific abdominal pain (NSAP) was the most common diagnosis. Most patients with this symptom probably have gastroenteritis.

The common causes of abdominal pain include *gastroenteritis, gastritis, peptic ulcer disease, reflux esophagitis, irritable bowel syndrome, dysmenorrhea, salpingitis, appendicitis, cholecystitis, cholelithiasis, intestinal obstruction, mesenteric adenitis, diverticulitis, pancreatitis, ureterolithiasis, incarcerated hernias, gas entrapment syndromes,* and *ischemic bowel disease* (particularly in the elderly). All these conditions can present with an acute or sudden onset of abdominal pain, many can cause recurrent abdominal pain, and a few require surgical intervention. Any acute abdominal condition requires the physician to make an early, precise diagnosis, since prognosis often depends on prompt initiation of therapy, particularly surgical treatment. The more serious the problem, the more urgent is the need for an accurate diagnosis.

The examiner can best establish a complete and accurate diagnosis by carefully noting the patient's age, gender, and past medical history; precipitating factors; location of the pain and of radiated discomfort; associated vomiting; altered bowel habits; chills and fever; and findings of the physical examination, particularly of the abdomen. **Abdominal pain without other symptoms or signs is rarely a serious problem.**

The physician must be especially aware of the conditions that cause abdominal pain and that usually require surgical intervention. According to one large study, the most common conditions requiring surgical intervention are *appendicitis, cholecystitis,* and *perforated peptic ulcer.* Others include *acute intestinal obstruction, torsion* or *perforation of a viscus, ovarian torsion, tumors, ectopic pregnancy, dissecting* or *ruptured aneurysms, mesenteric occlusion, bowel embolization,* and *bowel infarction.*

Several authors warn against the practice of "pattern matching" in the diagnosis of acute abdominal surgical conditions; they have found that typical findings occur in only 60% to 70% of patients. This means that if physicians attempt to match acute problems with patterns or stereotypes of the disease, they will fail to make the correct diagnosis in 30% to 40% of cases. Therefore, to improve diagnostic accuracy, physicians must know the standard and typical presentations and must also be aware of the subtleties involved in the differential diagnosis. The "best test" method is more accurate than "pattern matching" in establishing the diagnosis.

The "best test" method involves elicitation of specific information that correlates well with the correct diagnosis. This method suggests that when a specific symptom or physical sign is noted, its presence is highly useful in establishing the correct diagnosis. For instance, the finding of pain in the right upper quadrant (RUQ) most frequently suggests *cholecystitis.* Likewise, if pain is aggravated by movement, it most frequently indicates *appendicitis* but also suggests *perforated peptic ulcer* to a lesser degree. A "best test" question used to differentiate the most common causes of abdominal pain—NSAP and appendicitis—is whether the pain is aggravated by coughing or movement. The pain of appendicitis is aggravated by movement or coughing, whereas the pain of NSAP is not. Abdominal pain that is aggravated by movement or coughing is probably caused by peritoneal inflammation. "Best test" signs that are helpful in differential diagnosis include the presence of a *palpable mass* in diverticular disease, *hyperactive bowel sounds* in small bowel obstruction, *reduced bowel sounds* in perforation, and *involuntary guarding* in the right lower quadrant (RLQ) with appendicitis. The validity of "best test" findings has been supported by retrospective studies in which the diagnosis is known.

Nature of Patient

In elderly patients, it is often difficult for the physician to elicit an accurate description of the nature of the pain. These patients may be unable to distinguish new symptoms from preexisting complaints and concomitant illnesses. Many present late in their illnesses, often after treating themselves for indigestion or constipation. In contrast to the high frequency of appendicitis, cholecystitis, and perforated ulcers in most general surgical series, the most common causes of acute surgical abdomen in patients over 70 years of age are *strangulated hernias* (45%) and other forms of *intestinal obstruction* (25%).

The physician must remember that cancer is a common cause of abdominal pain in the elderly. In a study of patients over age 50 with NSAP, 10% had cancer. The majority of these patients with cancer had large bowel cancer. *Colonic cancer* is almost as common as perforated peptic ulcer, pancreatitis, and renal colic in patients over age 50. Cancer should be strongly suspected if the patient is older than 50 years and has had previous bouts of unexplained abdominal pain, if the present abdominal pain has lasted at least 4 days, and if constipation is present.

Elderly patients also have a higher frequency of uncommon causes of surgical abdomen, including *ruptured aortic aneurysm, acute mesenteric infarction,* and *inflammatory diverticular disease.*

The person's age also offers clues to diagnosis in other groups of patients. *Appendicitis* has its peak incidence in the second decade, although it can occur in patients older than 60 years as well as in infants. The incidence of *cholecystitis* increases with age and is the most frequent cause of acute abdominal pain in patients over 50.

Cholecystitis is more common in whites than in blacks, more prevalent in females than in males, and more common in women who take oral contraceptives or estrogens than in those who do not. Drugs that increase cholesterol saturation also increase the incidence of *cholelithiasis.* They include clofibrate (Atromid-S), conjugated estrogens, and estrogen-progestin combinations.

Nonspecific abdominal pain is an imprecise diagnosis, yet it is the most common diagnosis given to patients presenting to an emergency room with abdominal pain as their chief complaint. This diagnosis is most common in patients under the age of 40 years.

Irritable colon seems to be most common in young women, particularly those who have young children. This frequency has been attributed to the life pressures to which these women are subjected. Symptoms of irritable colon are also more frequent in others under stress, including children. The abdominal pain from an irritable colon may be a vague discomfort or pain in the lower left quadrant (LLQ), RLQ, or midabdomen. It occasionally radiates to the back. This pain may be relieved by defecation and may be associated with other well-recognized symptoms of irritable colon—mucus in the stool, constipation alternating with diarrhea, and small, marble-like stools.

Lower abdominal or pelvic pain in women is often difficult to evaluate. *Ectopic pregnancy, ovarian torsion, ruptured ovarian cyst, pelvic inflammatory disease, endometriosis,* and *mittelschmerz* must always be kept in mind. Surgical emergencies of gynecologic origin are more common in women of reproductive age and include *pelvic inflammatory disease with abscess, ectopic pregnancy, hemorrhage from an ovarian cyst,* and *adnexal* or *ovarian torsion.*

Peptic ulcer pain is most common between ages 30 and 50 years but may occur in teenagers and, rarely, in young children. It is considerably more common in men than in women. This diagnosis should not be entirely disregarded in women, however, because a significant incidence of perforated peptic ulcer among them may be a result of the physician's failure to consider peptic ulcer in the diagnosis. Although only 15% of patients with ulcer symptoms are older than 60 years, 80% of deaths from ulcers occur in this group, since ulcer disease in elderly patients is more likely to run a virulent course.

Acute intestinal obstruction occurs in all age groups. In the elderly, intestinal obstruction is usually caused by *strangulated hernias* or *cancer.* In any patient with severe abdominal pain and a history of abdominal surgery, however, adhesions are the most likely cause of intestinal obstruction.

Pancreatitis occurs most frequently in alcoholic patients and those with gallstones. *Sigmoid volvulus* is more common in males, mentally handicapped patients, and those with parkinsonism; *cecal volvulus* is more common in females. *Gallstone ileus* causes small bowel obstruction more often in the elderly and in women. *Mesenteric adenitis* is more common in children. *Peptic esophagitis* is more common in obese patients. The incidence of *diverticulitis* increases with age; this disorder is more common after age 60.

Nature of Pain

Classically, *biliary colic* develops in the evening and usually is a steady midepigastric or RUQ pain. Colicky or crampy pain that begins in the midabdomen and progresses to a constant pain in the RLQ suggests *appendicitis.* Other conditions that may begin in a crampy or colicky manner and progress to a more constant pain include *cholelithiasis* and *cholecystitis* (which tend to localize in the RUQ), *intestinal obstruction,* and *ureterolithiasis* (which involves excruciating pain that frequently radiates to the groin, testes, or medial thigh).

A constant, often annoying burning or gnawing pain located in the midepigastrium and occasionally associated with posterior radiation is seen with *peptic ulcer.* Peptic ulcer pain may be worse at night, although this is unusual. It is not ordinarily made worse by recumbency. The pain of peptic ulcer in elderly patients may be vague and poorly localized. Because of a lack of classic symptoms, an occasional absence of prior symptoms, and a confusing picture of abdominal pain, perforation associated with peritonitis is more common in older patients. It is particularly important to note that pain induced by percussion in the epigastrium may be the only physical finding to suggest ulcer disease in a person complaining of typical peptic ulcer pain. Likewise, severe exacerbation of pain that occurs when the physician percusses over the RUQ strongly suggests the presence of an *inflamed gallbladder.*

The diagnosis of abdominal pain caused by an *irritable colon* is fairly easy to make: the pain is usually dull, crampy, and recurrent. It is often associated with constipation that alternates with diarrhea, small stools, and mucus in the stools. In addition, moderate pain may be elicited when the physician palpates the colon. In elderly patients, however, severe diverticulitis may exist with similar symptoms.

Most abdominal pain, even when severe, usually develops over several hours. When the onset of severe abdominal pain is abrupt, it suggests *perforation, strangulation, torsion, dissecting aneurysms,* or *ureterolithiasis.* The most severe abdominal pain occurs with dissecting aneurysms and with ureterolithiasis. The pain of a dissecting aneurysm is often described as a "tearing" or "ripping" sensation and often radiates into the legs and through to the back. Patients with such pain usually present in profound shock. Individuals with the excruciating pain of ureterolithiasis may be writhing in agony but do not experience cardiovascular collapse. This pain is usually unilateral in the flank, groin, or testicle and is often associated with nausea and occasional vomiting.

Location of Pain

The location of the pain is one of the "best tests" for determination of a diagnosis (Fig. 1–1). RUQ pain is most frequently seen in *cholecystitis, cholelithiasis,* and leaking *duodenal ulcer* (Fig. 1–2). Another clue to gallbladder disease is the radiation of RUQ pain to the inferior angle of the right scapula. RUQ pain is also seen in patients with *hepatitis* or *congestive heart failure.* In the latter group the pain is thought to be caused by swelling of the liver that results in distention of

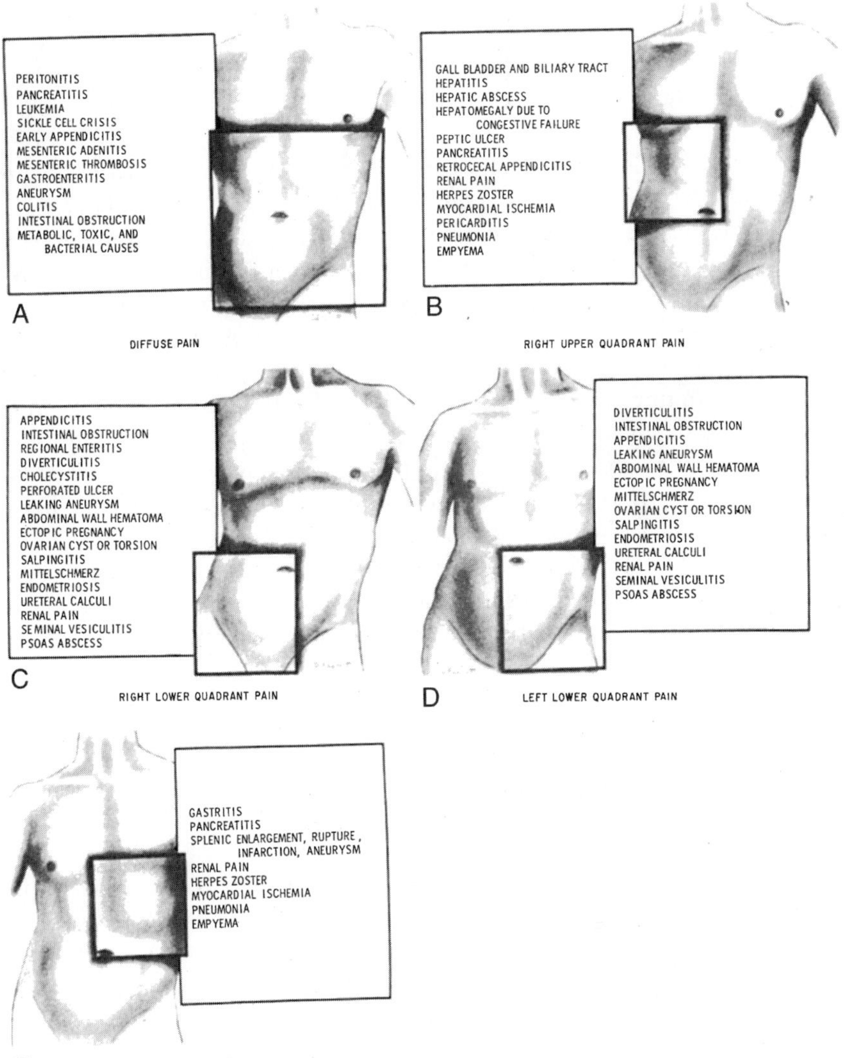

■ **Figure 1.1** Characteristic location of abdominal pain associated with various diseases. (From Schwartz S: Principles of Surgery, 2nd ed. New York, McGraw-Hill, 1974, p 972.)

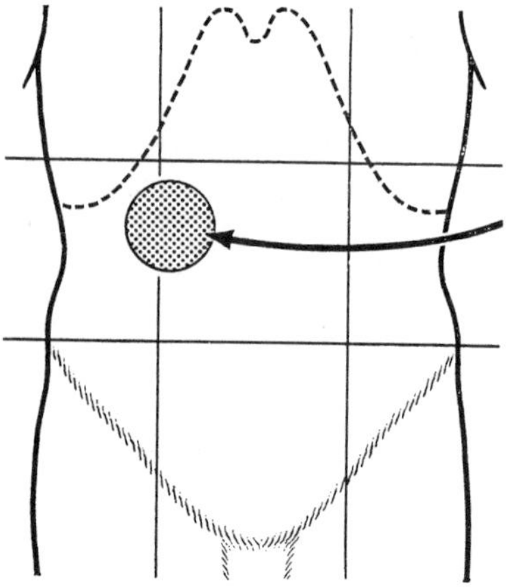

■ **Figure 1.2** Tenderness and rigidity in right hypochondrium. (From Cope Z: Early Diagnosis of the Acute Abdomen, 13th ed. London, Oxford University Press, 1968, p 43.)

Glisson's capsule. Less severe RUQ pain may be seen in patients with a *hepatic flexure syndrome* (gas entrapment in the hepatic flexure of the colon). If questioned carefully, these patients will admit to experiencing relief with the passage of flatus.

A gnawing, burning, midabdominal to upper abdominal pain suggests a condition with a peptic etiology—*ulcer, gastritis,* or *esophagitis.* Burning epigastric pain that radiates to the jaw is frequently seen in patients with peptic esophagitis. Severe upper abdominal pain that radiates into the back and is associated with nausea and vomiting suggests *pancreatitis.* Typically, this pain is worse when the patient is lying down and improves with leaning forward.

Left upper quadrant (LUQ) pain is most frequently seen in patients with *gastroenteritis* or *irritable colon* and less often in those with splenic flexure syndrome, splenic infarction, or pancreatitis. The pain from splenic flexure syndrome can be located in the LUQ or in the chest; therefore, it is also part of the differential diagnosis of chest pain. These pains tend to arise when the individual is bending over or wearing a tight garment, and they frequently are relieved by the passage of flatus.

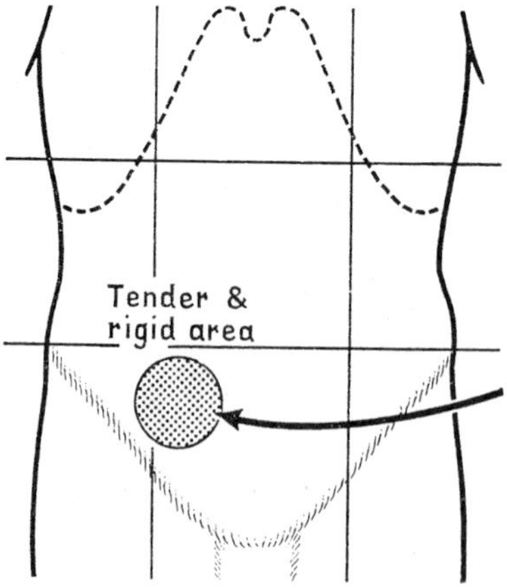

■ **Figure 1.3** Tenderness and rigidity in right iliac region. (From Cope Z: Early Diagnosis of the Acute Abdomen, 13th ed. London, Oxford University Press, 1968, p 45.)

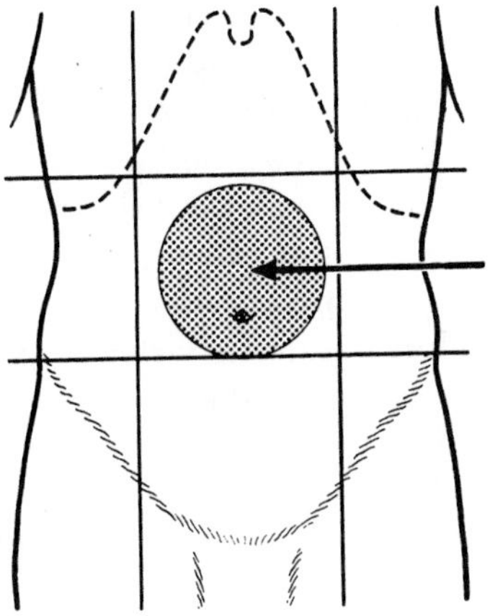

■ **Figure 1.4** Acute central abdominal pain without any other symptom. (From Cope Z: Early Diagnosis of the Acute Abdomen, 13th ed. London, Oxford University Press, 1968, p 38.)

Other causes of both RUQ and LUQ pain include supradiaphragmatic conditions with inflammation of the diaphragm, such as pneumonia, pulmonary embolism, pleurisy, and pericarditis.

RLQ pain is most often seen with *muscle strain, appendicitis, salpingitis,* and *diverticulitis* (Fig. 1–3). Diverticulitis pain, however, is more common in the LLQ. Less common causes of RLQ pain include ileitis, pyelonephritis, obturator hernia, carcinoma of the cecum, and colonic obstruction in patients with a competent ileocecal valve.

Other causes of RLQ or LLQ pain include *ureterolithiasis, salpingitis, ruptured ovarian cyst, ovarian torsion, ectopic pregnancy,* and *obturator hernia.* The pain of salpingitis usually is unilateral, although it may present bilaterally.

LLQ pain suggests *irritable colon* and *diverticulitis.*

Common causes of central abdominal pain include early *appendicitis, small bowel obstruction, gastritis,* and *colic* (Fig. 1–4).

Associated Symptoms

The abdominal pain seen with a truly *acute abdomen* is usually of such severity that patients overlook any associated symptoms they might have. Thus, it can be said that any additional complaint (e.g., headache) contradicts the diagnosis of an acute abdomen.

The timing of vomiting in relation to the onset of abdominal pain and associated symptoms may help the physician establish a precise diagnosis. The earlier the vomiting occurs in relation to the onset of abdominal pain, the less the abdominal distention. Patients with lower intestinal obstruction experience less vomiting and greater distention. Vomiting that precedes the onset of pain reduces the probability of an acute abdomen. Vomiting that begins after the onset of pain is more consistent with the diagnosis of an acute abdomen and frequently is seen in patients with *appendicitis.* The absence of vomiting, however, does not preclude the diagnosis of an acute abdomen.

If vomiting occurs soon after the onset of pain and the vomitus is light in color, the vomitus probably consists of digestive juices and bile; this suggests *gastritis, cholecystitis,* or *obstruction.*

Jaundice, dark urine, and light to acholic stools may be seen in patients with abdominal pain caused by *cholecystitis.* These symptoms suggest an obstructive etiology of the jaundice, and complete biliary obstruction should be suspected. **A history of occasional silver-colored stools alternating with normal or light-colored stools is virtually pathognomonic of *carcinoma of the ampulla of Vater.*** The production of silver-colored stools is a result of upper gastrointestinal blood from the ampullary carcinoma mixing with acholic stools.

Examination of vomitus from patients with acute abdominal obstruction may provide a clue to the location of the obstruction. Undigested food in the vomitus suggests that the obstruction is proximal to the stomach; this may result from *achalasia* or *peptic esophagitis.* Occasionally, undigested food may be seen in vomitus from patients with *pyloric obstruction.* This diagnosis is most likely if the vomiting persists and does not contain bile.

Brown vomitus with a fecal odor suggests mechanical or paralytic *bowel obstruction.* The more proximal the obstruction, the more frequent is the vomiting.

Constipation with small, dry stools—sometimes alternating with diarrhea or mucus in the stool—is frequently seen in patients experiencing increasing stress and suggests an *irritable colon.*

Precipitating and Aggravating Factors

The pain of *appendicitis* is aggravated by motion or coughing, as is the pain of *peritonitis,* regardless of its cause. The pain of *gastritis* is worsened by most foods, particularly alcoholic beverages. *Peptic ulcer* pain usually begins an hour or so after eating and is generally relieved by eating. If epigastric pain occurs primarily or is worsened in the recumbent position, *peptic esophagitis* should be suspected.

The pain of *salpingitis* and *endometriosis* is often worse during or before menstruation. Although patients may find that this pain is not exacerbated by limited movement in bed, more strenuous activity such as descending a flight of stairs will frequently increase the severity of the discomfort. The symptoms of NSAP are precipitated and exacerbated by problems in the individual's environment. They may also be part of a long-term psychiatric illness.

Ameliorating Factors

If the patient experiences relief after eating or taking antacids, *peptic ulcer* or *peptic esophagitis* is the probable cause of pain. The pain of *gastritis,* although worsened by the ingestion of food and alcoholic beverages, may be relieved by antacids. The pain of peptic esophagitis is often lessened when the patient is in an upright posture.

Pain relieved by defecation or the passage of flatus suggests an *irritable colon* or *gas entrapment* in the large bowel, whereas pain relieved by belching suggests *gaseous distention* of the stomach or esophagus. The pain of *gastroenteritis* is occasionally relieved by vomiting or diarrhea. Pelvic pain relieved by urination and associated with urinary frequency and dyspareunia suggests *interstitial cystitis,* which occurs most frequently in young women.

Physical Findings

Physical examination of the abdomen in patients with abdominal pain should include inspection, auscultation, palpation, and percussion as well as rectal and pelvic examinations. The physical examination should begin with inspection of the abdomen, with the physician standing at the foot of the patient's bed. This part of the examination often can provide major clues to the diagnosis because it allows the physician to note distention, abnormal pulsations, and abdominal movement with respiration. The second part of the examination should always consist of auscultation; it is preferable for the physician to listen to bowel sounds before beginning a manual investigation. When palpating the abdomen and vaginal area, the physician should be particularly attentive to lymph node enlargements or hernias and to the quality of femoral pulses.

Specific physical findings in appendicitis, cholecystitis, diverticulitis, and bowel perforation or infarction vary with the disease. If peritonitis is present, however, certain physical findings are common, regardless of the disease. The pain of peritonitis is severe, generalized, continuous, and of acute or gradual onset. The patient usually has abdominal tenderness with guarding, stabbing pain with gentle coughing, and pain on percussion. Abdominal rigidity occasionally is present. Decreased movement of the abdominal wall occurs with respiration. If rebound pain is present, it usually is found over the area of primary disease. Patients with peritonitis often are in shock, have fever or chills, and present with decreased or absent bowel sounds. The patient usually lies relatively motionless because movement aggravates the pain. Depending on the severity of the peritonitis and the prior cardiovascular status of the patient, hypotension, tachycardia, pallor, and sweating may also be present. Younger, healthier patients are relatively resistant to hypotension but easily develop tachycardia. In contrast, elderly patients with a decreased cardiovascular reserve more readily become hypotensive. The presence of cardiac disease may impair the development of tachycardia.

Appendicitis

Patients with acute appendicitis almost always have tenderness over the inflamed appendix, often with involuntary guarding as well as rebound tenderness over McBurney's point. Classically, a disproportionate rise in the pulse rate occurs with respect to the degree of fever.

Cholecystitis

Guarding in the RUQ and tenderness to palpation and percussion suggest cholecystitis. When gallbladder disease is suspected in patients with RUQ pain, the examiner should begin palpation very gently in other parts of the abdomen and end gently over the gallbladder. The goal of this careful palpation is detection of an enlarged (hydrops) gallbladder. An enlarged gallbladder may not be detected by deep palpation or percussion, since such aggressive examination may result in involuntary guarding, which prevents detection of the enlarged gallbladder. In all patients with abdominal pain, the physician should begin palpation away from the painful area and gradually move toward palpation over the most painful spot.

Peptic Ulcer

Patients with symptoms of peptic ulcer disease may show no abnormal physical findings except pain to gentle percussion over the midepigastrium or duodenal sweep. When peritonitis develops in patients with peptic ulcer disease, it is secondary to perforation of the involved viscus. If the viscus perforates anteriorly, extreme rigidity of the abdominal wall results. If the viscus penetrates posteriorly, back pain is a major symptom, and the symptoms of peritonitis are minimal. In the early stages of a penetrating or perforated peptic ulcer, bowel sounds may be increased or normal, but as the condition progresses, bowel sounds become diminished or absent.

Intestinal Obstruction

Auscultation of the abdomen may help the physician to diagnose obstruction. Classically, rushes of high-pitched, tinkling peristalsis are heard. These rushes are often associated with recurring crampy, colicky pain. The physician must listen for a succussion splash in all patients who complain of vomiting. This examination requires the examiner to place the stethoscope over the stomach and to shake the abdomen gently. A succussion splash may be heard over a stomach that is dilated or distended with air and fluid. This finding is normal in infants and adults immediately after eating. By 30 minutes after eating, the sound should not be heard unless an obstruction exists with an air-fluid level. Impaired gastric emptying occurs most often in patients with *pyloric obstruction* (congenital or acquired); it also occurs in patients with gastric tumors or gastric atony. Atonic gastric dilatation is most frequently seen in postoperative patients and in patients who have severe hyperkalemia or diabetic ketoacidosis.

The classic triad of physical findings in patients with acute intestinal obstruction consists of (1) sudden onset of colicky abdominal pain, (2) vomiting, and (3) obstipation. Bowel sounds are generally hyperactive and high pitched and occur in rushes; if perforation or peritonitis occurs, the bowel sounds become reduced. When the obstruction is in the large intestine, abdominal distention and general or local intestinal distention may occur. With *volvulus,* gross distention of the entire abdomen may occur early in the disease.

Salpingitis

The physical findings of salpingitis include unilateral or bilateral tenderness to palpation in the lower abdomen and increased bowel sounds. Involuntary guarding and rigidity are rare findings. Pelvic examination often elicits pain, particularly with lateral movement of the cervix and adnexal palpation. The patient frequently has a purulent cervical discharge.

Irritable Colon

Although most patients with an irritable colon have no significant physical findings (the diagnosis is made by careful history), a tender ascending or descending colon may be palpable.

Acute Diverticulitis

The classic triad for acute diverticulitis is (1) abdominal tenderness, (2) a palpable mass in the LLQ, and (3) fever. The mass or tenderness occasionally may be detected only by rectal examination. Diarrhea and rectal bleeding are uncommon, and bowel sounds are usually decreased.

Ureterolithiasis

Tenderness to percussion in the costovertebral angle and ileus may be the only physical finding in patients with ureterolithiasis. This diagnosis is usually confirmed by the presence of hematuria.

Diagnostic Studies

Although plain or flat abdominal radiographs frequently are ordered in patients with acute abdominal pain, they are diagnostic in less than 50% of cases. If an acute surgical abdomen is suspected and the diagnosis is unknown or dubious, the physician should obtain an electrocardiogram, chest and abdominal radiographs, complete blood count (CBC) with differential, electrolytes, blood urea nitrogen, serum amylase level (if pancreatitis is suspected), and urine and stool tests.

Rarely, laparotomy is necessary in patients with recurrent abdominal pain if the diagnosis is not apparent. In one series of 27 laparotomies for unexplained abdominal pain, carcinoma was found in 50% of patients. Laparoscopy and peritoneal cytology are helpful when surgical intervention is being considered. Recent studies have suggested routine use of laparoscopy in patients with an acute abdomen. In most situations it has replaced laparotomy. In equivocal cases of abdominal pain, laparoscopy may prevent unnecessary surgery. In patients over 50 years of age with *recurrent nonspecific acute abdominal pain,* the following laboratory tests should be done to detect cancer: (1) examination of stools for occult blood (this test should be done in all patients over age 50 regardless of the presence of abdominal pain); (2) sigmoidoscopy and, if necessary, colonoscopy; and (3) barium enema.

Text continued on page 15.

Differential Diagnosis of Abdominal Pain in Adults

CAUSE	NATURE OF PATIENT	NATURE OF PAIN	LOCATION OF PAIN	ASSOCIATED SYMPTOMS	PRECIPITATING AND AGGRAVATING FACTORS	AMELIORATING FACTORS	PHYSICAL FINDINGS	DIAGNOSTIC STUDIES
Gastroenteritis	Any age	Crampy	Diffuse	Nausea, vomiting Diarrhea Fever	Food	Occasional relief with vomiting or diarrhea	Hyperactive peristalsis	
Gastritis	Especially alcoholic patients	Constant Burning	Epigastrium	Hemorrhage Nausea, vomiting Diarrhea Fever	Alcohol NSAIDs Salicylates Food (occasionally)			
Appendicitis	Any age: peak age 10–20 yr M > F	Colicky Progressing to constant	Early: epigastrium, periumbilicus Later: RLQ	Vomiting (after pain has started) Constipation Fever	Pain worse with movement and coughing	Lying still	RLQ involuntary guarding Rebound to RLQ	CBC with differential Ultrasonography Laparoscopy CT scan
Cholecystitis, cholelithiasis	Adults F > M	Colicky Progressing to constant	RUQ Radiates to inferior angle of right scapula	Nausea, vomiting Dark urine, light stool Jaundice	Fatty foods Drugs, oral contraceptives Cholestyramine		Tenderness to palpation or percussion in RUQ	Liver function tests CBC, amylase Ultrasonography Isotopic gallbladder scan
Diverticulitis	More common in elderly	Intermittent cramping	LLQ	Constipation Diarrhea			Palpable mass in LLQ	Laparoscopy, especially in women
Pancreatitis	More common in alcoholic patients and those with cholelithiasis	Steady Mild to severe	LUQ, epigastric Radiates to back	Nausea, vomiting Prostration Diaphoresis	Lying supine	Leaning forward	Abdominal distention Decreased bowel sounds Diffuse rebound	Amylase Ultrasonography

Intestinal obstruction	Elderly Prior abdominal surgery	Colicky Sudden onset		Vomiting Obstipation			Hyperactive peristalsis in small bowel obstruction	Abdominal radiographs
Intestinal perforation Peritonitis	Elderly F > M	Sudden onset Severe Sudden or gradual onset	Diffuse	Guarding Rebound	Pain worse with movement or coughing	Lying still	Decreased bowel sounds Guarding Diffuse rebound	Abdominal radiographs Peritoneal lavage
Salpingitis	Menstruating females	Cramplike	RLQ LLQ Nonradiating	Chandelier sign	Pain worse while descending stairs and around time of menstruation		Adnexa and cervix tender to manipulation	Ultrasonography CT scan hCG to rule out ectopic pregnancy
Ectopic pregnancy	Fertile female with history of menstrual irregularity	Sudden onset Persistent pain	Lower quadrant	Tender adnexal mass (vaginal bleeding)				hCG
Peptic ulcer With perforation	30–50 yr M > F	Gnawing Burning Sudden onset	Epigastric radiating to sides, back, or right shoulder		Empty stomach Stress Alcohol	Food Alkali	Epigastric tenderness to palpation or percussion	Endoscopy Radiography
Mesenteric adenitis	Children Adolescents After respiratory infection	Constant	RLQ	Vomiting Rebound Constipation Diarrhea Fever				CBC with differential

Table continued on following page.

Differential Diagnosis of Abdominal Pain in Adults *Continued*

CAUSE	NATURE OF PATIENT	NATURE OF PAIN	LOCATION OF PAIN	ASSOCIATED SYMPTOMS	PRECIPITATING AND AGGRAVATING FACTORS	AMELIORATING FACTORS	PHYSICAL FINDINGS	DIAGNOSTIC STUDIES
Ureterolithiasis		Colicky Occasionally progresses to constant Severe Sudden onset	Lower abdomen Flank Radiating to groin	Nausea, vomiting Abdominal distention Chills, fever			Costovertebral angle tenderness Hematuria	Urinalysis Intravenous pyelography Ultrasonography
Dissection or rupture of aortic aneurysm	Elderly Hypertensive 40–70 yr	Unbearable Sudden onset	Chest or abdomen May radiate to back and legs	Shock			Shock Decrease or difference in femoral pulses	Radiography Ultrasonography CT scan
Reflux (peptic) esophagitis		Burning Gnawing	Midepigastrium Occasionally radiating to jaw		Recumbency	Antacids		Upper GI radiographs Endoscopy
Irritable colon	More common in young women	Crampy Recurrent	Most common in LLQ	Mucus in stools		Pain occasionally relieved by defecation	Colon tender to palpation	
Incarcerated hernia	More common in elderly	Constant	RLQ LLQ		Coughing Straining		Hernia or mass	Upper GI radiographs
Mesenteric infarction	Elderly	May be severe	Diffuse	Tachycardia Hypotension			Decreased bowel sounds Blood in stools	Abdominal radiographs

NSAIDs, Nonsteroidal antiinflammatory drugs; *M,* males; *F,* females; *hCG,* human chorionic gonadotropin; *GI,* gastrointestinal.

Specific laboratory tests may be ordered when certain diagnoses are suspected: *appendicitis*—CBC with differential, computed tomography (CT) scans, ultrasonography; *cholecystitis*—CBC with differential, isotopic and ultrasonographic scanning; *peptic ulcer*—upper GI radiographs; *perforated peptic ulcer*—radiographs to reveal free air; *acute intestinal obstruction*—abdominal radiographs; *ureterolithiasis*—intravenous pyelography, microscopic urinalysis; and *pancreatitis*—serum amylase level. Abdominal CT scans and abdominal ultrasonography are often helpful, especially when gallbladder, pancreatic, or pelvic disease is suspected. CT scans provide information concerning the bowel wall, mesentery, and intraperitoneal and retroperitoneal structures and are useful in surgical decision making. Endoscopic ultrasonography is useful in evaluating esophageal, gastric, and particularly pancreatic lesions.

Less Common Diagnostic Considerations

Abdominal pain may result from pneumonia, particularly of a lower lobe. Abdominal pain and vomiting may be the presenting symptoms in diabetes. RUQ pain can be caused by congestive heart failure resulting from stretching of Glisson's capsule. RUQ pain, jaundice, and anorexia may be the presenting symptoms of hepatitis.

Amebiasis can mimic appendicitis or diverticulitis or both. Abdominal or flank pain or both, when associated with nausea and vomiting, may be the presenting symptoms of a hydronephrosis.

An acute abdomen in a young black patient classically suggests the possibility of sickle cell crisis. Severe abdominal wall tenderness can result from a spider bite. Rarely, diffuse abdominal pain can be secondary to marked gaseous distention.

Severe pain in the back or flank or vague, poorly localized abdominal pain may be the first presenting symptom in patients with carcinoma of the pancreas. If abdominal pain is associated with thrombophlebitis (in the absence of trauma), migratory thrombophlebitis, or the development of diabetes, pancreatic carcinoma should be suspected. Carcinoma of the head of the pancreas usually presents with jaundice or abdominal pain early in the course of the illness.

Abdominal pain, sometimes associated with vomiting, that occurs in the middle of the menstrual cycle is called "mittelschmerz." It represents pain associated with the physiologic rupture of an ovarian follicle.

If a female of childbearing age suddenly develops severe, generalized abdominal pain, often associated with syncope or persistent dizziness, ectopic pregnancy must be considered. This is more common in younger women, in those of low parity, and in those with a history of prior pelvic sepsis or infertility. Physical findings include acute abdominal pain with guarding and rigidity, especially in the lower abdomen. Extreme tenderness to cervical manipulation has been reported in 85% of patients with an ectopic pregnancy. Laparoscopy, human chorionic gonadotropin, and ultrasonography may help the physician establish the diagnosis.

Vascular causes of abdominal pain include mesenteric thrombosis and acute mesenteric occlusion by embolism or torsion. The latter may have no associated signs or symptoms—only severe abdominal pain with bloody stools occurring later. Aortic aneurysm may cause constant low back pain, which may worsen with recumbency; dissection is characterized by severe, excruciating pain.

Purcell (1989) reviews other uncommon conditions simulating an acute abdomen.

Selected References

Birnbaum BA, Jeffrey RB: CT and sonographic evaluation of acute right lower quadrant abdominal pain. AJR Am J Roentgenol 170:361–371, 1998.

Burnett LS: Gyncologic causes of the acute abdomen. Surg Clin North Am 68:385–398, 1988.

Chung RS, Diaz JJ, Chari V: Efficacy of routine laparoscopy for the acute abdomen. Surg Endosc 12:219–222, 1998.

Cope Z: Cope's Early Diagnosis of the Acute Abdomen. New York, Oxford University Press, 1987.

De Dombal FT: Picking the best tests in acute abdominal pain. J R Coll Physicians Lond 13:203–208, 1979.

De Dombal FT: Acute abdominal pain in the elderly. J Clin Gastroenterol 19:331–335, 1994.

Diehl AK, Sugarek NJ, Todd KH: Clinical evaluation of gallstone disease: usefulness of symptoms and signs in clinical diagnosis. Am J Med 89:29–34, 1990.

Graham A, Henley C, Mobley J: Laparoscopic evaluation of acute abdominal pain. J Laparoendosc Surg 1:165–168, 1991.

Mayer IE, Hussain H: Abdominal pain during pregnancy. Gastroenterol Clin North Am 27:1–33, 1998.

Murtagh J: Acute abdominal pain: a diagnostic approach. Aust Fam Physician 23:358–374, 1994.

Paterson-Brown S, Vipond MN: Modern aids to clinical decision making in the acute abdomen. Br J Surg 77(1):13–18, 1990.

Phillips SL, Burns GP: Acute abdominal disease in the aged. Med Clin North Am 72:1213–1224, 1988.

Purcell TB: Nonsurgical and extraperitoneal causes of abdominal pain. Emerg Med Clin North Am 7:721–740, 1989.

Saegesser F: The acute abdomen, part 1: differential diagnosis. Clin Gastroenterol 10:123–144, 1981.

Spiro HM: An internist's approach to acute abdominal pain. Med Clin North Am 77:963–972, 1993.

Sturman MF: Medical imaging in acute abdominal pain. Compr Ther 17:15–21, 1991.

Trnka Y, Warfield CA: Chronic abdominal pain. Hosp Pract 19:201–209, 1984.

Wilson DH: The acute abdomen in the accident and emergency department. Practitioner 222:480–485, 1975.

CHAPTER 2

Abdominal Pain in Children

Since chronic abdominal pain is rare in children, the main emphasis of this chapter is the differential diagnosis of acute and recurrent abdominal pain. Because abdominal pain has many causes, a detailed history and a very careful physical examination are necessary. A small number of selected laboratory studies may also be required. Accurate diagnosis is essential because abdominal pain may be a manifestation of a surgical emergency; such cases must be identified promptly. Whenever significant concern exists about the presence of a surgical condition, the patient should be hospitalized to permit serial abdominal examinations and laboratory studies.

Gastroenteritis is the most common cause of acute abdominal pain in children. *Constipation,* another common cause of abdominal pain, may be acute but is more often recurrent. Other common nonsurgical causes of acute abdominal pain include *mesenteric adenitis, nonspecific abdominal pain, urinary tract infection, sickle cell disease, poisoning,* and *diabetes. Recurrent abdominal pain* is defined as three discrete episodes of abdominal pain occurring over 3 or more months. It is quite common over the age of 5 years and often has a psychosomatic cause.

The most common surgical causes of acute abdominal pain are *appendicitis, hernia strangulation,* and *intussusception.*

Nature of Patient

Presentation and causes of abdominal pain vary according to three age groups: (1) children under 5 years, (2) patients between 5 and 12 years, and (3) adolescents. The cause of abdominal pain in very young children is difficult to determine unless abdominal tenderness, guarding, doubling up, or vomiting is present. **With the exception of infantile colic, when children less than 3 years old complain of abdominal pain, it is usually organic in origin.** Physical examination is particularly important in this age group. *Intussusception* is likely when signs of intestinal obstruction are found in infants (peak incidence, 6 months). A lead point such as Meckel's diverticulum seldom is found. *Appendicitis* is uncommon in infants and children up to age 5 years, but it is the most common condition causing abdominal pain that requires surgery in this age group. Because appendicitis seldom is considered, the diagnosis is often missed or delayed. Perforation is therefore more common, and a disproportionately high percentage of deaths due to appendicitis occurs in children under 5 years of age. *Poisonings,* most common in children ages 1 to 4 years, are another frequent cause of abdominal pain.

In children between 5 and 12 years, the major dilemma involves *recurrent abdominal pain,* which can be a symptom of either psychosomatic or organic disease; it is usually due to psychological factors. Children with recurrent abdominal pain have a high incidence of behavioral and personality disorders. These patients tend to be "high-strung" perfectionists and are often apprehensive. Many have histories of colic and feeding problems in infancy and stressful family and school situations. Unexplained episodes of recurrent abdominal pain occur in 10% of school-age children, but an organic cause is found in less than 10% of these cases.

Inflammatory bowel disease frequently begins during adolescence and can be a cause of acute or recurrent abdominal pain. Growth failure in adolescents with abdominal pain is an important clue to this diagnosis, although it may also indicate *gluten-sensitive enteropathy. Sickle cell crises* occur almost exclusively in blacks but occasionally occur in people of Mediterranean descent. *Acute appendicitis* is most common in children ages 5 to 15 years, with a peak incidence between 10 and 15 years.

Nature of Pain

The timing of the first occurrence of abdominal pain in children may help to identify *psychological stress* as the cause. For example, abdominal pain that develops at a time of school problems, the birth of a sibling, or family discord suggests a psychological cause. *Functional abdominal pain* is usually central and nonradiating and rarely awakens the patient at night. It is rarely associated with recurrent vomiting or diarrhea but is often associated with headache and extremity pains.

In addition to observing the severity, duration, and location of abdominal pain, the examiner must note whether the onset is gradual or sudden. A gradual onset of cramping pain often suggests an intestinal cause, such as *appendicitis,* whereas a sudden onset of noncramping constant pain suggests *torsion of a viscus, intussusception,* or *perforation.* The pain of appendicitis classically precedes the development of vomiting and anorexia, begins gradually as a crampy epigastric or periumbilical pain, and progresses to a constant pain in the right lower quadrant (RLQ). In young children this pain may be mild or discontinuous or both. Because of frequent atypical presentations and a decreased incidence in young children, this diagnosis is often missed.

The pain of *mesenteric adenitis* often mimics appendicitis, although a child with adenitis is not quite as sick and is not necessarily anorexic. Mesenteric adenitis usually occurs after a viral or bacterial infection. The associated pain may be colicky in younger children and severe and episodic in older children. **The child has tenderness and guarding when the pain is present and usually shows no guarding when the pain is absent.** This is in contrast to appendicitis, in which the guarding persists despite the absence of pain. Guarding and abdominal tenderness are the symptoms most frequently associated with a surgical diagnosis.

Cramping diffuse abdominal pain that follows or coincides with the onset of diarrhea, nausea, or vomiting suggests *gastroenteritis.* Cramping pain occurring primarily after meals is often due to *constipation.* This diagnosis should be accepted only when an enema yields a large amount of feces and relieves pain. Sudden onset of severe, crampy, spasmodic pain that causes an infant to scream and draw up the legs should suggest *intussusception.* This spasmodic pain often recurs at 15- to 30-minute intervals, and the child may be normal, lethargic, or sleeping between attacks.

When abdominal pain is severe and colicky and radiates to the groin or flank, *urolithiasis* should be considered. Hematuria may confirm this diagnosis. Hematuria may also be noted when an inflamed retrocecal appendix overlies the ureter. Abdominal pain associated with tenderness to percussion in the costovertebral angle region may indicate *pyelonephritis.*

When the abdominal pain is relatively constant, located in the midepigastrium, and exacerbated by eating, *chronic gastritis* caused by *Helicobacter pylori* must be considered.

The abdominal pain of *diabetic acidosis* often is generalized, and ketosis is usually present. The abdominal pain of a *sickle cell crisis* is severe and usually associated with an ileus. This diagnosis should be considered in all black children with severe abdominal pain. Every black child in whom the diagnosis of appendicitis is considered should have a sickle cell test before surgery. When appendicitis is suspected in patients with a positive sickle cell test, an appendectomy should not be performed until the patient is clearly not responding to medical therapy for sickle cell crisis or shows progressive manifestations of sepsis. Recurrent abdominal pain suggests *sickle cell disease, inflammatory bowel disease, cystic fibrosis,* and *constipation.*

Location of Pain

The pain of *gastroenteritis* is poorly localized, whereas the pain of gas and constipation is usually located in the RLQ. The presumed mechanism of RLQ pain in *constipation* involves gaseous distention of the cecum. **Increasing localized tenderness in the RLQ associated with rebound to the RLQ is the most helpful finding favoring the diagnosis of appendicitis.** Subsequent to this localization of pain in the RLQ, paralytic ileus may develop. Classic findings often occur with the appendix in its usual location, but atypical symptomatology may result from an unusually located inflamed appendix. It is critical for the physician to perform a rectal examination because pain in the right upper quadrant may be due to a retrocecal appendicitis.

Associated Symptoms

A detailed evaluation of associated symptoms often helps establish the diagnosis. Some generally applicable rules concerning the differential diagnosis of acute abdominal pain are as follows:

1. When significant diarrhea is associated with abdominal pain, a surgical lesion is rare.
2. When abdominal distention, particularly with acidosis, is associated with abdominal pain, a surgical emergency is more likely.
3. When vomiting precedes abdominal pain, an extraabdominal cause is suggested; when abdominal pain precedes vomiting, an abdominal cause is likely.

When abdominal pain is diffuse and no localizing physical signs are found, associated diarrhea, nausea, or vomiting suggests *gastroenteritis.* A preceding upper respiratory infection (e.g., pharyngitis, tonsillitis, otitis media), a high fever, nausea or vomiting, and a good appetite suggest *mesenteric adenitis.*

Abdominal pain without systemic signs (e.g., fever, leukocytosis) or localized abdominal findings, especially with intense stress at home or school, suggests a *psychosomatic cause.* Some children with such findings also have nausea, vomiting, headaches, and diarrhea. Their pain is poorly localized, and they show no peritoneal signs.

A history of polyuria, polydipsia, weight loss, or diabetes in the patient or the family suggests that the abdominal pain may be caused by *diabetic ketoacidosis.*

Growth failure, particularly during adolescence, is an important clue suggesting *inflammatory bowel disease* or a *gluten-sensitive enteropathy.* Weight loss and anemia are other signs of organic disease.

Physical Findings

Jones (1979) and Gryskiewicz and Huseby (1980) provide excellent reviews of special techniques useful in pediatric abdominal examination. Physical examination should include general observation of the child and inspection of the abdomen for distention, masses, or abnormal pulsations. The abdomen should then be auscultated before palpation or percussion. Diffuse and generalized hyperperistalsis suggests *gastroenteritis,* whereas rushes of high-pitched peristalsis associated with crampy pains suggests an *obstructive process.*

Patients with *appendicitis* have tenderness over the inflamed appendix. Peritoneal inflammation, present in 97% of children with acute appendicitis, usually results in muscle guarding and rebound tenderness. Other signs of peritonitis include shallow breathing, absent peristalsis, low-grade fever with a disproportionate rise in the pulse rate, and leukocytosis (which may be absent during the first 24 hours). The child may lie quite still or move cautiously and often prefers to lie on the side with the right thigh flexed. With a retrocecal appendix the child may limp and demonstrate a positive psoas or obturator sign, although these signs are difficult to elicit in very young children. The following features of acute appendicitis apply distinctly to children:

1. Surgery should be performed within 24 hours of symptom onset; otherwise, perforation is likely.
2. The pain may be mild and discontinuous.
3. The pain may be atypically located when the appendix is not located in the right iliac area.

Both *mesenteric adenitis* and *nonspecific acute abdominal pain* can mimic appendicitis. It is very difficult for the physician to distinguish mesenteric adenitis from acute appendicitis by physical examination alone. **The value of serial abdominal examinations and serial laboratory tests, often performed in the hospital, cannot be overemphasized, particularly when the diagnosis is unclear.** With early inflammatory processes, irritation may be sufficient to make the abdomen diffusely tender but insufficient to produce peritoneal irritation. These patients may have no muscle guarding or rebound tenderness. In mesenteric adenitis the white blood cell count is usually not elevated, the temperature may be high (even higher than in acute appendicitis), and the history or physical findings often reveal a previous viral or bacterial respiratory infection. Mesenteric adenitis may also follow viral gastroenteritis. Crampy diffuse abdominal pain with nausea, vomiting, or diarrhea gradually changes to constant RLQ pain.

One long-term study of patients with *recurrent abdominal pain* revealed organic causes in only 2%, a finding that is not encouraging to the physician who is considering the possibility of early appendicitis. If the patient has a history of similar pain episodes and if the current episode subsides over 24 hours, the diagnosis of recurrent nonspecific abdominal pain is more likely. Until the diagnosis is clear, active serial observations are essential. Continued pain, tachycardia, anorexia, diarrhea, pain on movement, and especially rebound tenderness all warn that the pain is *not* nonspecific and that surgical intervention must be seriously considered. When the temperature, blood count, sedimentation rate, urinalysis, and stool examination for occult blood and ova and parasites are normal, recurrent nonspecific abdominal pain is most likely.

A bulge in the inguinal area or the presence of an undescended testicle suggests an *inguinal hernia.* A lump may be palpated either rectally or abdominally in infants with *intussusception.* When intussusception is ileocecal (most common), a lump may be palpated in the right upper quadrant or the epigastrium. Rectal examination classically reveals bloody mucus on the examining finger. The "currant jelly" stool of dark blood is a late sign of intussusception. A barium enema not only may reveal the intussusception but also may alleviate it.

Palpation of fecal material in the colon and tenderness over the course of the colon suggest pain from *obstipation.* A firm inspissated stool may be palpated rectally. This diagnosis is confirmed if an enema yields a large amount of stool and relieves the pain. Occasionally an enlarged kidney is detected by palpation, suggesting hydronephrosis as the cause of abdominal pain.

Physical findings associated with abdominal pain from *diabetic ketoacidosis* include Kussmaul's respiration, diffuse abdominal pain, and sweet, fruity breath. The presence of Kussmaul's respiration and the absence of shallow respiration (which is usually seen with peritonitis) also suggest diabetic ketoacidosis.

Diagnostic Studies

Many indications for diagnostic studies have already been reviewed. Studies useful in the differential diagnosis of abdominal pain include complete blood count with differential, erythrocyte sedimentation rate, abdominal radiographs, ultrasonography, stool examination for occult blood, urinalysis, and urine culture and sensitivity. **Every child should have a blood sugar test and urinalysis before abdominal surgery. All black patients should have a sickle cell test.** Frequent serial tests may be necessary with acute pain. With recurrent abdominal pain the tests should be repeated, but less frequently. **When recurrent abdominal pain is the chief complaint, when no additional symptoms suggest organic disease, and when a thorough history and physical examination are negative, only simple diagnostic studies should be performed.** In special instances, gastrointestinal barium studies, cholecystography, ultrasonography, intravenous pyelography, computed tomography, endoscopy, proctoscopy, and small bowel biopsy may be helpful.

Less Common Diagnostic Considerations

Congenital intestinal obstruction, Hirschsprung's disease, duodenal atresia, midgut volvulus, and necrotizing enterocolitis may occur in the neonate. Abdominal distention, food refusal, and vomiting are typically present in all these conditions. Likewise, radiographs are usually diagnostic. Neonates with Hirschsprung's disease fail to pass meconium. Many with duodenal atresia or midgut volvulus demonstrate visible gastric peristalsis.

A twisted ovarian cyst should be considered in cases of acute lower abdominal pain in girls. A mass usually is palpable, but a thorough rectal examination may be difficult unless it is performed with the patient under general anesthesia. Ultrasonography may help detect an ovarian cyst. A history of mittelschmerz also suggests that the pain may be due to an ovarian cyst. In older girls, salpingitis and pelvic inflammatory disease must be considered whenever a fever is observed in association with lower abdominal pain. The fever is usually higher than that observed with appendicitis, and a vaginal discharge is usually present. If a Gram stain of the vaginal secretion reveals gonococci, the diagnosis is clear.

Complete or incomplete intestinal obstruction resulting from adhesions should be considered as a cause of abdominal pain in any patient with an abdominal scar. This pain is usually cramping and typically accompanied by bilious vomiting. Physical examination may reveal abdominal distention, and distended loops of bowel occasionally may be identified clinically or radiographically. In the early phase, high-pitched tinkling bowel sounds may occur in rushes. If the obstruction continues, peristalsis becomes lower in pitch and less frequent.

Peptic ulceration and occasional perforation may develop in children experiencing major stress as the result of serious physical trauma (e.g., burns, severe head injuries). Unfortunately, diagnosis is frequently delayed because of the severity of the other associated problems. Peptic ulceration and perforation should be considered whenever children with abdominal symptoms have undergone major stress. Upright or decubitus radiographs may demonstrate free air in the peritoneal cavity.

Differential Diagnosis of Abdominal Pain in Children

CONDITION	NATURE OF PATIENT	NATURE OF PAIN	LOCATION OF PAIN	ASSOCIATED SYMPTOMS	PHYSICAL FINDINGS	DIAGNOSTIC STUDIES
Gastroenteritis	All ages	Crampy	Diffuse	Diarrhea Vomiting	Hyperperistalsis Low-grade fever	
Intussusception	Under 5 yr; peak incidence 6 mo	Severe, crampy			Rushes of high-pitched peristalsis "Currant jelly" stools Walnut-size mass, palpated abdominally or rectally	Barium edema Abdominal radiographs
Constipation	Any age; peak incidence 5–12 yr	Recurrent, crampy (especially after meals)	Often RLQ		Feces in rectum Feces may be palpable in colon	Enema yields large amount of feces and relieves pain
Psychosomatic cause	Frequently 5–12 yr High-strung, perfectionist History of colic	Recurrent (3 or more episodes of central, nonradiating pain in 3 mo)		Psychological stress Headaches No vomiting or diarrhea	Absence of systemic signs	Laboratory studies and radiographs within normal limits

Table continued on following page.

Differential Diagnosis of Abdominal Pain in Children *Continued*

CONDITION	NATURE OF PATIENT	NATURE OF PAIN	LOCATION OF PAIN	ASSOCIATED SYMPTOMS	PHYSICAL FINDINGS	DIAGNOSTIC STUDIES
Appendicitis	Uncommon in young children Peak incidence 5–15 yr	Atypical in children Precedes anorexia and vomiting Worse with movement	Begins gradually in epigastrium or periumbilical area Progresses to constant RLQ pain	Poor appetite	Serial examinations useful Fever Guarding persists when pain is not present Rebound in RLQ Decreased peristalsis	Leukocytosis Abdominal radiographs Ultrasonography
Mesenteric adenitis	As in appendicitis	As in appendicitis	RLQ	Symptoms of recent upper respiratory infection Good appetite	No guarding when pain is not present Fever Similar to appendicitis	Complete blood count with differential Lymphocytosis
Inflammatory bowel disease	Adolescence			Diarrhea	Growth failure Diffuse abdominal tenderness, often without rebound	Upper and lower gastrointestinal radiographs Elevated erythrocyte sedimentation rate
Inguinal hernia			Lower quadrant	Undescended testicle Abdominal distention	Bulge in inguinal area	

Gallstones are rare in children and are most likely to occur in those with hemolytic anemias. Abdominal pain may be the presenting complaint in children with lower lobe pneumonias. Children with migraine headaches also may complain of abdominal pain.

Lactose intolerance can cause recurrent abdominal pain in children and should be considered if the onset of pain coincides with heavy lactose ingestion. Before invasive procedures are performed or a psychogenic origin is assumed, a lactose-restricted diet should be attempted. Blunt, nonpenetrating abdominal trauma can cause rupture of the spleen, liver, intestines, or kidneys and result in abdominal pain. Crohn's disease should be considered in adolescents who have abdominal pain associated with weight loss, anemia, rectal bleeding, diarrhea, or passage of mucus from the rectum.

Acute pancreatitis, although rare in children, can be caused by trauma, viral infection (especially mumps), prolonged steroid therapy, or obstruction of the common bile duct due to a stone or an inflammatory process. Patients with this condition usually have marked nausea, vomiting, low-grade fever, and severe, constant upper abdominal pain radiating to the back.

Allergies to foods and drugs occasionally cause abdominal pain. Lead poisoning should be suspected if the child has paroxysms of diffuse abdominal pain alternating with constipation. A history of pica may or may not be obtained from the parents or patient.

Urinary tract infections, kidney stones, and ureteropelvic junction obstruction may cause abdominal pain. Children with ureteropelvic junction obstruction often have recurrent unilateral pain that often occurs at night after ingestion of large quantities of fluid.

Selected References

Alford BA, McIlhenny J: The child with acute abdominal pain and vomiting. Radiol Clin North Am 30:441–453, 1992.

Finelli L: Evaluation of the child with acute abdominal pain. J Pediatr Health Care 5:251–256, 1991.

Forbes D: Abdominal pain in children. Aust Fam Physician 23:347–357, 1994.

Galler JR, Neustein S, Walker WA: Clinical aspects of recurrent abdominal pain in children. Adv Pediatr 27:31–53, 1980.

Gryskiewicz JM, Huseby TL: The pediatric abdominal examination. Postgrad Med 67:126–138, 1980.

Jones PF: The acute abdomen in infancy and childhood. Practitioner 222:473–478, 1979.

Lake AM: Acute abdominal pain in childhood: finding the cause. Postgrad Med 65:119–127, 1979.

Lebenthal EB: Recurrent abdominal pain in childhood. Am J Dis Child 134:347–348, 1980.

Macarthur C, Saunders N, Feldman W: *Helicobacter pylori,* gastroduodenal disease, and recurrent abdominal pain in children. JAMA 273:729–734, 1995.

Mason JD: The evaluation of acute abdominal pain in children. Emerg Med Clin North Am 14:629–643, 1996.

Shrand H: Problems in family practice: acute abdominal pain in children. J Fam Pract 2:131–134, 1975.

Stevenson RJ: Abdominal pain unrelated to trauma. Surg Clin North Am 65:1181–1215, 1985.

CHAPTER 3

Backache

Low back pain causes countless visits to physicians, including 5% of all visits to family physicians. Two percent of the population consult a physician each year because of back pain. More than 80% of adults have had at least one episode of back pain, and many have had recurrent episodes since adolescence. It is the most common cause of disability in patients under age 45, and by age 50, 80% to 90% show evidence of degenerative disc disease at autopsy.

Despite the frequency of low back syndrome, it is poorly understood; physical examination is often unrewarding; and diagnostic tests are often negative or falsely positive. **Some patients have local or radicular signs but no evidence of morphologic abnormalities, even after testing with all available diagnostic technologies.** On the other hand, 50% to 60% of asymptomatic individuals reveal degenerative changes, and 20% have disc herniation without symptoms. To complicate matters even more, patients may change from one low back syndrome to another (e.g., from sciatica to chronic low back pain). **Therefore, low back pain should be considered a symptom that is rarely attributable to a specific disease or pathologic lesion.**

Low back pain most often has a mechanical origin. Mechanical causes include *acute lumbosacral strain, postural backache,* and *degenerative lumbosacral arthritis,* all of which may be caused by problems with muscles, tendons, ligaments, and discs. Other common causes include *sciatica* (often associated with a *herniated disc*), *lumbar spinal stenosis,* and *chronic low back pain.* Social and psychological factors are more pronounced in patients with *chronic low back pain,* and the severity of their symptoms does not match documented abnormalities.

Nature of Patient

Backaches in children are relatively uncommon. **In young children, backache represents serious disease more often than in adults, although the most common cause of backache in children is lumbosacral sprain.** This type of sprain usually results from participation in sports. A sprained back occasionally is caused by *trauma* (e.g., injuries sustained during a motor vehicle accident or during participation in gymnastics).

Because low back pain may represent serious illness in children, a thorough history and physical examination should be performed. *Infection* should be a strong diagnostic consideration, especially in suspected intravenous (IV) drug users. *Spondylolisthesis* and *spondylolysis* occur more often in teenagers than in younger patients. In these patients, pain usually develops after strenuous athletic activity, and the cause can best be detected with single-photon emission computed tomography (SPECT), since plain radiographs may not detect an early stress fracture.

Regardless of the cause, backache is most common in patients between 20 and 50 years of age. It occurs more often in people such as industrial workers and farmers who do heavy manual labor. In young adults who complain of persistent backache, *nonbacterial inflammatory disease,* such as *Reiter's syndrome* and *ankylosing spondylitis,* should be considered. It is particularly important for the examiner to ask these patients about other inflammatory changes that may be associated with Reiter's syndrome (e.g., iritis, pharyngitis, urethritis, arthritis). Even if the patient has spondylolisthesis, the physician must rule out inflammatory causes of backache. *Postural backaches* are more common in multigravida patients and individuals who are obese or otherwise in poor physical condition. *Herniated discs* occur in young adults but are relatively uncommon.

The number of backaches caused by *disc disease* increases as age increases from 25 to 50 years. Disc syndromes are more common in men, particularly older ones. In older patients, backache is a common symptom but not a common chief complaint. When it is the chief complaint in patients over 50 years of age, serious illness such as *lumbar spinal stenosis* with or without *cauda equina syndrome* must be considered, although the most common cause is *lumbosacral osteoarthritis.* Everyone probably develops some degenerative joint disease in the low back, but as a rule, clinical problems arise only when this degeneration reaches a moderate degree. It is then usually preceded by some traumatic incident, possibly minor, that precipitates the onset of symptoms. **In patients over 50 years who present with backache without significant history of prior backaches, serious conditions such as cancer and multiple myeloma must be considered.**

Nature of Symptoms

To determine the cause of backache, the physician must consider important historic factors such as age, location of pain, possible radiation of pain, effects of back or leg motion, and previous trauma (Table 3–1).

The pain of *acute lumbosacral strain* is characterized by a sudden onset often related to turning, lifting, twisting, or unusual physical activity. It is usually well localized at the lumbosacral region.

The pain of a *musculoskeletal strain* and a *postural backache* is often described as dull and persistent and associated with stiffness. Patients have difficulty locating a precise point of maximum pain, although the pain is usually centered in the lower lumbar region. After trauma, this pain may have an immediate or delayed onset. Patients may state that they felt something "give way." The pain typically radiates across the lower back and occasionally into the buttocks, but rarely into the lower extremity. **Radiation does not always indicate nerve root compression.**

The low back pain of *degenerative lumbosacral arthritis* has a gradual onset, is not usually precipitated by physical activity, and is usually associated with a

TABLE 3.1 Differential Features of Common Causes of Pelvic Girdle Pain

CAUSE	SITE OF PAIN	AGGRAVATING AND RELIEVING FACTORS	PHYSICAL FINDINGS	OTHER FINDINGS
Degenerative disc disease with facet impingement	Buttock, posterior thigh	Worse with spinal extension; relieved by rest in fetal position	Restricted spinal movement, tender spinal segment	Radiographs abnormal
Degenerative disc disease with nuclear prolapse	Buttock, posterior thigh	Worse with spinal extension; relieved by rest in fetal position	Restricted spinal movement, tender spinal segment, nerve root dysfunction	Radiographs abnormal; prolapse shown on film or magnetic resonance imaging
Sacroiliitis	Buttock, posterior thigh	Worse at rest; relieved with activity	Restricted spinal movement	Radiographs abnormal
Osteoarthritis of hip	Groin, occasionally buttock or knee	Worse with activity; relieved with rest	Restricted hip movement	Radiographs abnormal
Meralgia paresthetica	Lateral thigh paresthesia	Worse at night	Tenderness just below antero-superior iliac spine	Relieved by local infiltration of anesthetic and steroids
Trochanteric bursitis	Lateral thigh	Worse at night and with activity	Tenderness over greater trochanter	Relieved by local infiltration of anesthetic and steroids

From Little H: Trochanteric bursitis, Can Med J 120:456–458, 1979.

history of morning stiffness. Many patients with this condition complain that their lumbosacral motion is limited by pain and stiffness that is often worse in the morning but improves an hour or so after arising. Radiation of pain to the knee, calf, or lower leg is uncommon.

Many patients with *herniated disc syndrome* have a history of previous, less severe episodes. The pain usually has a sudden onset and often radiates into the buttock, down the posterolateral aspect of the leg, and sometimes to the foot. The pain of a disc syndrome has been compared with a toothache—sharp, lancinating, radiating pain that may be associated with paresthesias and muscle weakness (caused by nerve root pressure). Remitting pain usually indicates a posterolateral disc protrusion, but an intermittent backache also can be caused by a disc that does not produce significant root irritation. More than 90% of lumbar disc herniations occur at L4–L5 or L5–S1. If root irritation is present, neurologic findings (sensory loss, motor weakness, or hyporeflexia) are diagnostic. The patient may also have tenderness to palpation in the sciatic notch.

The qualitative characteristics of low back pain can be of considerable practical diagnostic importance. Variable, diffuse, and intense sensations of pressure often occur in patients without demonstrable organic disease. When the pain is described consistently and specifically, it is easier for the physician to demonstrate organic disease. Inflammatory disease (e.g., ankylosing spondylitis) and infectious processes (e.g., tuberculosis) are *not* likely if pain is related to posture, trauma, or overly strenuous activities; if it is episodic and intermittent; if it is aggravated by action; and if it is relieved by rest and recumbency.

Back pain in *sacroiliac syndromes* tends to be localized over the posterosuperior iliac spine. In *sacroiliitis* (an inflammatory arthritis of the sacroiliac joints), the pain may alternate from side to side, although it is usually felt in the low back and buttocks, and may radiate into the posterior thigh. **Sacroiliitis pain does not have a radicular distribution.**

Occasionally, low back pain may be a manifestation of the *irritable bowel syndrome.* In these cases, there often is associated midback pain, abdominal pain, and a history characteristic of an irritable colon. This pain does not radiate into the leg. The low back pain from *prostatitis* is usually a vague ache that is not affected by movement or coughing and is not associated with muscle spasm or limited mobility.

Rarely, the acute pain of *renal colic* presents with excruciating pain in the back rather than in the flank or groin. These patients show a gradual shift in the location of pain to the flank with radiation into the groin. With renal colic the straight leg–raising test usually is negative, and the urinalysis generally shows hematuria.

Some patients with *depression* may experience chronic low back pain. It is often described as diffuse, accompanied by a sensation of severe pressure. When somatic pain is a manifestation of depression, the severity of the pain varies with the mental state: pain increases with anxiety and depression and often decreases with extreme fear. If an elderly patient describes a burning or aching back pain, particularly if it is superficial and unilateral, *herpes zoster* should be suspected, since this pain often precedes the herpetic skin lesions.

Associated Symptoms

With *lumbar osteoarthritis,* patients often have pain in other joints. Patients with *herniated disc syndrome* usually have neurologic symptoms such as sciatica, paresthesias, dysesthesias, hypoesthesias, anesthesias, paresis, sphincter problems, and impotence. **Pressure on the unmyelinated fibers may cause *cauda equina syndrome,* a rare surgical emergency whose signs include central back pain associated with weakness of the leg muscles, impotence, urinary frequency, urinary retention (sometimes with overflow), incontinence, saddle anesthesia, and loss of sphincter tone.**

Low back pain associated with vaginal discharge suggests a *gynecologic* cause. In men, back pain associated with burning on urination, difficulty in urination, or fever suggests *prostatitis.* If herpes zoster is associated with back pain, underlying *cancer* should be strongly considered.

Precipitating and Aggravating Factors

Spondylolysis in adolescents is often precipitated by athletic activity. **It often presents as low back pain that is aggravated by activity and leads to an erroneous diagnosis of lumbosacral strain.**

Acute lumbosacral strain usually is precipitated by lifting, twisting, unusual physical activity or position, or trauma. Many patients are older and overweight and have not been physically active. When acute lumbosacral strain occurs in athletes, it may be caused by poor equipment, inadequate coaching, insufficient warm-up or conditioning, or any body position that unnecessarily exaggerates lordosis. Acute lumbosacral strain in adolescent athletes may be precipitated or aggravated during periods of rapid growth, since the soft tissues, ligaments, and musculotendinous units do not keep up with bone growth. Patients with acute lumbosacral strain experience pain with motion but not with coughing and straining. *Postural backaches* worsen as the day progresses.

In patients with *herniated disc syndrome,* pain can be precipitated by trauma or certain types of movement, particularly twisting in the bent-back position, as when starting a lawn mower or outboard engine. Aging also facilitates the development of this syndrome; herniation of the nucleus pulposus is the result of degenerative changes that occur with aging of the disc. The pain of a disc syndrome may be exacerbated by coughing, laughing, straining at stool, sneezing, sitting, and lateral bending; in acute cases it may be aggravated by almost any activity that results in the movement of the lower back, particularly hyperextension. The pain caused by *degenerative lumbosacral arthritis* also may be increased by lateral bending and extension of the lumbar spine. The polyradicular pain of *spinal stenosis* worsens with lumbar extension. Backaches that worsen during or just after menstruation suggest a *gynecologic* cause.

Ameliorating Factors

Inflammatory back pain often improves with exercise, whereas mechanical pain worsens. Many patients with an *acute lumbosacral strain* state that lying prone and motionless relieves the pain. Most acute back pain relieved by rest is of mechanical origin. This can be a significant point in differential diagnosis if the malingerer, the neurotic patient, or one with strong secondary gain can be ruled out. Many patients with low back pain from *osteoarthritis* state that their pain diminishes when they lie on the floor or on a firm mattress. Likewise, some patients with disc syndrome are relieved by lying down. This variable therefore is not helpful in the differential diagnosis of low back pain. Some patients with *disc syndrome* inform the physician that they feel better when walking or lying on their sides with their knees flexed (fetal position). This latter finding strongly suggests that the pain is caused by disc disease. Patients with inflammatory, infectious, or tumorous spinal disease usually have constant pain in all positions.

The back discomfort from *irritable colon* may be relieved by defecation. The pain of *spinal stenosis* improves with lumbar flexion.

Physical Findings

The investigation of low back pain should include a general medical, personal, sociologic, occupational, and sexual history. Special attention should be paid to previous backaches and factors that precipitate, aggravate, or ameliorate the pain, as well as to a history of trauma or heavy physical activity. This section outlines a satisfactory examination of a patient with low back pain. **Physical examination should include a rectal and a pelvic evaluation, especially in patients over age 40 years and in those without a history or physical findings characteristic of the common causes of backache.** Particular attention should be paid to observations made during examination of the breast, prostate, thyroid, lymph nodes, and peripheral pulses. Any evidence of systemic inflammatory disease such as iritis, urethritis, or arthritis should be noted. Examination of the spine should include determination of range of motion anteriorly, posteriorly, and laterally, as well as inspection for pelvic tilt.

Examination of the back also should include observation of the patient in the anatomic position, determination of range of motion of both the trunk and the lumbar spine, cervical flexion with and without trunk flexion, and gait. With the patient sitting, knee and ankle reflexes should be checked, as should extension of each leg. In teenagers with low back pain, a "one-legged hyperextension test" should be performed because it may suggest a pars stress fracture or spondylolysis. The examiner also should determine the strength of dorsiflexion of toes and ankles, sensation to touch and pinprick in the lower extremity, and integrity of proprioception (Figs. 3–1 to 3–4) while the patient is in this position.

With the patient supine, five tests should be performed: straight leg raising, Lasègue's compression (Fig. 3–5), bowstring, knee compression, and pelvic pressure. The range of motion of hip joints must be established, and painful areas of extremities must be palpated. With the patient prone, the spine should be palpated, as should the sacroiliac joints; the hips should be hyperextended and the knees flexed.

Physical findings in patients with *acute lumbosacral strain* usually are limited to the lower back, which demonstrates some limitation of motion. The patient may have local swelling and tenderness to palpation as well as spasm of the paraspinal muscles. The neurologic examination is negative, unlike with a herniated disc, which often is associated with spasm of the hamstring muscles and neurologic findings in the lower leg. Palpation over the sciatic notch may reveal pain or tenderness with some radiation to the knee or upper calf, but sensory and motor examination is intact. The lumbar lordotic curve often increases and may change minimally with bending. The patient frequently has limited range of motion of the lower back, particularly anteriorly and posteriorly, but not as much laterally. Although a straight leg–raising test may cause back pain, it does not induce pain with a sciatic distribution.

When *osteoarthritis* causes low back pain, the patient may have symmetric restriction of movement, unlike with a *herniated disc,* which usually causes

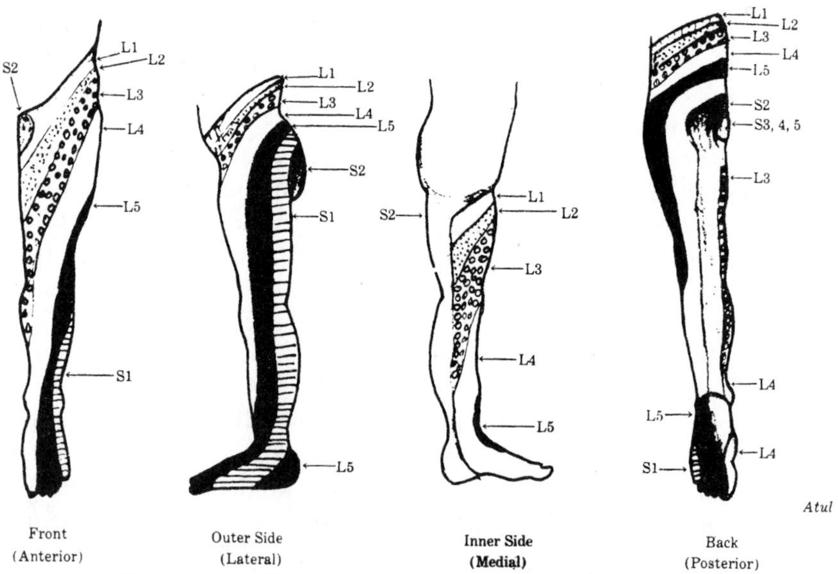

■ **Figure 3.1** Dermatomes of skin. (From Lane F, ed: Medical Trial Technique Quarterly, 1980 annual issue, pp 456–466.)

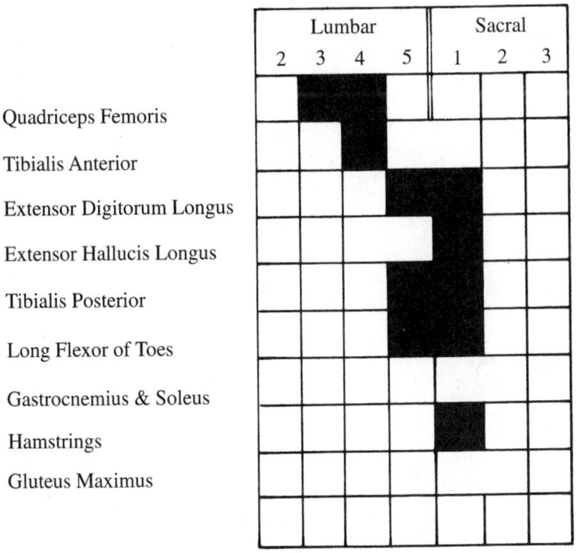

■ **Figure 3.2** Nerve supply of various muscles (main nerve roots are shaded). (From Lane F, ed: Medical Trial Technique Quarterly, 1980 annual issue, pp 456–466.)

asymmetric limitation of motion. The patient also may have tenderness to palpation in the lumbosacral region or at L4, L5, or S1.

When low back pain results from a *disc syndrome,* the physical findings often differ from those of a lumbosacral strain or osteoarthritis. Instead of increasing the lumbar lordotic curve, a disc syndrome usually reverses it, often with forward or

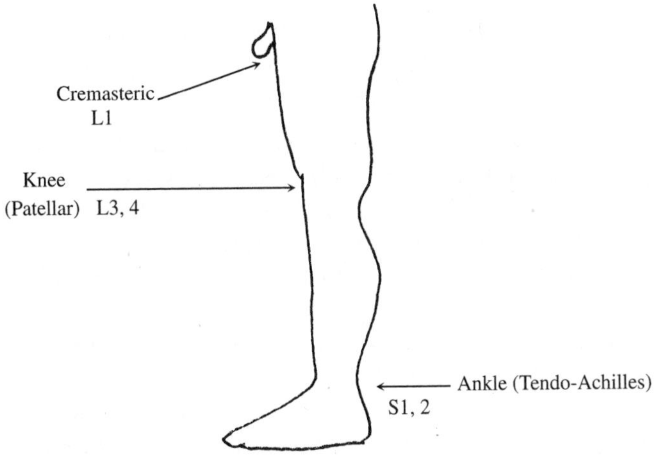

■ **Figure 3.3** Root origin of reflexes. (From Lane F, ed: Medical Trial Technique Quarterly, 1980 annual issue, pp 456–466.)

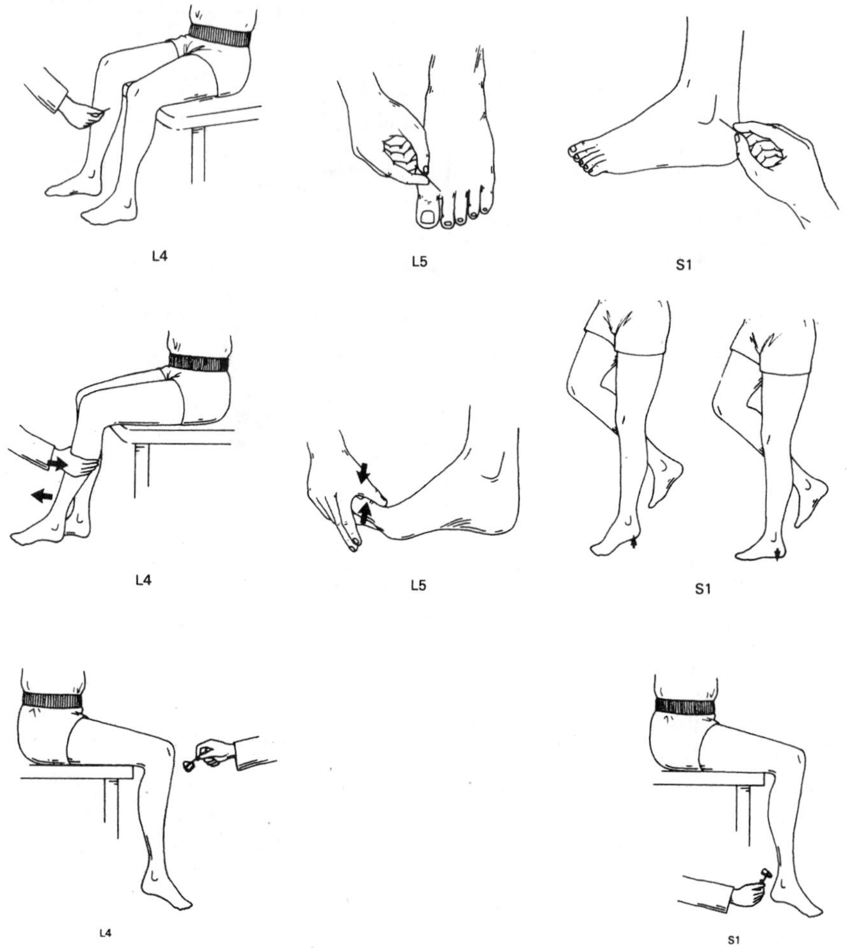

■ **Figure 3.4** Neurologic screening examination of lower extremity in patients with low back pain. (From Birnbaum JS: The Musculoskeletal Manual, 2nd ed. Philadelphia, WB Saunders Co, 1986, p 124.)

lateral tilt or both. As with osteoarthritis and lumbosacral strain, spinal movement is limited with a disc syndrome. The distinguishing features are the production of sciatic pain after hyperextension or lateral tilt and diminished or absent knee jerks in patients with disc syndrome. As with other causes of low back pain, the patient may have spasm of the paraspinal muscles and tenderness to palpation in the sciatic notch.

Restricted straight leg raising implies root irritation and is suggestive, but not diagnostic, of a herniated disc. Positive crossed, straight leg raising usually indicates a massive or central herniated disc or a mass lesion. The location of pain elicited by straight leg raising often suggests the area of nerve root irritation. Pain in the back or lumbosacral region suggests a higher lesion than pain in the calf or along the distribution of the sciatic nerve. Another clue to a ruptured disc may be asymmetric hamstring tightness.

Most patients with sciatic nerve root irritation, regardless of its cause, experience pain in the calf with straight leg raising. They usually demonstrate a positive Lasègue's sign as well.

Patients with herniated disc syndrome seldom present a surgical emergency. **Three basic factors influence the outcome of pressure on a nerve root: the amount of pressure on the nerve root, the duration of pressure, and the amount of myelin surrounding the nerve axon.** Mild pressure with local edema and inflammation causes nerve root irritation with some pain and paresthesias. Stretching the root aggravates the pain, as occurs with a positive straight leg–raising test or a Lasègue's sign. With increased pressure the patient has impaired conduction, motor weakness, reflex diminution, and some sensory loss in addition to pain. Severe pressure produces marked motor paralysis, loss of reflexes, and anesthesia. Mild to moderate pressure for short periods is tolerated fairly well by myelinated fibers. Prolonged pressure, however, is poorly tolerated, particularly by minimally myelinated nerves. **If paralysis following compression of myelinated fibers persists for 24 hours, it may be irreversible.** Myelin

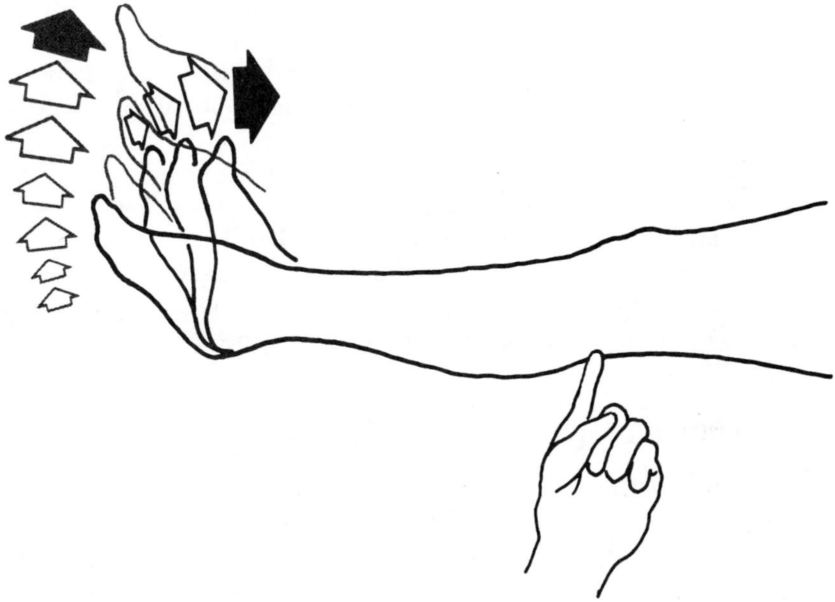

■ **Figure 3.5** Sciatic nerve stretch test. Examiner uses Lasègue's test to invoke pain down leg by raising limb with knee extended. If this fails to induce pain, compression of posterior tibial nerve in lateral popliteal space is painful if nerve root involvement is present, or pain may be invoked by sharp dorsiflexion of foot (Bragard's test). (From Jacobs B: American Family Physician, October 1978, p 13 [monograph].)

protects nerves from compression; the central parasympathetic nerve fibers to sphincters, however, are unmyelinated. **Therefore, loss of sphincter tone or urinary retention is a surgical emergency. If pressure on these unmyelinated fibers is not relieved immediately, permanent damage may ensue.**

Diagnostic Studies

In patients with osteoarthritis or a mechanical cause of their low back pain, the erythrocyte sedimentation rate (ESR) and alkaline phosphatase (ALP) level are within normal limits. The ESR is elevated in *multiple myeloma, infectious spinal disease,* and *ankylosing spondylitis.* The ALP level is elevated in patients with *Paget's disease.*

Plain radiography seldom is indicated in otherwise healthy patients ages 20 to 50 who present with acute low back pain. Structures such as muscles, ligaments, and discs are often responsible for back pain but are not visualized on plain films. Radiographic examination is normal or may show increased lumbar lordosis in patients with an acute lumbosacral or low back strain. When osteoarthritis causes low back pain, radiography frequently shows narrowing of the lumbar spaces with spurring and often sclerosis of the vertebrae. Radiography may assist in the diagnosis of compression fractures, cancer, Paget's disease, and multiple myeloma.

Magnetic resonance imaging is the most sensitive test for herniated discs and the most comprehensive way of evaluating degenerative changes and detecting tumors, fibrosis, cysts, and arachnoiditis. Computed tomography scans (with or without contrast media) are helpful in locating herniated discs and spinal tumors. **Imaging studies should not be used to make a diagnosis, but to confirm diagnoses made by history and physical examination.** These studies should be performed after 7 weeks of conservative management in patients with low back pain unless evidence of motor, sensory, reflex, sphincter, or autonomic deficit is present or if major trauma, infection, or neoplasia is suspected.

Less Common Diagnostic Considerations

Although most backaches are caused by lumbosacral strain, disc disease, osteoarthritis, or postural backache, innumerable less common causes exist. Backaches can result from disease of almost any system and have been classified as viscerogenic, vascular, neurogenic, psychogenic, spondylogenic, genitourinary, musculoskeletal, and secondary to metastatic or primary tumors of bone or soft tissue. They also may be caused by functional-mechanical derangement in the musculoskeletal system resulting from poor posture or obesity. Back pain in children is a rare complaint and may have a serious, organic cause. In older patients in whom back pain is a major complaint, particularly if it is the first attack, the physician must consider serious diseases such as metabolic disorders (osteoporosis, osteomalacia, chondrocalcinosis, Paget's disease), compression fractures, infections, and metastatic cancer from the breast, lung, or prostate. Infection and cancer are the most common diseases that cause back pain.

Ankylosing spondylitis most often occurs in young to middle-aged males. It has an insidious onset and lasts at least 3 months. Classically, it is associated with marked morning stiffness. In contrast to more common causes of backache, ankylosing spondylitis is associated with a significantly elevated ESR and, rarely, with fever. There may be a family history of the same illness. Other joints may be involved, and the pain is frequently worse at night. The human leukocyte antigen (HLA) B27 test seldom is positive. Fifty percent of patients with ankylosing spondylitis develop transient arthritis of larger peripheral joints; sometimes they develop conjunctivitis or urethritis.

Vertebral fractures, or *compression fractures,* may occur with severe trauma or more often with osteoporosis of the vertebrae in elderly patients. In these patients, vertebral fractures may occur after minor trauma. They also can occur after prolonged immobilization or steroid use. The back pain usually is at the level of the fracture and radiates locally across the back and around the trunk, but seldom into the lower extremities. Vertebral fractures occur more frequently in the middle and lower dorsal spine. Radiography is useful in confirming the diagnosis.

Infectious diseases of the spine, more common in children and intravenous drug users, also cause backaches. Many patients with such infections have an elevated ESR and may be febrile. An infectious cause of backache should be considered in cachectic individuals or patients undergoing prolonged steroid or immunosuppressive therapy. Uncommon causes of disc space infection include actinomycosis, tuberculosis, brucellosis, and fungal infections.

Neoplastic disease can cause backache, particularly in elderly patients. Although primary neoplasms are rare, myeloma and metastatic disease are more common. In a patient with a known cancer the onset of back pain should suggest spinal metastases. Metastatic carcinoma is more common in older patients and should be particularly suspected if they have a history of cancer. Often, after an insidious onset, waist-level or midback pain becomes progressively more severe and more persistent. The pain usually is unrelieved by lying down and frequently worsens at night. Unexplained weight loss with severe back pain aggravated by rest should suggest metastatic carcinoma in the spine. Multiple myeloma can cause severe, unremitting backaches; these are present at rest and may worsen with recumbency. This diagnosis can be confirmed with radiography of the spine, pelvis, and skull; elevated ESR; and abnormal serum protein electrophoretic patterns.

The back pain of *acute pancreatitis* is invariably associated with marked gastrointestinal symptoms. Chronic low-grade pancreatitis, however, may cause vague back pain without noticeable abdominal symptoms. Patients with posterior penetrating *ulcers* may have pain in the high midback as their chief complaint. This pain usually is not in the lumbar area and occasionally is relieved by antacids. Frequently, the patient has tenderness to epigastric palpation. Pain can be referred to the back from the urinary tract, uterus, prostate, and retroperitoneal structures.

Text continued on page 42.

Differential Diagnosis of Backache

CONDITION	NATURE OF PATIENT	NATURE OF SYMPTOMS	ASSOCIATED SYMPTOMS	PRECIPITATING AND AGGRAVATING FACTORS	AMELIORATING FACTORS	PHYSICAL FINDINGS	DIAGNOSTIC STUDIES
Acute lumbosacral strain	*Adults* (ages 20–50): especially those who do strenuous work *Children:* often caused by trauma or sports	Sudden onset Pain usually localized to lumbosacral region		Precipitated by lifting, twisting, and unusual physical activity Aggravated by motion but not by coughing or straining	Lying prone and motionless	**Neurologic examination negative** Paraspinal muscle spasm and pain Straight leg raising causes back but not leg pain Limitation of motion in lumbosacral region anteriorly and posteriorly Increased lumbar lordosis	Usually not indicated
Postural backache (low back strain)	Obese, physically unfit adults	Vague low back pain Difficult to locate point of maximum pain Occasional radiation into buttocks		Worsens as day progresses		**Neurologic examination negative** Limitation of motion anteriorly and posteriorly Increased lumbar lordosis Straight leg raising causes back pain, not leg pain	

Degenerative lumbosacral arthritis	Over age 50	Gradual onset, not precipitated by physical activity Lumbosacral spine motion limited Pain worse in morning Pain radiation into leg uncommon	Often arthritis in other joints	Aggravated by lateral bending and extension of lumbar spine	Lying on back on floor Better 2 hr after arising	**Neurologic examination negative** Symmetric restriction of movement	Radiograph shows disc space narrowing and spurring
Lumbar disc disease	More common in males age 40 or older Rare in children	Sudden onset, previous less severe episodes Pain often radiates down posterolateral aspect of leg Buttock pain or paresthesia pain possibly lancinating or resembling pain of severe toothache	Hypesthesia Dysesthesia Weakness of some leg muscles	Coughing Sneezing Hyperextension of lumbar spine	Lying on side with knees flexed	Neurologic signs in lower leg Asymmetric limitation of motion Hamstring spasm Tender to palpation in sciatic notch Reversal of lumbar lordotic curve Forward or lateral tilt Pain of sciatic distribution after hyperextension of lateral tilt Restricted straight leg raising	MRI CT scan

Table continued on following page.

Differential Diagnosis of Backache *Continued*

CONDITION	NATURE OF PATIENT	NATURE OF SYMPTOMS	ASSOCIATED SYMPTOMS	PRECIPITATING AND AGGRAVATING FACTORS	AMELIORATING FACTORS	PHYSICAL FINDINGS	DIAGNOSTIC STUDIES
Chronic low back pain	All ages	Pain lasts longer than 6 mo Symptoms and disability dissociated from physical findings	Psychological and social dysfunction	Trauma of sciatica may be initial event	Few	Few	Usually negative **Abnormalities may not represent cause of pain**
Spinal stenosis	More common in elderly males	Gradual onset Often mimics intermittent claudication except pain usually in buttocks or thighs Often bilateral		Pain worse with spinal extension Exercise Not precipitated by exercise with spine flexed (e.g., bicycling)	Spinal flexion Pain slowly improves with cessation of walking	Polyradiculopathy Good pedal pulses	MRI CT scan
Gynecologic disorders			Vaginal discharge	Worse around menstruation or ovulation	Lying supine with knees flexed	Abnormal pelvic examination	
Prostatitis	Older men	Constant low back pain	Urinary hesitancy	Change in sexual frequency		Prostate tender to palpation No limitation of back motion No muscle spasm	White blood cells in prostatic secretion

Irritable colon	Young women Stressed individuals	Pain occurs in midback	Mucus in stools Abdominal pain	Stress	Defecation	Colon tender to palpation	
Depression	Adults	Severity of pain varies with mental state Diffuse, pressure-like pain	Early-morning wakefulness Fatigue Constipation Anorexia	Some "loss" or other event		Depressed affect	
Neoplasm (usually backache caused by metastases)	History of cancer especially of breast and prostate First episode of backache occurs after age 50	Gradual onset of pain	Weight loss	May be worse lying down		Rectal, pelvic, or breast examination may reveal primary tumor	Radiographs CT scan MRI
Herpes zoster	Elderly patients	Burning superficial pain	Herpetic lesions appear after onset of pain			Herpetic vesicles	

MRI, Magnetic resonance imaging; *CT*, computed tomography.

Spinal stenosis can cause central low back pain that may radiate into one or both legs. The pain has the character of intermittent claudication: the patient is forced to rest after walking one or two blocks. An important diagnostic feature is that the pain also is relieved by flexion of the spine. It may occur at night, and the patient may find relief by walking, especially in a stooped position.

Spondylolisthesis and *spondylolysis* occur infrequently in the general population but are common causes of back pain in growing individuals. These conditions are caused by repetitive flexion and extension forces, particularly in congenitally predisposed individuals, and are more common in gymnasts and football linemen. The pain is severe, worse with activity, and relieved by rest. Diagnosis is confirmed by appropriate radiographic studies.

Selected References

Alvarez JA, Hardy RH: Lumbar stenosis: a common cause of back and leg pain. Am Fam Physician 57:1825–1834, 1998.

Bernard TN Jr, Kirkaldy-Willis WH: Recognizing specific characteristics of nonspecific low back pain. Clin Orthop 217:266–280, 1987.

Bueff HU, Van Der Reis W: Low back pain. Prim Care 23:345–364, 1996.

Bunnell WP: Back pain in children. Orthop Clin North Am 13:587–604, 1982.

Clancy WG: Low back pain in athletes. Am J Sports Med 7(6):361–369, 1979.

Deyo RA: Early diagnostic evaluation of low back pain. J Gen Intern Med 1:328–338, 1986.

Grabias SL, Mankin HJ: Pain in the lower back. Bull Rheum Dis 30(8):1040–1045, 1979–1980.

Katz JN: The assessment and management of low back pain: a critical review. Arthritis Care Res 6(2):104–114, 1993.

Kaushal SP: The aching back—the history and physical examination. Med Trial Tech Q 26(4):456–466, 1980.

Kirkaldy-Willis WH: Five common back disorders: how to diagnose and treat them. Geriatrics 33:32–41, 1978.

Lazaro L, Quinet RJ: Low back pain: how to make the diagnosis in the older patient. Geriatrics 49:48–53, 1994.

Payne WK, Ogilvie JW: Back pain in children and adolescents. Pediatr Clin North Am 43:899–917, 1996.

Practice parameters: Magnetic resonance imaging in the evaluation of low back syndrome (summary statement). Report of the Quality Standards Subcommittee of the American Academy of Neurology. Neurology 44:767–770, 1994.

Ralston S, Weir M: Suspecting lumbar spondylolysis in adolescent low back pain. Clin Pediatr 37:287–294, 1998.

Russo R, Cook P: Diagnosis of low back pain: role of imaging studies. Occup Med 13:83–96, 1998.

CHAPTER 4

Belching, Bloating, and Flatulence

In this chapter, *belching* is defined as the eructation of gas through the mouth; *bloating* is gaseous abdominal distention; and *flatulence* is the passage of intestinal gas through the rectum.

Belching

Belching is not a symptom of organic disease. The only cause of belching is swallowing of air *(aerophagia).* Air is swallowed or, more accurately, sucked into the stomach and released in the form of a belch. Air swallowing may occur with eating or drinking; more air is swallowed with liquids than with solids. Aerophagia also occurs as a conscious or, more often, as an unconscious nervous habit unassociated with food ingestion. It also can be associated with mouth breathing, gum chewing, orthodontic appliances, and poorly fitting dentures. Chronic, repetitive, "unintentional" belching usually is caused by repetitive inhalation of air and regurgitation of it from the stomach or esophagus in the form of a belch. Some patients who demonstrate these findings consciously or unconsciously relax the upper esophageal sphincter during inspiration.

Nature of Patient

Excessive belchers tend to be nervous, anxious, and tense. Belching often is normal in infants, although excessive belching may be the result of excessive air swallowing during feeding. If the seal of the infant's lips is inadequate around the real or artificial nipple, air may be ingested during nursing. This may be exaggerated if, during feeding, the child is held in a position that is too horizontal.

Some patients with gastric or biliary disorders develop a habit of trying to relieve abdominal discomfort by swallowing (sometimes unconsciously) air and belching it up again; they believe that this provides some relief of their abdominal discomfort.

If associated pathology can be confidently ruled out, patients must be reassured that nothing serious is wrong. It may help to describe how a patient with a laryngectomy can be trained to swallow air; accordingly, a patient with a belching problem can be *un*trained. Simply instructing some patients not to belch when they feel the urge to do so may gradually stop their habit of swallowing air and belching it back. Antifoaming agents have not been particularly helpful. Rather, patients should be instructed to avoid chewing gum, eating quickly, smoking, and drinking carbonated beverages.

Associated Symptoms

The most common associated symptom is abdominal distention, representing gas in the stomach. Most swallowed air that is not belched up is reabsorbed in the small intestine. Usually, intestinal gas is derived by fermentation of intestinal contents. Some patients who swallow large amounts of air may experience or perceive abdominal discomfort until they belch. An urge to belch accompanied by chest pain on belching is a rare finding that may indicate an inferior wall myocardial infarction.

Precipitating and Aggravating Factors

The most common precipitating factor is air swallowing and subsequent relaxation of the esophageal sphincter to produce a belch. Nervous concern about belching can initiate a vicious cycle of unconscious air swallowing and more belching. For some individuals, a supine position prevents swallowed gastric air from escaping into the esophagus, and an upright position facilitates belching. *Emotional stress* increases the likelihood of air swallowing. Ingestion of carbonated beverages, gum chewing, and poorly fitting dentures may also aggravate belching.

Diagnostic Studies

Although belching is invariably caused by swallowing air, this does not rule out coexisting unrelated pathology. If other symptoms warrant further tests, cholecystography, upper gastrointestinal (GI) studies, and chest radiography should be considered.

Less Common Diagnostic Considerations

Rarely, oral eructation of intestinal gas occurs. In these patients the odor is offensive, resembling that of methane or hydrogen sulfide. This suggests fermentation in stagnating gastric contents secondary to gastroparesis, vagotomy, or pyloric obstruction from an ulcer or tumor.

Bloating and Flatulence

Bloating and flatulence are two common complaints reported to physicians. The problem has been recognized since the time of Hippocrates, who taught that "passing gas is necessary to well-being." In the days of early Rome, it was noted that "all Roman citizens shall be allowed to pass gas whenever necessary." Because swallowed air is reabsorbed in the small bowel, most of the gas in the distal small bowel and colon is produced within the bowel by fermentation. In most instances, flatulence is not of any clinical significance, but because various pathologic conditions may be associated with it, their presence should be investigated if the flatulence is excessive.

Bloating may be caused by gaseous distention of the stomach, small bowel, or colon. This occurs more frequently in patients with *gastroparesis, malabsorption* of various sugars and fat, and *colonic bacterial fermentation* of unabsorbed foods. In some patients, disturbed visceral motility and increased sensitivity to normal luminal distention may cause the sensation of bloating.

Flatulence is usually caused by excessive production of gas in an otherwise normal individual or increased discomfort from normal amounts of abdominal gas in healthy individuals. If bloating and flatulence have persisted for several years without the development of signs of serious organic pathology (e.g., weight loss, ascites, jaundice), the patient can be reassured that the flatulence is not of great clinical significance. It must always be remembered, however, that some patients with *gallbladder disease, colon carcinoma, diverticulitis,* and *diverticulosis* may present with a chief complaint of abdominal discomfort, bloating, and occasionally flatulence. Patients with colon carcinoma may present with vague abdominal discomfort or distention.

Nature of Patient

Flatulence is particularly common in infants up to age 3 months. This is referred to as "3-month colic" and is caused by immature nervous control of the gut, which permits gas to become trapped in bowel loops.

Malabsorption may lead to excessive fermentation of unabsorbed nutrients; this may produce an increase in flatulence. This can occur in patients with pancreatic insufficiency, pancreatic carcinoma, biliary disease, celiac disease, or bacterial overgrowth in the small intestine.

Native Americans and other patients, particularly of African or Mediterranean descent, complaining of excess bloating or flatulence may have malabsorption and subsequent fermentation due to *lactose intolerance.* Lactose intolerance does not usually occur in infants or preschool children unless they develop a lactase deficiency secondary to other disorders such as bacterial or viral infections of the small bowel, giardiasis, or sensitivity to cow's milk or gluten (celiac disease). This diagnosis is confirmed if diarrhea develops or if the bloating or flatulence is exacerbated after ingestion of a lactose load (found in milk, ice cream, or other dairy products).

Flatulence also may be seen in patients with *diverticulitis* or *diverticulosis.* Flatulence is common in patients on a diet high in fiber or legumes, often recommended for hypercholesterolemia.

Nature of Symptoms

Most gas that passes from the rectum has an unpleasant, foul odor. The gases that cause this odor are produced by intestinal bacteria. Because of their odor, these gases are detectable in minute quantity.

Associated Symptoms

Flatulence of no clinical significance may be associated with abdominal distention, bloating, borborygmi, abdominal discomfort, and cramping pain. When flatulence or bloating occurs, moderate abdominal pain may be associated, even in the absence of organic disease. Patients may be unable to obtain relief by passing flatus. In some individuals, this is caused by disordered motility of the gut; it cannot propel the gas forward through the bowel. This is not caused by an increased volume of gas but rather by the patient's inability to propel the gut gas forward. Some individuals have an exaggerated pain response to bowel distention despite a normal volume of intestinal gas.

Diverticulitis should be suspected if flatulence is accompanied by lower abdominal pain, constipation, or diarrhea. *Giardiasis* should be suspected as the cause of flatulence, particularly if it is accompanied by foul-smelling, watery, or semisolid stools or abdominal distention.

Precipitating and Aggravating Factors

The symptoms of bloating and flatulence are exacerbated by the ingestion of unabsorbable carbohydrates, including sorbitol, a sugar used as a noncaloric sweetener for candy and other dietetic foods. These provide a substrate for the intestinal bacterial production of carbon dioxide and hydrogen.

Flatulogenic foods include milk, onions, dry beans, celery, carrots, raisins, bananas, apricots, prune juice, apple juice, pretzels, bagels, wheat germ, Brussels sprouts, and ice cream. Patients with a lactase deficiency may develop bloating and flatulence from ingesting many dairy products. The flatulogenic properties of these foods vary greatly among individuals.

Constipation may also aggravate the symptoms of abdominal distention. This can be explained by the increased smooth muscle spasm in the colon around the gas bubbles. **Although constipation may aggravate abdominal bloating, diarrhea usually does not relieve such distention.**

Many patients with *gas entrapment syndromes* experience a worsening of the pain when bending over to tie their shoes or when wearing a tight garment. Occasionally this pain is exacerbated by flexion of the leg on the abdomen.

Ameliorating Factors

Factors that may be associated with decreasing symptoms are diets low in undigestable carbohydrates or lactose, failure of the patient to recline after meals, exercise, and ingestion of buttermilk or broad-spectrum antibiotics. Passage of flatus often relieves the sensation of abdominal bloating, at least temporarily. Any abdominal pain syndrome that is greatly relieved by passage of flatus should suggest gas entrapment.

Physical Findings

When gas is trapped in the splenic flexure, palpation of the left upper quadrant (LUQ) can cause abdominal pain or pain in the chest (pseudoangina). With gas entrapment in the hepatic flexure, the pain most frequently is in the right upper quadrant (RUQ) and may simulate gallbladder discomfort.

Differential Diagnosis of Belching, Bloating, and Flatulence

CONDITION	NATURE OF PATIENT	NATURE OF SYMPTOMS	ASSOCIATED SYMPTOMS	PRECIPITATING AND AGGRAVATING FACTORS	AMELIORATING FACTORS	PHYSICAL FINDINGS	DIAGNOSTIC STUDIES
Belching							
Aerophagia	Nursing infants Nervous, anxious, and tense children and adults	Occurs with eating or drinking Conscious or unconscious nervous habit	Abdominal distention	*Infants:* nursing while in horizontal position Mouth breathing Gum chewing Orthodontic appliances Emotional stress Poorly fitting dentures Supine position Gastric or biliary disorders	Behavior modification: avoidance of gum chewing, eating quickly, smoking, and drinking carbonated beverages Upright position	Those of gas in stomach	
Bloating and flatulence							
Excessive intestinal bacterial fermentation causing increased gas	Most common cause at any age, especially in elderly adults	Flatulence Bloating	Abdominal discomfort or pain	Ingestion of nonabsorbable carbohydrates	Avoidance of all carbohydrates, particularly nonabsorbable ones		
Increased awareness of normal amount of gas					Passage of flatus		

Table continued on following page.

Differential Diagnosis of Belching, Bloating, and Flatulence *Continued*

CONDITION	NATURE OF PATIENT	NATURE OF SYMPTOMS	ASSOCIATED SYMPTOMS	PRECIPITATING AND AGGRAVATING FACTORS	AMELIORATING FACTORS	PHYSICAL FINDINGS	DIAGNOSTIC STUDIES
Malabsorption	Pancreatic insuffiency Pancreatic carcinoma Biliary disease Celiac disease Bacterial overgrowth in small intestine	Increased flatulence	Diarrhea	Nonabsorbable carbohydrates		Greasy, foul-smelling stools	Stool analysis GI radiographs
Lactase deficiency	Common in patients of African or Mediterranean descent and Native Americans	Bloating Excess flatulence	Diarrhea	Lactose load (from dairy products)	Avoidance of lactose Lactase supplement		Mucosal biopsy Lactose load Hydrogen breath test
Giardiasis	Campers and hikers at higher risk	Increased flatulence	Abdominal distention Watery diarrhea, often foul-smelling	Drinking water infested with *Giardia*			Stool analysis for *Giardia* Duodenal aspirate for *Giardia*
Gas entrapment							
Splenic flexure			Pseudoangina	Abdominal pain worsened by bending or wearing tight garments	Passage of flatus	LUQ pain on palpation Pain worsened by flexion of left leg on abdomen	Fluoroscopy for trapped gas
Hepatic flexure			Pain resembling gallbladder discomfort		Passage of flatus	RUQ pain on palpation Pain worsened by flexion of right leg on abdomen	

Diagnostic Studies

The physician should consider the following studies when appropriate: upper and lower GI radiographic examination, proctosigmoidoscopy, cholecystography, and stool analysis for fat and occult blood. If these tests do not reveal organic disease, the patient should be reassured and dietary modification recommended. Likewise, a diagnostic trial of a lactose load can be used to determine, presumptively, if a lactase deficiency is present. If this exacerbates bloating, flatulence, or diarrhea, the patient should avoid foods with lactose. Analysis of breath hydrogen before and after a lactose load is a more specific test for lactase insufficiency.

More complicated tests can be performed, such as D-xylose absorption, mucosal biopsy, and the analysis of flatus for the volume and composition of the various intestinal gases. Large quantities of carbon dioxide or hydrogen suggest malabsorption and fermentation of unabsorbable carbohydrates such as fruits and beans. Lactase deficiency also can lead to excessive quantities of hydrogen in the flatus.

Less Common Diagnostic Considerations

Incomplete or intermittent bowel obstruction, malabsorption syndromes, small bowel diverticula, maldigestion due to pancreatic or biliary disease, and short bowel syndrome may cause bloating or flatulence.

Selected References

Bouchier IAD: Flatulence. Practitioner 224:373–377, 1980.

Clearfield HR: Clinical intestinal gas syndromes. Prim Care 23:621–628, 1996.

Levitt MD, Bond JH: Flatulence. Annu Rev Med 31:127–137, 1980.

Moutes RG, Perman JA: Lactose intolerance: pinpointing the source of nonspecific gastrointestinal symptoms. Postgrad Med 89:175–178, 181–184, 1991.

Rao SSC: Belching, bloating and flatulence. Postgrad Med 101:263–278, 1997.

Raskin JB: Intestinal gas. Geriatrics 38(12):77–93, 1983.

Van Ness MM, Cattau EL: Flatulence: pathophysiology and treatment. Am Fam Physician 31:198–208, 1985.

CHAPTER 5

Breast Lumps

Over their lifetime, most women will detect a lump in their breasts. Approximately 80% of breast masses are discovered by the patient before mammography or physician examination. Most of these lumps are benign cysts. An estimated 1 in 10 women will develop carcinoma of the breast, however, and about 50% of these women will die of their disease. Therefore, it is crucial to be able to separate benign from malignant lesions. Benign breast disease is a continuum of entities, from fibroadenoma and cysts with atypia to cystic changes with marked atypia.

Breast cancer is the second most common cancer in women, after lung cancer. **Breast cancer is the most common cause of death in women ages 40 to 50.** The most common breast lesions are *fibrocystic breasts, fibroadenomas, breast cancer, mastitis* (especially in lactating women), *fat necrosis,* and *gynecomastia,* which by definition occurs only in males. Breast lumps occur in as many as 50% of premenopausal women. Most of these lumps are benign, but because breast cancer is part of the differential, this is a problem of great concern.

Breast lumps are masses in the breast noted on physical examination and may be either benign or malignant. *Benign breast disease* is a pathologic diagnosis and usually applies to masses that have undergone tissue sampling. It includes fibrocystic disease, fibroadenoma, and uncommon conditions such as mastitis, lipoma, traumatic fat necrosis, and galactocele. At biopsy, 90% to 95% of all benign breast disease is fibrocystic disease or fibroadenoma. *Fibrocystic disease* is a poorly defined group of pathologic breast lesions that includes cysts, fibrosis, adenosis, ductal ectasia, hyperplasia, and papilloma.

Nature of Patient

Breast masses are rare in children and are seen more often in adolescents, but malignancy is rare in both groups. Benign breast disease is common in women under age 30. Of women with benign breast disease, 45% have fibrocystic disease, whereas about 45% have fibroadenomas. After age 30, 85% of those with benign breast disease have fibrocystic breasts, and 10% have fibroadenomas. In other words, fibroadenomas become less common with increasing age. Breast cysts are uncommon in elderly patients, but when they occur, 50% of the patients are using estrogen supplements.

Menstrual status, previous history of breast-feeding, parity, family medical history, and drug use are also important in assessing the risk of breast cancer. Users of oral contraceptives have a lower incidence of breast cancer. Factors that increase the risk for breast cancer include a mother or sister who had breast cancer, early menarche, late menopause, and nulliparity. There is twice the risk of breast cancer in patients whose mother or sister had breast cancer and three times the risk if both mother and sister had breast cancer. Also, a rare genetic type of familial breast cancer appears to be inherited as an autosomal dominant trait. Other factors that increase the risk for breast cancer include age greater than 50, first pregnancy after age 35, obesity, and benign proliferative breast disease (ductal and lobular hyperplasia or atypia).

Gynecomastia is normal in the neonatal period, during puberty, and in older males. It also occurs in certain familial syndromes and various pathologic states (cirrhosis, prolactinoma, ulcerative colitis, orchitis, cryptorchidism) and among users of many drugs. Gynecomastia in neonates is probably related to the high levels of estrogen in the placental and fetal circulation. In neonatal gynecomastia, involvement is usually bilateral, and fluid occasionally may be expressed from the nipple. Forty percent of pubertal boys (ages 13–14) develop gynecomastia. When bilateral and mild, it may be diagnosed by the physician, but the patient or family do not recognize it unless it is marked. Unilateral gynecomastia is a more frequent patient complaint.

Nature of Symptoms

The most common breast complaints are nipple discharge, breast pain, and a lump in the breast. Nipple discharge, usually bilateral, can be caused by drugs such as oral contraceptives or phenothiazines. Discharges that are unilateral, pink or bloody, nonmilky, or associated with a mass are suggestive of cancer.

Fibroadenoma is the most common breast lump that occurs during adolescence, but because it is asymptomatic, it usually is detected on physical examination by the patient or physician. These lumps usually are single, unilateral, and located in the upper outer quadrant, although they may be multiple or bilateral in 25% of patients. Fibroadenomas do not vary in size with the menstrual cycle, whereas the lumps of fibrocystic breast disease often enlarge premenstrually.

Associated Symptoms

Pain in the breast *(mastodynia)* in young women suggests fibrocystic disease, especially if the pain is bilateral and increases premenstrually. **Pain in one breast in postmenopausal women is highly suggestive of a malignant process.** Cyclic breast pain that increases premenstrually suggests a benign condition, especially fibrocystic breast disease. Mastodynia also may be caused by papillomas, sclerosing adenosis, ductal ectasia, sporadic puerperal mastitis, breast lipomas, traumatic fat necrosis, and galactoceles. Other causes of chest wall pain include pectoral or intercostal muscle sprain, mastitis, costochondral separation, and costochondritis.

If the lump is fixed to the skin or if nipple discharge or axillary adenopathy is present, cancer is probable. Although nipple discharge, particularly if it is bloody,

Differential Diagnosis of Breast Lumps

CONDITION	NATURE OF PATIENT	NATURE OF SYMPTOMS	ASSOCIATED SYMPTOMS	PRECIPITATING AND AGGRAVATING FACTORS	AMELIORATING FACTORS	PHYSICAL FINDINGS	DIAGNOSTIC STUDIES
Fibroadenoma	Usually age 20–40 Rare in postmenopausal women unless taking estrogen	Usually asymptomatic	May enlarge, especially during adolescence and pregnancy			Usually solitary Multiple or bilateral in 15%–25% Firm, mobile, smooth, rubbery	Mammography Biopsy
Fibrocystic breasts	Frequency increases with age, peaks around menopause, then resolves	Cyclic breast pain, especially around menstruation Usually bilateral	Rare nipple discharge, usually not bloody	Pain and tenderness worsen premenstrually	Menopause Reduction in ingestion of methylxanthines in tea, coffee, cola, and chocolate Oral contraceptives	Multiple tender breast lumps Usually bilateral and in upper outer quadrants Occasionally single or unilateral	Mammography Ultrasonography

Cancer	Usually over age 40 1 in 10 women	Usually none until late in disease	Occasional pain in one breast in postmenopausal patient Bloody nipple discharge Axillary adenopathy	Increased incidence if mother and/or sister had breast cancer Early menarche Late menopause Over age 50 Nulliparous	Decreased incidence in users of oral contraceptives	Hard, irregular, fixed lump	Mammography Biopsy Fine-needle aspiration
Fat necrosis	Older women More common in large pendulous breasts	Painful, tender to palpation		Trauma; surgical trauma		Firm, solitary, irregular lump May be attached to skin	
Gynecomastia	Males, especially pubertal and elderly Alcoholics	Breast enlargement Unilateral or bilateral, often tender	Adrenogenital syndrome	Drugs: oral and topical estrogens, marijuana, spironolactone, methyldopa, phenytoin, cimetidine, digitalis, finasteride		Under nipple	

suggests cancer, it occasionally occurs with fibrocystic disease and in males with adrenogenital syndrome.

If lactation is associated with a breast lump, a *prolactinoma* or pregnancy should be suspected.

Precipitating and Aggravating Factors

Risk factors for breast cancer are discussed earlier in this chapter. The pain and tenderness of fibrocystic breasts often worsen during the premenstrual period. Gynecomastia is exacerbated by several drugs, including marijuana, spironolactone, methyldopa, phenytoin, cimetidine, finasteride, diazepam, tricyclic antidepressants, phenothiazines, histamine H_2-receptor blockers, and digitalis. Fat necrosis may be precipitated by external trauma as well as surgical trauma.

Ameliorating Factors

Cyst size is reduced and pain decreases in patients with fibrocystic breast disease when they become menopausal. Oral contraceptives, pregnancy, and reduction in the ingestion of methylxanthines contained in coffee, tea, cola, and chocolate also often alleviate the symptoms of fibrocystic disease.

Physical Findings

Fibroadenomas usually are unilateral and occur in the upper, outer quadrant. They usually present as a smooth, oval, occasionally irregular, 3- to 4-cm firm to elastic lump that is freely movable. Fibrocystic disease usually is bilateral, symmetric, with multiple, tender, soft, or cystic round lumps that have regular borders. They occasionally are single or unilateral. In contrast, malignant breast lumps are typically hard, irregular, fixed, and associated with a nipple lesion or discharge, adenopathy, and occasionally pain.

All suspicious lesions must be biopsied to obtain a histologic diagnosis, even though mammography is negative and not all the typical findings of cancer are present.

Gynecomastia usually is unilateral but may be bilateral. In contrast to breast tissue from gynecomastia, cancerous lesions are not usually palpable under the male nipple. The lumps of fat necrosis usually are firm, solitary, and irregular and may be attached to the overlying skin.

Diagnostic Studies

Various organizations have different recommendations for mammography. Generally it is recommended that mammography be performed yearly after age 50. At least one mammogram should be done between ages 35 and 40, but more frequently in patients at greater than usual risk, such as those with a mother or sister or both with a history of breast carcinoma. Fine-needle aspiration, fine-needle biopsy, and excisional biopsy are all useful techniques for determining the histologic character of a breast lump. Biopsies are indicated when the mammogram suggests cancer or a suspicious lesion is palpable on physical examination.

Mammographic signs of cancer include (1) irregularity of the mass, (2) mass appearing smaller on mammogram than on physical examination, (3) nipple retraction, (4) increased stromal density on sequential examinations, and (5) calcification appearing on the mammogram. Biopsy should be performed on all suspicious lesions to obtain a histologic diagnosis. **Because mammograms can miss 10% to 15% of lesions, biopsies should be performed on any suspicious mass that is palpable on physical examination.** Ultrasound examination and fine-needle aspiration are helpful in differentiating cystic from solid lesions.

Newer methods for breast imaging include magnetic resonance imaging (MRI), digital mammography, computer-aided diagnosis, positron emission tomography (PET), and single-photon emission computed tomography (SPECT). Their specific roles in screening and diagnosis have yet to be determined.

Less Common Diagnostic Considerations

Less common causes of benign breast lumps include papillomas, sclerosing adenosis, duct ectasia, lobular neoplasia, and apocrine metaplasia. Solitary *papillomas* are the most common benign cause of nipple discharge and bleeding. They usually are unilateral and located in the subareolar region. They most often occur in perimenopausal women and do not increase their cancer risk. In contrast, multiple papillomas increase cancer risk fourfold and most often occur in premenopausal women. With multiple papillomas, nipple discharge is rare. They are bilateral in 25% of patients and occur distal to the nipple.

Ductal ectasia results from ductal dilatation and stasis of ductal contents with a subsequent inflammatory reaction. It often is associated with nipple discharge and, occasionally, ductal calcification. In women over age 55, nipple discharge is most often caused by ectasia, although one third of patients with nipple discharge have a ductal papilloma.

Mondor's disease is a superficial thrombophlebitis of the anterolateral portion of the breast and chest wall. It may occur spontaneously or secondary to injury or surgery. The skin may be retracted along the course of the thrombosed vein.

Sporadic puerperal mastitis, which seldom occurs in lactating mothers, may result in a breast abscess presenting as a lump. Fever, chills, and tenderness usually are present.

Selected References

Bland KI, Love N: Evaluation of common breast masses. Postgrad Med 92:95–108, 1992.

Conry C: Evaluation of a breast complaint: is it cancer? Am Fam Physician 49:445–450, 1994.

Donegan WL: Evaluation of a palpable breast mass. N Engl J Med 327:937–942, 1992.

Eddy DM: Screening for breast cancer. Ann Intern Med 11:389–399, 1989.

Grady D, Hodgkins ML, Goodson WH III: The lumpy breast. West J Med 149:226–229, 1988.
Greydanus DE, Parks DS, Farrell EG: Breast disorders in children and adolescents. Pediatr Clin North Am 36:601–638, 1989.
Hindle WH: The diagnostic evaluation. Obstet Gynecol Clin North Am 21:499–517, 1994.
Hutchins LF, Broadwater R Jr, Lang NP, et al: Breast cancer. Dis Mon 36:63–125, 1990.
Neuman JR: Evaluation and treatment of gynecomastia. Am Fam Physician 55:1835–1844, 1997.
Scott EB: Fibrocystic breast disease. Am Fam Physician 36:119–126, 1987.
Steering Committee on Clinical Practice Guidelines for the Care and Treatment of Breast Cancer: The palpable breast lump: information and recommendations to assist decision-making when a breast lump is detected. Can Med Assoc J 158(suppl 3):S3-S8, 1998.
Winchester DP: Evaluation and management of breast abnormalities. Cancer 66:1345–1347, 1990.

CHAPTER 6

Chest Pain

Chest pain is one of the most common complaints of adult patients. Whether they admit it or not, they are usually concerned that this pain is caused by some type of cardiac disease. Therefore, the physician must be thoroughly familiar with the differential diagnosis of chest pain. Although the physician must realize that it is in the patient's interest not to overlook any acute cardiac illness, it is just as essential that cardiac disease not be incorrectly diagnosed or inferred, because such misdiagnosis may cause some patients to become "iatrogenic cardiac cripples."

Common causes of chest pain include *angina pectoris; myocardial infarction;* musculoskeletal chest wall conditions, including *costochondritis, benign overuse myalgia, fibrositis,* and *referred pain; trauma; cervicodorsal arthritis; psychoneurosis; esophagitis; esophageal spasm; pleuritis;* and *mitral valve prolapse* (Table 6–1). Less common causes of chest pain include *lung tumors, gas entrapment syndromes, pulmonary hypertension, pulmonary embolus,* and *pericarditis.* Persons with biliary disease, including *cholelithiasis, cholecystitis,* and *common duct stones,* may also present with pain in the chest.

Nature of Patient

Chest pain due to *coronary artery disease* (CAD) or other serious organic pathology is rare in young people. In children, chest pain most likely results from *musculoskeletal system trauma* (e.g., strain, overuse, costochondritis), an *inflammatory process* (e.g., pleurisy), or a *psychiatric problem* (e.g., anxiety, conversion disorder, depression). When pain similar in quality to angina pectoris occurs in a child or adolescent, *reflux esophagitis, mitral valve prolapse,* or *cocaine abuse* should be suspected. Although uncommon, myocarditis and pericarditis may cause cardiac chest pain in children. Rarely, children with congenital anomalies of the coronary arteries may have ischemic pain. Although *pulmonary embolism* is uncommon in children, it should be suspected in any postoperative, immobilized, or bedridden patient. Likewise, females of any age are at increased risk for pulmonary embolism if they are taking oral contraceptives.

In adults, any cause of chest pain may occur. Some patients experience chest wall pain after *aortocoronary bypass* using internal mammary artery grafts. In older patients, *CAD, cervicodorsal arthritis, tumors, esophagitis,* and *pulmonary embolism* are the most common causes.

TABLE 6.1 Noncardiac Causes of Chest Pain

RESEMBLES ANGINA SLIGHTLY	NOT TYPICAL OF ANGINA
Psychoneurosis*	Psychoneurosis*
Pulmonary hypertension*	Costochondritis
Esophagitis, esophagospasm*	Nonspecific myositis
	Radiculitis
	Cervicodorsal arthritis
	Bursitis
	Shoulder disease
	Pericarditis
	Pneumonia
	Aneurysm
	Gastrointestinal distention with gaseous entrapment*
	Peptic ulcer
	Gallbladder disease*
	Diaphragmatic or paraesophageal hernia*

*Relieved by nitroglycerin.
From Seller RH: *In* Rakel RE, Conn HF: Family Practice, 2nd ed. Philadelphia, WB Saunders Co, 1978.

Nature of Pain

Although the physician must differentiate chest pain of cardiac origin from other types of pain, it is not sufficient to establish whether or not the pain is of cardiac origin. Patients with pain of cardiac origin should receive varying forms of therapy and will have a different prognosis, depending on whether their pain is caused by *angina pectoris, Prinzmetal's angina, hypertrophic cardiomyopathy, mitral valve prolapse,* or *pericarditis.* An accurate diagnosis usually can be made by a precise history. In eliciting the history of chest pain, the examiner should note five specific characteristics of the discomfort: location of pain, quality of pain, duration of pain, factors that precipitate or exacerbate the pain, and ameliorating factors.

The distinctive clinical characteristics of *angina pectoris* are that the pain is paroxysmal (lasting 30 seconds to a few minutes), dull, pressing, squeezing, or aching; it is located substernally; and it may radiate to the precordium, upper extremities, neck, or jaw. The term *anginal salute* refers to the way patients hold a clenched fist over their sternum to describe their pain. Some patients experience no chest pain and only neck, arm, or jaw discomfort. The location of pain in patients with angina pectoris may vary greatly from person to person, but it differs little with recurrent episodes in the same patient. Thus, if the patient complains of chest pain in different locations during separate episodes, the pain is probably not caused by angina pectoris. Pain of biliary tract or esophageal origin is likely to be substernal, whereas the pain of pericarditis is likely to be precordial.

Patients with angina pectoris describe their pain as a tightness, pressure, or heaviness, and infrequently as a burning sensation. Burning is relatively uncommon and suggests the possibility of *peptic esophagitis,* the most frequent imitator of CAD. **Rarely, if ever, is anginal pain described as knifelike, sharp, or sticking.**

Although some patients describe the pain as "sharp," they usually mean that it is severe in intensity rather than knifelike in quality. The pain of *pulmonary hypertension,* which often occurs in patients with mitral stenosis or primary pulmonary disease, may be indistinguishable from the pain of angina pectoris. It is usually described as a dull, pressing, substernal pain. It is precipitated by exertion and relieved by rest or administration of nitroglycerin. Although this pain may radiate to either arm, it radiates more often to the right arm. Patients with pulmonary hypertension and CAD may experience chest pain as a result of pulmonary hypertension, CAD, or both.

Dull, achy, or burning chest pain also may be experienced by patients with *peptic esophagitis* or *esophagospasm, pulmonary hypertension, cervicodorsal arthritis, gallbladder disease, diaphragmatic* or *paraesophageal hernias,* and *mitral valve prolapse.* The associated exacerbating or ameliorating factors are most helpful in establishing the diagnosis.

Sharp, sticking pains, especially if they last only a few seconds, are more characteristic of *psychoneurosis, costochondritis, cervicodorsal arthritis, mitral valve prolapse, chest wall syndrome, pericarditis,* and *pleuritic processes.* The location of the pain usually is not helpful in differentiating the cause of the chest pain in these conditions, with a few exceptions. Pain on the side of the chest, particularly if it is exacerbated by respiration, is more likely to be pleuritic. Pain localized to the costochondral junction or specific intercostal spaces is most likely caused by *costochondritis* or *intercostal myositis.* The pain of *chest wall syndrome* may occur during exercise or at rest; occasionally, it is nocturnal. The pain may be described as "sticking," but also as "dull" and "pressing." The most critical finding in the diagnosis of chest wall syndrome is detection of chest wall tenderness on physical examination. It frequently is located substernally, at the left parasternal region, near the shoulder, and in the fourth or fifth left intercostal space (Fig. 6–1). Pain

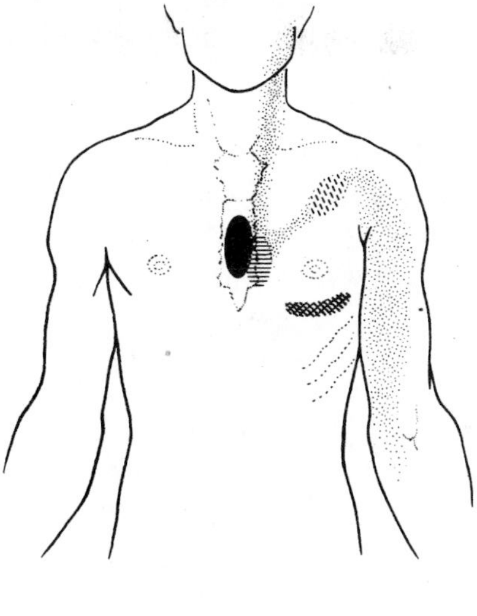

■ **Figure 6.1** Regions of anterior chest where spontaneous pain is most often experienced and where tenderness can be elicited. Circumscribed areas represent primary site of pain and of tenderness; stippled areas represent radiation of pain. (From Epstein SE, et al: Chest wall syndrome: a common cause of unexplained cardiac pain. JAMA 241:2793–2797, 1979.)

that is positional, pleuritic, sharp, or reproduced by palpation means a much lower probability of ischemic heart disease.

The presence of cervicodorsal arthritis or reflux esophagitis does not rule out the possibility that chest pain is caused by coronary disease. Patients may have two conditions, each of which contributes to their chest pain. For example, a patient may have pain from esophagitis as well as pain from angina pectoris. When two conditions coexist, the patient may be able to distinguish between the two types of chest pain. If questioned carefully , for example, a patient may describe a dull substernal pain often induced by exercise and relieved by nitroglycerin but not antacids, as well as another dull substernal pain radiating to the neck and arms that is not as thoroughly relieved by nitroglycerin but occasionally is ameliorated by antacids. When further investigated, this patient may have documented CAD and reflux esophagitis.

Associated Symptoms

The pain of *mitral valve prolapse* occasionally may be indistinguishable from that of CAD, in that it may occur with exertion and seldom can be relieved by nitroglycerin. More often the chest pain of mitral valve prolapse has features not typical of angina that should alert the physician to the pain not being of coronary origin. The chest pain of mitral valve prolapse usually occurs during rest. Although it may last for a few minutes, it also may last for several hours. It often is described as "sticking" and is not substernally located. It frequently is alleviated by lying down; the pain of *angina pectoris* often is worsened by recumbency, as is the pain of *reflux esophagitis.* **If atypical chest pain is associated with arrhythmias (particularly tachyarrhythmias) and lightheadedness or syncope, mitral valve prolapse should be suspected.**

Patients with *pneumonia* or *pulmonary embolism* may have chest pain but usually also have fever, cough, or hemoptysis. Patients who have protracted or vigorous coughing may experience chest pain resulting from intercostal muscle or periosteal trauma. Local chest wall tenderness usually is present.

Patients with *hypertrophic cardiomyopathy* (HCM) may have typical angina pectoris, but their chest pain is not necessarily caused by CAD. **In patients with HCM the most common symptom is dyspnea, which usually precedes the development of chest pain.** In any patient with angina pectoris who has coexisting or antecedent dyspnea, a careful search for HCM should be made.

Although the pain from *esophagitis* often is similar to anginal pain, the associated symptoms are helpful in establishing the differential diagnosis. The pain of esophagitis usually is not related to exertion but is related to overeating and recumbency. The pain typically awakens the patient at night. This symptom is rare in patients with angina pectoris unless they have angina decubitus. Patients with angina decubitus usually have congestive heart failure, and their pain often is precipitated by minimal exertion.

Cervicodorsal arthritis may produce chest pain. This pain seldom is similar to that of angina pectoris. More often it is sharp and piercing but occasionally may be described as a deep, boring, dull discomfort. The major characteristics of *root pain* are (1) pain with body movement, (2) pain on coughing and sneezing, and (3) pain after prolonged recumbency. The pains may occur in any part of the chest or shoulder girdle, may radiate down the arms, and may be bilateral or unilateral. Chest pain may be precipitated by bending or hyperextension of the upper spine or neck. Usually the pain is not related to exercise and is fleeting and thus is not truly relieved by rest.

The chest pain associated with *pericarditis* may be pleuritic or heavy and steady.

Precipitating and Aggravating Factors

Anginal pain often is precipitated by physical exertion, emotional stress, sexual activity, exposure to cold, and occasionally, eating (Table 6–2). *Prinzmetal's angina* occurs at rest. Chest pain due to pulmonary hypertension also is induced by exertion.

Chest pain from *peptic esophagitis* often is precipitated by overeating and recumbency. It frequently awakens the patient at night. Chest pain from *esophageal spasm* can be precipitated by swallowing certain substances, particularly cold liquids and anything that stimulates the production of endogenous gastrin. Thus, chest pain that follows ingestion of alcohol should suggest esophageal spasm. Chest pain during exercise such as jogging may be caused by esophageal reflux rather than angina pectoris. The former is relieved by antacids.

If the pain is exacerbated or reproduced when pressure is applied over the painful area, *costochondritis, Tietze's syndrome, rib fractures, chest wall syndrome,* and *nonspecific myositis* are more likely. Reproduction or exacerbation of pain with chest wall pressure does not usually occur in patients with ischemic cardiac pain.

Although a few patients with chest pain due to *hypertrophic cardiomyopathy* obtain relief with nitrates, the pain of HCM usually is exacerbated and the murmur intensified by nitroglycerin. **Just as chest pain associated with dyspnea should alert the physician to the possibility of HCM, chest pain exacerbated by nitrates should suggest HCM, as should the associated lightheadedness, dizziness, or syncope.**

Ameliorating Factors

Nitroglycerin usually relieves *angina pectoris* within 2 to 4 minutes; rest alone usually brings relief in less than 10 minutes. Unfortunately, a positive response to nitroglycerin does not confirm CAD as the cause of pain. Nitroglycerin works primarily by relaxing smooth muscle. **Nitroglycerin also may relieve chest pain due to peptic esophagitis and esophageal spasm, biliary dyskinesia and cholelithiasis, gas entrapment syndrome, pulmonary hypertension, mitral valve prolapse, and occasionally, psychoneurotic chest pain** (see Table 6–1).

Pain can be caused by CAD and yet not be relieved by nitroglycerin. The pain

TABLE 6.2 Diagnosis of Chest Pain

CONDITION	CHEST PAIN		DIZZINESS, VERTIGO, SYNCOPE	RESPONSE TO		CARDIAC AUSCULTATION	ABNORMAL ECG		STRESS ECG	SYMPTOMS REPRODUCED AT BEDSIDE
	TYPICAL	ATYPICAL		NITRATES	PROPRANOLOL		QRS COMPLEX	ST SEGMENT–T WAVE		
Coronary heart disease	+++	+	Rare	++++	++++	– to +++	Common	Common	+++	–
Angina with normal coronary arteries	++	++	Rare	++	++	–	Occasional	Common	+++	–
Hypertrophic cardiomyopathy	+++	+	++	+	+++	– to +++ Variable	Common	Common	+++	Rare
Mitral valve prolapse	+	+++	++	+	+++	– to +++ Variable	Rare	Common	++	Rare
Hyperventilation syndrome	+ Rare	++	++	–	+	–	–	Rare	+	++
Esophageal disease	+ (?)	+++	–	+	–	–	–	–	–	–
Radicular syndromes	+	+++	+	+ (?)	–	–	–	–	–	+++
Chest wall syndromes	–	+++	–	–	–	–	–	–	–	+++

ECG, Electrocardiogram.

From Levine HJ: Difficult problems in the diagnosis of chest pain. Am Heart J 100:108–117, 1980.

may be too severe or the nitroglycerin may be outdated or administered improperly. If the symptoms suggest CAD and sublingual nitroglycerin does not provide relief, the physician should determine whether the patient is taking the medication properly. A helpful method is to take a tiny piece of paper, crumple it into the size of a nitroglycerin tablet, and have the patient place it under the tongue. The patient should be instructed (1) to let the nitroglycerin dissolve and remain under the tongue unswallowed, (2) to expect a warm flushing feeling, and (3) to keep the saliva under the tongue until the pain is relieved. At this point the patient may either swallow the saliva or expectorate it.

Valsalva's maneuver also may give prompt relief of angina pectoris, but it does not usually relieve the chest pain of obstructive HCM. Occasionally, patients with HCM obtain relief of chest pain by squatting, which decreases outflow obstruction.

If antacid relieves a patient's chest pain, this strongly suggests that the discomfort is caused by *reflux esophagitis.* Relief of chest pain by recumbency suggests *mitral valve prolapse,* whereas relief by squatting suggests *HCM.* Relief of chest pain by passage of flatus suggests *gas entrapment* in the hepatic or splenic flexure.

Physical Findings

Few physical findings are diagnostic of *angina pectoris.* A sinus tachycardia or a bradycardia may coincide with anginal pain. Signs of *congestive heart failure* in patients with chest pain suggest that the pain probably is caused by myocardial ischemia. If a careful examination performed during an episode of ischemic heart pain reveals a palpable systolic bulge near the apex, a paradoxic splitting of the second sound, a diastolic filling sound (S_3 or S_4), or a transient mitral regurgitant murmur, this strongly suggests that ischemic heart disease is the cause of chest pain. Likewise, *hypertension, diabetic retinopathy,* or the presence of cutaneous manifestations of atherosclerosis such as *xanthomas* increases the probability of CAD as the cause of chest pain.

Squatting decreases outflow tract obstruction and thus diminishes the characteristic midsystolic murmur of *hypertrophic cardiomyopathy.* The systolic murmur of HCM is increased with the patient in the upright position and during Valsalva's maneuver. Atrial and ventricular arrhythmias (dysrhythmias) are common in HCM and occasionally may be the earliest manifestation. Chest wall tenderness to palpation or auscultation of a pericardial friction or a pleural friction may assist in diagnosis.

Tenderness in the region of spontaneous pain, especially if the quality of pain can be reproduced by pressure on the area, strongly suggests *chest wall syndrome.* Certain maneuvers (e.g., horizontal arm flexion, "crowing rooster" maneuver) also may cause the pain of chest wall syndrome. *Mitral valve prolapse* is suggested by auscultation of a midsystolic "click," late systolic murmur, or both. Patients may have mitral valve prolapse with absent or transient auscultatory findings.

Diagnostic Studies

Resting electrocardiograms (ECGs) may be normal in 50% of patients with angiographically confirmed CAD. An ECG obtained during a bout of chest pain is more likely to be abnormal. Some studies have revealed that even during an episode of chest pain, ST-segment depression occurs in only 50% of patients. **An appropriately administered exercise ECG is probably the most useful and noninvasive test in the diagnosis of CAD.**

Stress echocardiography, myocardial perfusion scanning, and radionuclide cineangiography have greatly enhanced the ability to diagnose CAD using noninvasive tests. Coronary angiography should be reserved for patients who will probably need and who consent to have coronary artery surgery, as well as for other select patients.

The ECG of *mitral valve prolapse* may show changes similar to those of CAD. ECG changes, if present, usually include ST-segment depression and T-wave inversion or abnormalities in leads II, III, and AVF and occasionally in the precordial leads. The ST-segment–T-wave changes of mitral valve prolapse may be differentiated from those of CAD by the oral administration of 40 mg of propranolol. The ST-segment–T-wave abnormalities seen in some patients with mitral valve prolapse (and in some athletes) may diminish or disappear 1 to 2 hours after propranolol administration, whereas patients with angina pectoris are unaffected.

The ECG usually is abnormal in patients with *obstructive hypertrophic cardiomyopathy,* although a normal ECG may be obtained. The most common ECG abnormalities include those of left ventricular hypertrophy, intraventricular conduction defects, and nonspecific ST-segment–T-wave changes. The ECG findings (P-wave abnormalities) most helpful in the diagnosis of HCM are those not generally seen in patients with CAD. These P-wave abnormalities suggestive of atrial enlargement are common in patients with HCM and uncommon in patients with CAD. An ECG picture of transmural infarction (Q waves in the anteroseptal or inferior leads) also may be seen in some patients with HCM.

The echocardiogram is the preferred study for the diagnosis of both mitral valve prolapse and obstructive HCM.

Less Common Diagnostic Considerations

The pain of *costochondritis* and *costochondrodynia* usually is localized to the costochondral junction. The pain may be constant or may be exacerbated by movement of the chest wall, including respiratory motion. The physician may confirm the diagnosis by applying pressure over the painful area, thus replicating the pain.

Cervical angina, also called *pseudoangina,* is a rare cause of chest pain, which is similar to that of angina pectoris in quality, location, and radiation. The pain is not brought on by exertion but is often precipitated by cervical motion, sneezing,

Text continued on page 68.

■ Differential Diagnosis of Chest Pain

CONDITION	NATURE OF PATIENT	NATURE OF PAIN	ASSOCIATED SYMPTOMS	PRECIPITATING AND AGGRAVATING FACTORS	AMELIORATING FACTORS	PHYSICAL FINDINGS	DIAGNOSTIC STUDIES
Angina pectoris	Adult	Achy, dull, tight, severe, pressing Not usually sharp or sticking Substernal		Exertion Cold exposure Emotional stress	Nitroglycerin Rest Valsalva's maneuver	Sinus tachycardia, bradycardia, or apical systolic bulge coincident with pain Xanthomas Signs of heart failure	Exercise ECG Coronary arteriography Radionuclide tests
Prinzmetal's angina	Adult	Achy, dull, tight, severe, pressing Not usually sharp or sticking Substernal		Often occurs at rest	Nitroglycerin Rest		ECG during attack Coronary arteriography
Esophagitis	Any age	Burning Tightness May be identical to that of angina	Water brash "Heartburn" after alcohol	Overeating Recumbency (may awaken from sleep) Occasionally precipitated by exertion	Antacids		Esophagoscopy Infusion of dilute acid into esophagus (Bernstein's test)
Esophageal spasm	Especially obese adults	May be identical in quality to angina		Often induced by ingestion of alcohol or cold liquids	Occasionally relieved by nitroglycerin		Esophageal manometry

Table continued on following page.

Differential Diagnosis of Chest Pain *Continued*

CONDITION	NATURE OF PATIENT	NATURE OF PAIN	ASSOCIATED SYMPTOMS	PRECIPITATING AND AGGRAVATING FACTORS	AMELIORATING FACTORS	PHYSICAL FINDINGS	DIAGNOSTIC STUDIES
Mitral valve prolapse	Any age	Not usually substernal Often has sticking quality May last several hours Not typical of angina	Palpitations Arrhythmias Often occurs at rest Syncope		Beta blockers Recumbency	Click/late systolic murmur	Echocardiogram Phonocardiogram
Hypertrophic cardio-myopathy	Any age	Pain may be similar to that of angina	Dyspnea Arrhythmias Lightheadedness	Pain may be aggravated by nitroglycerin	Beta blockers Squatting	Murmur intensified by nitroglycerin and Valsalva's maneuver Decreased by squatting	Echocardiogram
Intercostal myositis	Any age	May be sticking in quality		May intensify with inspiration		Localized tenderness to palpation No pleural friction	
Cervicodorsal arthritis	Adult	May be sharp or sticking Duration only a few seconds		May be precipitated by certain movements (e.g., neck exercises and twisting) Not related to stress			Radiographs of cervicodorsal spine

Chest wall syndrome	Adult	Often sharp and sticking Fleeting		May be aggravated by recumbency and certain positions		Local tenderness to palpation "Crowing rooster" maneuver may precipitate pain	
Pericarditis	Any age	Sharp or dull Protracted duration	Fever Recent viral infection			Pericardial friction	ECG Echocardiogram CBC
Myocardial infarction	Adult	Severe Crushing Precordial Protracted duration	Sweating Fatigue Nausea		Not relieved by nitroglycerin		ECG Serial CK-MB levels Radionuclide studies
Gas entrapment syndrome	Any age Often obese	Dull, achy	Flatulence	Aggravated by bending and tight garments	Passage of flatus Nitroglycerin	Flexing thigh and palpation of colon may elicit pain	Gas in hepatic or splenic flexure on radiographs

CBC, Complete blood count; *CK-MB,* creatine kinase, muscle-brain subunits (CK_2, found primarily in cardiac muscle).

or coughing and aggravated by tilting the head laterally. The diagnosis is confirmed by finding cervical disc disease on magnetic resonance imaging (MRI).

Gas entrapment syndromes (gas trapped in the hepatic or splenic flexure) are suggested by a history of chest pain when the patient bends over or wears a tight garment. The pain may be exacerbated by bending, flexing the thigh on the chest, or palpating the colon. The pain may be relieved by passage of flatus or by ingestion of sublingual nitroglycerin.

The pain of *pulmonary hypertension* may be indistinguishable from that of angina pectoris and other causes of exercise-induced chest wall pain. It also can be relieved by sublingual nitroglycerin. It should be suspected in patients with mitral stenosis or other causes of pulmonary hypertension, pulmonary disease, an accentuated pulmonary second sound, or ECG signs of right atrial disease (peaked P waves) or right ventricular overload. The pain of a pulmonary embolus in the acute phase may be caused by pulmonary hypertension. Subsequently, the pain is related to pulmonary infarction with associated pleurisy. The pain usually is not related to exercise and tends to become more constant (often with a pleuritic component) in the later stages.

Pericarditis should be suspected in the patient with continual chest pain associated with diffuse ECG changes. This pain tends to be aggravated by changes in position. A pericardial friction rub confirms the diagnosis.

Lung and mediastinal tumors often present with chest pain, which tends to be constant, especially in the later stages. **Whenever the diagnosis of chest pain is not clear, particularly in adult patients, the examiner should obtain a chest radiograph to detect possible tumors.**

Selected References

ACC/AHA Guidelines for the Clinical Application of Echocardiography: Executive summary. J Am Coll Cardiol 29:862–868, 1997.

Anselmino M, Clark GWB, Hinder RA: Esophageal chest pain: state of the art. Surg Annu 25(part 1):193–210, 1993.

Anzai AK, Merkin TE: Adolescent chest pain. Am Fam Physician 53:1682–1688, 1996.

Chambers J, Bass C: Atypical chest pain: looking beyond the heart. Q J Med 91:239–244, 1998.

Diagnosis of chest pain. Lancet 1:129–130, 1977 (editorial).

Epstein SE, Gerber LH, Borer JS: Chest wall syndrome: a common cause of unexplained cardiac pain. JAMA 241:2793–2797, 1979.

Fam AG: Approach to musculoskeletal chest wall pain. Prim Care 15:767–782, 1988.

Levine HJ: Difficult problems in the diagnosis of chest pain. Am Heart J 100:108–117, 1980.

Murata GH: Evaluating chest pain in the emergency department. West J Med 159:61–68, 1993.

Pellikka PA: Stress echocardiography in the evaluation of chest pain and accuracy in the diagnosis of coronary artery disease. Prog Cardiovasc Dis 39:523–532, 1997.

Schroeder JS, Lamb IH, Hu M: The prehospital course of patients with chest pain: analysis of the prodromal, symptomatic, decision-making, transportation and emergency room periods. Am J Med 64:742–748, 1978.

Sharkey AM, Clark BJ: Common complaints with cardiac implications in children. Pediatr Clin North Am 38:657–666, 1991.

Zoob M: Differentiating the causes of chest pain. Geriatrics 33:95–101, 1978.

CHAPTER 7

Colds, Flu, and Stuffy Nose

The differential diagnosis of colds, flu, and stuffy nose might appear unimportant, since most of these conditions have no specific cures. Because upper respiratory infections (URIs) are the most common affliction of adults and children, however, the sheer case volume requires the physician to be particularly expert in the diagnosis and symptomatic treatment of these conditions.

Many different *viruses* are responsible for causing colds, URIs, and flu. The physician must be able to differentiate these viral infections from *allergic rhinitis* (both perennial and seasonal), *chronic rhinitis,* and the common complications of these viral infections, which include *sinusitis, otitis media, bronchitis,* and *pneumonia.* These last four complications usually are secondary to superimposed bacterial infections, which will respond to appropriate antibiotic therapy. The constitutional complaints often associated with URI also may represent the prodrome of other viral infections, such as *infectious mononucleosis, measles,* and *mumps.*

Nature of Patient

Children typically experience more severe constitutional symptoms with URIs or colds than do adults. After a *common cold,* adults with a history of bronchitis, allergies, asthma, heavy cigarette smoking, or immune incompetence and children with a history of recurrent bronchitis, allergies, or cystic fibrosis develop lower respiratory tract infections more frequently than other people.

Influenza tends to be milder in neonates and children; severity increases with age. Many elderly patients develop a superimposed *bacterial pneumonia.* More than 70% of deaths recorded during known influenza epidemics have occurred in patients over age 65. Other high-risk groups include patients with acquired immunodeficiency syndrome (AIDS), chronic cardiorespiratory disease, chronic renal disease, diabetes, and third-trimester pregnancies. *Rhinitis medicamentosa* should be suspected in patients who frequently use nasal drops, sprays, or inhalers.

The physician must be especially alert for the development of complications of common URIs. *Sinusitis* is more likely to occur in a patient with a history of recurrent sinusitis. *Otitis media* is more common in young children, *bronchitis* in smokers and those with underlying *pulmonary disease,* and *pneumonia* in older and diabetic patients.

Nature of Symptoms and Associated Symptoms

Symptoms of common *viral upper respiratory infections* are well known. These symptoms largely depend on the particular infective viral agent, the patient's age, and the underlying medical conditions. The incubation period is 1 to 3 days. Usually, patients have profuse nasal discharge and congestion and complain of stuffy nose, sneezing, postnasal drip, cough, and sore throat. They also may complain of headache, fever, malaise, and hoarseness and may note pharyngeal exudates, oropharyngeal vesicles, and lymphadenopathy. Children may experience vomiting, diarrhea, abdominal pain, and wheezing.

Although a URI is the most frequent cause of nasal airway obstruction, other causes must be considered, including polyps, foreign body, herpes simplex, furuncle (folliculitis of nasal vibrissae), and less common infections. In neonates, unilateral nasal obstruction may be caused by a congenital abnormality (e.g., choanal atresia). In a child with unilateral nasal obstruction as the presenting symptom, the physician should consider a foreign body.

Although the symptoms of influenza and common URI may be similar, *influenza viral infections* often can be differentiated from the symptoms of a common cold by the sudden onset of typical signs of flu: shivering, chills, malaise, insomnia, marked aching of the limb and back muscles, dry cough, retrosternal pain, and loss of appetite. A patient with *type A influenza* may not have coryza (profuse nasal discharge).

In addition to acute stuffy nose, chronic stuffy nose is a common complaint. *Chronic rhinitis* is most frequently caused by *allergy* (both seasonal and perennial), *nonallergic rhinitis with eosinophilia* (NARES), drugs (topical and systemic), and *vasomotor rhinitis.* Chronic rhinitis is characterized by nasal congestion, postnasal drip, rhinorrhea, sneezing, and nasal itchiness. It is difficult to determine the specific cause on the basis of the symptoms alone.

The physician must especially recognize *allergic rhinitis* and *chronic rhinitis* as causes of nasal stuffiness. The two types of allergic rhinitis are perennial and seasonal. Patients with *perennial rhinitis* usually complain of nasal airway blockage with a persistent watery mucoid drainage. Their nasal turbinates are pale and boggy. Patients with *seasonal rhinitis* usually complain of sneezing, itchy eyes, lacrimation, and a watery nasal discharge. Their symptoms have a seasonal variation, unlike those of the perennial group.

Chronic, or idiopathic, rhinitis is not known to have a specific cause. Most patients have persistent engorgement of the nasal turbinates, which leads to nasal obstruction and a profuse watery rhinorrhea. They often complain of persistent nasal obstruction that may alternate from side to side. Sneezing is not as common as it is in allergic rhinitis.

When symptoms of a cold and cough persist longer than the patient's fever, the URI may have subsided, and the persistent symptoms may be caused by a sinusitis of bacterial origin.

Precipitating and Aggravating Factors

Nasal sprays, antihypertensive drugs, hormones, and psychotropic agents often cause chronic nasal congestion. The more frequent offenders are reserpine, methyldopa, prazosin, beta blockers, estrogens, oral contraceptives, thioridazine, chlordiazepoxide, amitriptyline, and perphenazine. Aspirin and nonsteroidal antiinflammatory drugs (NSAIDs) can cause nasal stuffiness, rhinorrhea, asthma, and nasal polyposis.

Symptoms of chronic rhinitis are exacerbated by allergy, stress, hormonal changes (e.g., those associated with menstruation and menopause), marked temperature variations, and chemical irritants.

Ameliorating Factors

Ameliorating factors are not particularly helpful in differential diagnosis.

Physical Findings

The physical examination is most helpful in the detection of complications such as otitis media, sinusitis, pneumonia, and other bacterial infections. The physician should suspect something more serious than a simple URI if the temperature is greater than 102°F (38.8°C). If the patient has severe sore throat, exudative pharyngitis, earache, severe head or neck pain, or wheezing, the physician must exclude complications such as *streptococcal pharyngitis, otitis media, sinusitis, meningitis,* and *bacterial pneumonia,* since these conditions respond well to appropriate antibiotic therapy.

Patients with *acute sinusitis* often have pain over the involved sinuses that usually is unilateral and dull in the early stages but that may become bilateral and more severe later. Coughing, sneezing, and percussion over the involved sinuses often exacerbate the pain. Percussion of the teeth may produce pain when the maxillary sinuses are infected. Some patients may even have a toothache as an early manifestation of sinusitis. Patients with ethmoid sinusitis often experience retro-orbital pain on coughing or sneezing. They also may demonstrate chemosis, proptosis, extraocular muscle palsy, or orbital fixation. A mucopurulent nasal discharge, with or without blood, frequently is present.

Examination should include not only palpation and percussion over the sinuses but also careful observation of the pharynx, cranial nerves, eyes (including evaluation of visual acuity), ears, nose, and mouth. Visual loss, cavernous sinus thrombosis, and brain abscesses are serious potential sequelae. When correctly performed, transillumination may be helpful in the diagnosis of frontal and maxillary sinusitis.

Text continued on page 75.

Differential Diagnosis of Colds, Flu, and Stuffy Nose

CONDITION	NATURE OF PATIENT	NATURE OF SYMPTOMS AND ASSOCIATED SYMPTOMS	COMPLICATIONS	PRECIPITATING AND AGGRAVATING FACTORS	PHYSICAL FINDINGS	DIAGNOSTIC STUDIES
Common cold/viral upper respiratory tract infections	Anyone	Constitutional symptoms worse in children Incubation period 1–3 days Profuse nasal drainage Nasal congestion Sneezing Postnasal drip Cough Sore throat Headache Fever (<102°F) Hoarseness General malaise	Lower RTI, especially in adults with history of bronchitis, allergies, asthma, heavy cigarette smoking, immune incompetence Sinusitis, especially in patients with history of recurrent sinusitis Bronchitis in smokers and patients with pulmonary disease Pneumonia in elderly and diabetic patients Nasal airway obstruction Streptococcal pharyngitis Meningitis		Mucopurulent nasal discharge Nasopharyngeal mucosal infection and swelling Temperature usually <102°F Pharyngeal exudates less frequent than with bacterial infections Lymphadenopathy	Throat culture (to rule out streptococcal infection and pharyngitis) Monospot (to rule out infectious mononucleosis)
	Children	Vomiting Diarrhea Abdominal pain Wheezing	Lower RTI in children with history of recurrent bronchitis, allergies, cystic fibrosis Otitis media		Fever, may be >102°F Wheezing when bronchiolitis is associated	

Allergic rhinitis Perennial	Onset before age 20 Family history of allergic disease	Nasal airway blockage Persistent watery nasal discharge No seasonal variation			Pale boggy nasal turbinates Watery nasal discharge	Nasal smear: eosinophils
Seasonal		Sneezing Itchy eyes Lacrimation Watery nasal discharge Seasonal variation		Allergens Dust Pollen Spores	Pale boggy nasal turbinates	
Chronic (idiopathic) rhinitis		Persistent nasal obstruction May alternate sides Profuse watery rhinorrhea Sneezing not common		Allergy Stress Hormonal changes Marked temperature changes Chemical irritants	Swollen nasal turbinates	
Sinusitis	Prior history of sinusitis	Often recurrent pain over sinuses Early: unilateral dull Later: bilateral severe		Coughing Sneezing Percussion of involved sinuses		Sinus CT scan Transillumination of sinuses
Maxillary		May present as toothache			Pain with percussion of teeth	
Ethmoid		Retro-orbital pain Mucopurulent nasal discharge (may be bloody)	Visual loss Cavernous sinus thrombosis Brain abscess	Coughing and sneezing may cause retro-orbital pain	Chemosis Proptosis Extraocular muscle palsy Orbital fixation	

Table continued on following page.

Differential Diagnosis of Colds, Flu, and Stuffy Nose *Continued*

CONDITION	NATURE OF PATIENT	NATURE OF SYMPTOMS AND ASSOCIATED SYMPTOMS	COMPLICATIONS	PRECIPITATING AND AGGRAVATING FACTORS	PHYSICAL FINDINGS	DIAGNOSTIC STUDIES
Rhinitis medicamentosa	Frequent users of nasal drips, sprays, or inhalants	Nasal congestion		Nasal medications	Mucosa injected	Nasal smear: no eosinophils
	Hypertensive patients taking certain antihypertensive drugs	Nasal stuffiness		Reserpine Beta blockers Clonidine Hydralazine Methyldopa Prazosin Estrogens Oral contraceptives Chlordiazepoxide Amitriptyline		

RTI, Respiratory tract infection.

Diagnostic Studies

Throat cultures may be useful in diagnosing streptococcal pharyngitis. The monospot test is helpful in the diagnosis of infectious mononucleosis. Nasal smears allow detection of eosinophils in allergic rhinitis. Computed tomography (CT) permits visualization of the sinuses, deviated septa, and intracranial lesions. Allergy skin testing should be performed in patients with rhinitis and when the diagnosis is not clear.

Less Common Diagnostic Considerations

Frequent respiratory infections should alert the physician to the possibility of an anatomic abnormality, immune incompetence, or mucoviscidosis. Less common causes of nasal blockage include nasal polyps, sick building syndrome, tumors, foreign bodies, collagen vascular disorders, and congenital malformations in neonates.

Selected References

Beare AS: Upper respiratory infections. Practitioner 227:953–961, 1983.

Busse WW: Chronic rhinitis: a systemic approach to diagnosis and treatment. Postgrad Med 73:325–335, 1983.

Durham SR: Medical approach to rhinitis. Br J Hosp Med 50:458–462, 1993.

Kirkpatrick GL: The common cold. Prim Care 23:657–675, 1996.

Knight A: The differential diagnosis of rhinorrhea. J Allergy Clin Immunol 95:1080–1083, 1995.

Newman RK, Johnson JT: Nasal airway obstruction: approach to diagnosis and management. Postgrad Med 68:184–191, 1980.

Reed SE: The common cold. Practitioner 223:753–757, 1979.

Solomon WR: Newer approaches to the diagnosis of rhinitis. Ear Nose Throat 65:42–46, 1986.

Stevenson J: Influenza. Practitioner 223:759–763, 1979.

CHAPTER 8

Constipation

Constipation is common in Western society. The frequency of constipation diagnoses depends on both the patient's and the physician's definitions of the problem. One bowel movement each day is what most patients consider normal. Many physicians, however, may accept two to three hard and dry stools a week as normal if this is usual for the individual. Some experts believe that anyone who strains to defecate or who does not effortlessly pass at least one soft stool daily is constipated. By this definition, constipation is very common.

Constipation may also be defined as a change in the person's normal bowel pattern to less frequent or more difficult defecation. In this chapter, *constipation* is defined as straining with bowel movements or as bowel movements that occur fewer than three times per week. Constipation has been attributed to the deficiency of dietary fiber in the customary Western diet, which has replaced fiber with excessive ingestion of refined carbohydrates.

Constipation usually is not caused by a serious disease. In most patients it can be corrected by decreasing the amount of refined carbohydrates and increasing the amount of fiber ingested. It is particularly important for the examiner to ask whether the constipation is of recent onset and constitutes a change in previous bowel habits, since such findings may indicate serious disease.

The most common causes of constipation are *laxative habit, diets high in refined carbohydrates and low in fiber, change in daily habits or environment, drug use, irritable bowel syndrome,* and *painful defecation due to a local anorectal problem.* In many cases, multiple factors contribute to the patient's constipation. Less common causes include *bowel tumors, fecal impaction, pregnancy,* and *metabolic disorders* (e.g., *hypothyroidism, diabetes, hypercalcemia*).

The common causes of constipation can be divided into three categories: simple constipation, disordered motility, and secondary constipation. *Simple constipation* usually results from a diet that contains excessive refined carbohydrates and is deficient in fiber. It may be influenced by environmental factors. *Disordered motility,* the next most common category, is seen with idiopathic slow transit (most common in elderly persons), idiopathic megacolon and megarectum (more common in children), irritable bowel syndrome, and uncomplicated diverticular disease. *Secondary constipation* can be a response to drugs, chronic laxation, prolonged immobilization, and organic disease of the anus, rectum, or colon (anal fissures, strictures, and carcinoma).

Nature of Patient

Constipation is uncommon in neonates and is usually caused by *anal fissures* or *feeding problems.* Rarely, it results from congenital problems such as *Hirschsprung's disease.* In children the most common cause of constipation is a change in daily habits or environment. The earlier that constipation begins in childhood, the greater is the likelihood of an organic cause.

Disorders of defecation in children are common, difficult to manage, and negatively perceived by the family. Approximately 85% to 95% of constipation in children is functional. In children ages 6 months to 3 years, it frequently results from some *psychological cause.* Early diagnosis of psychological causes of constipation in children facilitates treatment. Toilet training may have occurred recently, for example, or constipation may have developed because the child had a condition, such as a rectal fissure, that caused painful defecation. Fearing painful defecation, the child suppressed the urge to defecate, perpetuating the production of hard, dry stools, which continued to irritate the rectal fissure.

In adults, most constipation is caused by *dietary fiber deficiency* or *laxative habit.* Laxative use is more common in women than men. Constipation is a common complaint in elderly persons, although 80% to 90% of patients over age 60 have one or more bowel movements per day. Despite this, 50% of patients over 60 use laxatives. This apparent discrepancy may be a result of older persons' greater preoccupation with bowel function compared with younger people. Constipation in elderly patients most often is caused by inappropriate diet, decreased activity, poor dentition, use of constipating medications, and impaired motility. Constipation ranks with joint pain, dizziness, forgetfulness, depression, and bladder problems as one of the major causes of misery in older patients.

Obstipation (regular passage of hard stools at 3- to 5-day intervals) and *fecal impaction* are most common in elderly patients. Some patients with fecal impaction will have continuous soiling (liquid passing around hard stools), which they describe as diarrhea. Elderly patients who are confined to bed, drink small amounts of fluid, or take constipating drugs are particularly vulnerable to fecal impaction. Although fecal impaction is more common in elderly persons, the physician must be aware that it can occur in any patient subjected to sudden immobility, bed rest, or a marked change in diet or fluid consumption.

Tumors of the bowel are uncommon in children and young adults, but their frequency increases after age 40. **In any patient over age 40 who presents with recent constipation or marked change in bowel habit, the physician must rule out carcinoma of the colon and rectum.**

Nature of Symptoms

The most important factor in determining whether constipation should be investigated for a serious cause or treated symptomatically and by dietary modification is whether it is chronic or of recent onset. Patients who have longstanding constipation and those whose constipation developed with a recent depressive illness, change in diet, recent debility, or ingestion of constipating medicine can be treated symptomatically. Their clinical status should be reassessed after a few weeks of appropriate therapy. **Patients with unexplained constipation of recent onset or a sudden aggravation of existing constipation associated with abdominal pain, passing of blood or mucus, a progressive decrease in the number of movements per day, or a substantial increase in laxative requirements should be investigated even in the absence of abnormal physical findings.** These patients should have colonoscopy, and stools should be tested for occult blood. **Constipation occurs in less than one third of patients with carcinoma of the colon and is less common than diarrhea in these patients.**

Ribbonlike stools suggest a motility disorder. They can also be caused by an organic narrowing of the distal colon or sigmoid. A progressive decrease in the caliber of the stools suggests an organic lesion. If the patient complains of stools that have a toothpaste-like caliber, a fecal impaction should be suspected.

Tumors of the descending colon are more common in older adults with right-sided lesions, increasing in frequency as the patient grows older. One third of colon cancers in patients over 80 are right sided, and fewer than one half of these patients have altered bowel habits. They usually present late with an anemia or a palpable mass on the right side of the colon.

Associated Symptoms

In children, simple constipation often is associated with abdominal distention, decreased appetite, irritability, reduced activity, and soiling. Obstipated children (i.e., those who pass hard, dry stools every 3 to 5 days) also may have overflow soiling. If soiling persists after the constipation or obstipation has improved, the physician should search for some *psychological disturbance;* fecal impaction is relatively rare in children. When children have abdominal distention associated with constipation, it usually is caused by improper diet or decreased motility; intestinal obstruction is a rare cause of constipation in children. Acting out, school problems, and difficulties with interpersonal relationships should suggest that the constipation has a psychological cause.

If constipation is associated with steatorrhea and greenish yellow stools, a *small bowel* or *pancreatic lesion* should be suspected. Constipation with early-morning rushes, hypogastric cramps, tenesmus, and passage of blood all suggest that the constipation is of colonic origin.

In adults, colicky pain, abdominal distention, anemia, decreased effectiveness of laxatives, weight loss, anorexia, and blood, pus, or mucus in the stool should suggest a *colonic tumor.* Weight loss, anorexia, and anemia usually are observed only in the late phases of colonic tumors. Rectal discomfort, leakage of stool, bleeding, urgency, tenesmus, diarrhea alternating with constipation, and rectal prolapse all suggest a *rectosigmoid tumor.* In contrast, abdominal distention and sudden onset of obstipation suggest a more proximal colon lesion.

If it alternates with diarrhea or is accompanied by passage of hard scybala or intermittent left- or right-sided iliac pain that occasionally radiates through to the back, constipation is probably caused by *irritable bowel syndrome.* A change in stool frequency or consistency associated with abdominal pain also suggests an irritable colon, as do abdominal distention and mucus in the stools.

Fecal incontinence, which some patients actually describe as diarrhea, should suggest a *fecal impaction.* Most patients with this condition must strain at stool, do not have normal-formed stools, often have a toothpaste-like stool, and often have continuous soiling. Rectal examination usually reveals large quantities of hard feces in the rectal ampulla.

Constipation that develops after painful *hemorrhoids* suggests that the constipation is secondary to suppression of defecation because it induces pain. Patients with this condition, as well as others with local anorectal problems, often report blood in the bowel movements. When questioned, they usually recognize that the blood is on the surface of their stool, on the toilet paper, or in the toilet bowel rather than mixed in with the stool.

Precipitating and Aggravating Factors

Patients and their family members should be questioned about stressful problems such as divorce, death of a spouse, or loss of a job. Twenty percent of children have moderate constipation when they begin to become effectively toilet trained. Functional constipation may be precipitated by hospital admission, traveling, suppression of the urge to defecate, uncomfortable lavatory environment (e.g., latrine), and immobilization. Reduction in laxative dose or change in brand of laxative occasionally precipitates constipation.

In elderly patients, constipation can be aggravated by limited variety in meals, decreased fluid or fiber intake, poor dentition, increased costs of fresh high-fiber foods (e.g., fruits, vegetables), impaired motility, debilitating illnesses, confinement to bed, and frequent ingestion of constipating drugs.

Certain drugs typically cause constipation. These include antacids that contain aluminum hydroxide or calcium, anticholinergics, antiparkinsonian drugs, diuretics, tricyclic antidepressants, opiates, phenytoin, codeine (in analgesics or cough medicine), cough mixtures, morphine-containing drugs, calcium channel blockers, iron-containing compounds, and certain antihypertensive and antiseizure drugs. The patient may be taking one of these constipating agents but may develop symptoms only when a second drug is added.

Ameliorating Factors

A diet high in fiber (e.g., whole-grain cereals, bran or vegetable fiber) and low in refined sugar often alleviates constipation. Many patients find that weight reduction diets that are low in carbohydrates and high in fiber relieve constipation. Increased fluid intake, particularly in patients who do not drink enough fluids or

Text continued on page 84.

Differential Diagnosis of Constipation

CONDITION	NATURE OF PATIENT	NATURE OF SYMPTOMS	ASSOCIATED SYMPTOMS	PRECIPITATING AND AGGRAVATING FACTORS	AMELIORATING FACTORS	PHYSICAL FINDINGS	DIAGNOSTIC STUDIES
Simple constipation							
Low dietary fiber	Most common cause of constipation in adults	Dry, hard stools Stool frequency less than 5 times/wk Straining at stool	*Children:* may be associated with abdominal distention	Excessive intake of refined carbohydrates	Increased dietary fiber Decreased intake of refined carbohydrates	Ascending or descending colon tender to palpation Feces palpable in sigmoid colon	
Functional (environmental and daily-habit changes)	Most common cause of constipation in children Common cause in adults	Vague abdominal discomfort	*Children:* Abdominal distention Decreased appetite Irritability Decreased activity Soiling	Toilet training Traveling Uncomfortable lavatories Immobilization	Resume prior habits		
Disordered motility							
Irritable bowel syndrome	Any age, especially young adults	Change in stool frequency and consistency Constipation alternates with diarrhea Mucus in stools	Abdominal distention Abdominal pain	Stress	Increased dietary fiber Decreased environmental stresses	Colon tender to palpation	

Obstipation/fecal impaction	Most common in elderly and those subject to sudden immobility, bed rest, or decreased fluid consumption	Regular passage of hard stools at 3- to 5-day intervals Continuous soiling patients describe as diarrhea Toothpaste-caliber stools Fecal incontinence Straining at stool				Large quantities of hard feces in rectal ampulla	
Idiopathic slow transit	Most common in elderly people	Dry, hard stools Decreased stool frequency		Decreased exercise Decreased dietary fiber Decreased fluid intake	Increased exercise Increased dietary fiber Increased fluids Improved dentition		
Hirschsprung's disease (aganglionic megacolon)	Rare cause of constipation in children	Present from birth Soiling absent				Rectum empty	Barium enema
Secondary constipation							
Anal fissure	Affects any age	Patient suppresses painful defecation Hard stools	Blood on surface of feces, on toilet paper, or in toilet			Anal fissure	Anoscopy

Table continued on following page.

Differential Diagnosis of Consipation *Continued*

CONDITION	NATURE OF PATIENT	NATURE OF SYMPTOMS	ASSOCIATED SYMPTOMS	PRECIPITATING AND AGGRAVATING FACTORS	AMELIORATING FACTORS	PHYSICAL FINDINGS	DIAGNOSTIC STUDIES
Secondary constipation *Continued*							
Hemorrhoids	Adults	Patients suppress painful defecation	Blood on surface of feces, on toilet paper, or in toilet	Pregnancy Prior hemorrhoid problems		Hemorrhoids	Anoscopy
Drug-induced constipation	Chronic laxative users Patients taking other medications Most common in elderly patients			Laxatives Codeine Morphine Analgesics Aluminum-containing antacids Antiparkinsonian drugs Cough mixtures Antidepressants Iron and calcium supplements Antihypertensives Calcium channel blockers			

Bowel tumors	Uncommon in children Frequency increases after age 40	Constipation in less than third of patients with colon cancer; diarrhea more common Early-morning rushes Decreased laxative effectiveness Blood, pus, or mucus in stool	Elderly patients with right-sided lesions may present late with anemia Weight loss Anorexia Colicky abdominal pain and distention	Possible palpable mass	Rectal examination Stool examination for occult blood Colonoscopy Barium enema
Rectosigmoid tumors		Rectal discomfort Stool leakage Urgency, tenesmus Progressive narrowing of stool caliber	Rectal bleeding Rectal prolapse		Sigmoidoscopy
Proximal colon tumors		Sudden onset Obstipation	Abdominal distention	Anemia	Colonoscopy Barium enema

who take diuretics, often is helpful. Relief of painful anorectal problems frequently alleviates constipation. If a change in daily routine (e.g., rushing off to work, giving up the morning cigarette) has caused constipation, instructing the patient to readjust daily activities to permit bowel movements at the time of the urge to defecate often is effective.

Physical Findings

A rectal examination should be performed in all patients with a significant complaint of constipation. This examination allows the physician to determine whether the rectum is full or empty, whether an anorectal problem exists (e.g., fissure, hemorrhoids), and whether a rectal mass is present. A stool specimen should be obtained to check for occult blood.

The physician also should conduct an abdominal examination, with special attention to the colon, to detect palpable masses (fecal or otherwise) or abdominal tenderness. Normally, the colon is neither palpable nor tender. If the colon can be palpated and if it is tender, particularly over the descending or ascending regions, an irritable or spastic colon is probable. Stigmata of myxedema and abdominal distention should suggest that the constipation is secondary to hypothyroidism. Anemia, manifested by tachycardia and conjunctival pallor, should suggest a right-sided colonic lesion.

Diagnostic Studies

Examination of stools for occult blood, hematocrit or hemoglobin, and erythrocyte sedimentation rate are appropriate, inexpensive, and noninvasive tests to evaluate constipation. Anoscopy, sigmoidoscopy, colonoscopy, and barium enema also are helpful.

Less Common Diagnostic Considerations

In neonates, *Hirschsprung's disease* (aganglionic megacolon) is the most prevalent of the less common causes of constipation. Early diagnosis is important. To differentiate between Hirschsprung's disease and chronic constipation, the physician should be aware that each condition is associated with characteristic symptoms. In Hirschsprung's disease, symptoms usually date from birth, soiling is absent, and the rectum is empty. With chronic constipation, onset may occur from ages 6 months to 3 years, soiling is common, and the rectum is usually full of feces.

Other less common causes of constipation in children include anorectal stenosis, chronic lead poisoning, hypothyroidism, hyperparathyroidism, medication, anal fissures, allergy to cow's milk, and neurologic abnormalities such as spina bifida.

If constipation is associated with nausea, polyuria, fatigue, and sometimes a history of kidney stones, *hypercalcemia,* although uncommon, may be the cause. Other metabolic and endocrinologic causes of constipation include diabetes, pregnancy, and hypothyroidism. Constipation may be the presenting symptom in patients with classic *myxedema.* Myxedematous patients frequently have an adynamic bowel with moderate abdominal distention. Adynamic bowel also occurs with senility, scleroderma, and spinal cord injuries and diseases. Idiopathic megacolon and megarectum also can produce severe constipation.

Psychiatric causes of constipation include depressive illness and anorexia nervosa. Occasionally, constipation is induced in depressed patients as the result of the anticholinergic effect of antidepressant drugs.

Marked prostatic enlargement may contribute to constipation. Disease or weakness of the abdominal muscles, neurologic diseases, diverticular diseases, occult rectal prolapse, pancreatic carcinoma, and lead poisoning are all rare causes of constipation.

Selected References

Abi-Hanna A, Lake AM: Constipation and encopresis in childhood. Pediatr Rev 19:23–31, 1998.

Bonapace ES, Fisher RS: Constipation and diarrhea in pregnancy. Gastroenterol Clin North Am 27:197–211, 1998.

Castle SC: Constipation—endemic in the elderly? Gerontopathophysiology, evaluation, and management. Med Clin North Am 73:1497–1509, 1989.

Floch MH, Wald A: Clinical evaluation and treatment of constipation. Gastroenterologist 2:50–60, 1994.

Loening-Baucke V: Encopresis and soiling. Pediatr Clin North Am 43:279–298, 1996.

Murtagh J: Constipation. Aust Fam Physician 19:1693–1697, 1990.

Nivatvongs S, Hooks VH: Chronic constipation: important aspects of workup and management. Postgrad Med 74:313–323, 1983.

Painter NS: Constipation. Practitioner 224:387–391, 1980.

Pettei MJ: Chronic constipation. Pediatr Ann 16:796–813, 1987.

Romer Y, Evans JM, Fleming KC, Phillips SF: Constipation and fecal incontinence in the elderly population. Mayo Clin Proc 71:81–92, 1996.

Thompson WG, Heaton KW: Functional bowel disorders in apparently healthy people. Gastroenterology 79:283–288, 1980.

CHAPTER 9

Cough

When evaluating patients with a cough, the physician should remember that (1) most healthy people seldom cough, and (2) the main function of coughing is airway clearance. The complaint of cough should be taken seriously, since it is one of the few ways by which abnormalities of the respiratory tree manifest themselves.

Cough can be initiated by irritation of upper or lower airways. The most common causes of an acute cough are *infections* (most often *viral upper respiratory tract infection, bronchitis,* and *laryngitis*), *allergies* (often seasonal), and *postnasal drip.* The most common causes of a chronic cough (longer than 3 weeks) are *chronic bronchitis, postnasal drip, asthma,* and *gastroesophageal reflux.* Other common causes include *chronic obstructive pulmonary disease* (COPD), *heart failure, tuberculosis, lung tumor,* and *habit.* The most common causes of recurrent cough in children are *recurrent viral upper respiratory tract infections, reactive airway disease, asthma, viral bronchitis,* and *allergies.*

Nature of Patient

Viral infections are the most common cause of acute cough at all ages. This is particularly true of preschool children and even more likely if they are in close daily contact with many other children. In school-age children, *mycoplasmal pneumonias* are quite common. Because the incubation period is long (approximately 21 days), infection spreads slowly. *Bacterial pneumonias* also cause coughing and have their highest incidence in winter months. **Recurrent viral bronchitis is most prevalent in preschool and young school-age children and is the most common cause of a persistent cough in children of all ages.** There may be a genetically determined host susceptibility to frequently recurring bronchitis. Young patients with recurrent cough often are asthmatic. Physicians should be suspicious of underlying asthma contributing to a recurrent cough when there is a family history of allergies, atopy, or asthma.

A chronic cough in children frequently is caused by *allergic rhinitis, chronic sinusitis,* or *enlarged adenoids.* Although rare, chronic cough in very young children (under age 12 months) should suggest congenital malformations or neonatal infections, including viral and chlamydial pneumonias. Other relatively rare causes of chronic cough in young infants include recurrent aspiration of milk, saliva, or gastric contents and cystic fibrosis. A chronic cough in children between ages 1 and 5 years should suggest bronchiectasis or cystic fibrosis after the more common causes have been ruled out. **In both children and adults, chronic cough may be the only manifestation of gastroesophageal reflux.**

Chronic cough in adults most often is caused by *chronic bronchitis* (especially in smokers), *gastroesophageal reflux disease* (GERD), *postnasal drip, asthma, environmental irritants, allergies,* and *habit.* Chronic cough resulted from GERD, postnasal drip, or asthma in 99% of nonsmokers with a normal chest radiograph in one study. In older adults, any chronic cough without an obvious explanation should suggest *tumor* or *tuberculosis.*

Nature of Symptoms

When the cough is of sudden onset and associated with fever or symptoms of an acute infection, a *viral* cause is most likely. The cough is noisy, produces minimal sputum, and is often worse at night. With *bacterial* and *mycoplasmal infections,* cough is often the most prominent symptom. Its onset may occur over hours or days, and the sputum produced is usually thick and yellowish. In mycoplasmal infections, the cough may be severe and persist for 1 to 4 months, although all other signs and symptoms abate within 7 to 10 days.

The cough caused by a viral upper respiratory infection (URI) or viral bronchitis usually lasts for 7 to 10 days. If the cough persists for longer than 14 days, a secondary bacterial infection may exist. If the cough is associated with shortness of breath and bilateral wheezing, asthma is likely. The cough of asthma usually is nonproductive or productive of minimal clear mucoid secretions. An asthmatic cough is often worse at night, is associated with wheezing, is brought on by specific irritants, and is more common in patients with a family history of asthma, allergies, or atopy.

Patients with an acute or chronic cough secondary to *postnasal drip* may not be aware of this condition. They should be questioned about swallowing mucus, frequent throat clearing, "hawking," or cough that is worse in the morning. Examination may reveal mucoid secretions in the posterior pharynx, a cobblestone appearance of the mucosa, or signs of sinusitis.

A nocturnal cough associated with shortness of breath should suggest *paroxysmal nocturnal dyspnea* or *congestive heart failure.* A nocturnal cough without associated dyspnea indicates an *allergic origin.* A cough that recurs in late afternoon or early evening also is often of allergic origin. This type of cough may occur in people who work in the city (where the pollen count is low) and then return in late afternoon or evening to their suburban homes (where the pollen count is higher). A seasonal incidence of cough is highly suggestive of an allergic cause.

In smokers a chronic minimally productive cough, often worse in the morning, probably is related to the irritant effect of inhaling tobacco smoke. Although more common in cigarette smokers, it also can occur in cigar and pipe smokers who inhale.

The evaluation of all patients whose chief complaint is cough should include a complete history, with particular attention to duration and character of the cough, smoking history, environmental and occupational experiences, antecedent allergies, asthma, sinusitis, symptoms of URIs, heartburn, and shortness of breath or fainting while coughing ("tussive syncope"). *Gastroesophageal reflux* should also be considered if cough is precipitated by chocolate, caffeine, or other foods (e.g., onions) that facilitate reflux. Exercise-induced cough may also be caused by reflux.

Associated Symptoms

If a runny nose, sore throat, or generalized aches and pains are present, the cough probably has an *infectious* cause. The presence of fever, chills, exudative or nonexudative pharyngitis, conjunctivitis, otitis, abdominal pain, headache, or pleuritic chest pain suggests the presence of *bacteria* or *mycoplasma.* Because postnasal drip (one cause of cough) may coexist with other conditions that produce chronic cough (e.g., bronchiectasis, heart failure, bronchogenic carcinoma, tuberculosis), the physician should not automatically assume that the postnasal drip is the only cause of the cough. If episodic wheezing or shortness of breath occurs in a patient complaining of cough, asthma is likely. When a cough is associated with heartburn or a sour taste in the mouth, gastroesophageal reflux is likely.

If sneezing, a boggy edematous nasal mucosa, conjunctivitis, tearing, itching of the roof of the mouth, or itching of the eyes is present, an *allergic* cause of an otherwise unexplained cough is most likely.

Elderly patients, whose physical activity may be restricted by arthritis or other associated disease, may not present with the usual symptom of dyspnea on exertion. The chief complaint instead may be a chronic unexplained cough that may occur only at night while the patient is recumbent or that may worsen at night. **Therefore, any unexplained nocturnal cough in elderly patients should suggest congestive heart failure.**

Precipitating and Aggravating Factors

In all cases of unexplained cough (particularly in children) when exercise precipitates the cough, an asthmatic cause should be suspected, even with no typical wheezing. Some coughs are precipitated by exposure to very dry, superheated air, as frequently occurs in patients whose homes are heated with forced hot air. This cough may be exacerbated by sensitivity to spores in the dry, superheated air.

Chronic debilitating conditions such as alcoholism, malnutrition, diabetes, uremia, leukemia, and antitumor therapy may facilitate the development of infections that produce coughing. Long-term *cigarette smoking,* chronic exposure to *industrial irritants,* or *chronic respiratory disease* in childhood predisposes the patient to the development of lung disease and cough.

Patients with *allergic rhinitis* and *chronic sinusitis* are predisposed to postnasal drip and its resultant cough. This cough may be worse at night when the patient is recumbent because more mucus drips into the throat when in this position.

Cough due to *gastroesophageal reflux* may also be worse when the patient is recumbent and may be precipitated by coffee, tea, caffeine, chocolate, alcohol, and exercise. Other coughs that worsen in the recumbent position or at night include those caused by allergies, paroxysmal nocturnal dyspnea, asthma, and breathing dry hot air.

Ameliorating Factors

In patients with allergic rhinitis, antihistamine therapy may ameliorate coughing by reducing secretions in the nose and paranasal sinuses. If smokers with chronic cough stop smoking, the cough usually abates. In one study, 77% of patients who ceased smoking lost their cough, most after 1 month of not smoking. Coughing was greatly reduced in 13%.

Physical Findings

The ears, nose, mouth, throat (including indirect laryngoscopy), sinuses, neck, lungs, and cardiovascular system should be examined. The patient should always be asked to cough so that the cough characteristics may be heard and the sputum examined. A mucopurulent sputum suggests *infection,* although some *allergic* coughs are productive. If a large number of eosinophils are observed in a stained sputum specimen, an allergic cause is probable.

In patients with an acute cough secondary to infection, the chest examination often is normal, but the pharynx may be injected or pale, boggy, and swollen. The sinuses should be palpated, percussed, and transilluminated for evidence of *sinusitis.* When the mucosa of the nose and oropharynx has a cobblestone appearance (from chronic stimulation of submucosal lymphoid follicles), *postnasal drip* probably is causing the cough. If the lung fields are hyperresonant to percussion, and if auscultation reveals distant breath sounds, scattered rhonchi or wheezes, or prolonged expiration, *COPD* should be suspected.

Cough may be the earliest symptom of *heart failure,* particularly in patients with pulmonary hypertension or mitral stenosis. Cough may occur before the usual findings of chronic congestive heart failure (rales, edema, tachycardia, and gallop) are evident.

Diagnostic Studies

Tests used to determine the cause of cough include a complete blood count, an eosinophil count, sinus and chest radiographs, and cytologic and microscopic sputum examination. Pulmonary function tests, bronchoscopy, and cardiovascular studies may help in some cases.

The chest radiograph may be negative in some patients with diffuse infiltrative lung disease. Approximately 5% of patients with sarcoidosis have normal chest films. Likewise, patients with cough due to a tracheobronchial lesion may have a normal chest radiograph.

Text continued on page 93.

Differential Diagnosis of Cough

CONDITION	NATURE OF PATIENT	NATURE OF SYMPTOMS	ASSOCIATED SYMPTOMS	PRECIPITATING AND AGGRAVATING FACTORS	AMELIORATING FACTORS	PHYSICAL FINDINGS	DIAGNOSTIC STUDIES
Acute cough							
Viral upper respiratory tract infections	Most common cause of acute cough in all ages	Acute onset of noisy cough (over hours or days) Cough worse at night and may persist for 7–10 days Sputum thick and yellowish, but minimal amount produced	Fever Runny nose Sore throat General aches and pains			Pharynx injected or pale, boggy, and swollen Coarse rhonchi	
Mycoplasmal bronchitis or pneumonia	Common cause of acute cough in school-age children Frequent cause of persistent cough in adults	Long incubation period (about 21 days) Severe cough may persist for 1–4 months Other symptoms (e.g., fever) abate within 10 days	Same as for bacterial pneumonia but not usually as severe			Scattered rales Signs of pneumonia	Chest radiograph Cold agglutinins Complement fixation
Viral bronchitis	Recurrent infections are most common cause of persistent cough in children, who are often asthmatic	Cough may persist 7–10 days	Fever				

Allergies	History of allergy in family	Minimally productive May be nocturnal Recurrent cough without dyspnea May have seasonal incidence	Sneezing Conjunctivitis Tearing Itching of eyes and roof of mouth Postnasal drip		Antihistamines	Boggy, edematous nasal mucosa	Stained sputum smear for eosinophils
Bacterial pneumonia		Noisy cough Incidence highest in winter Acute onset Cough worse at night	Fever, chills Signs of acute infection Pharyngitis Conjunctivitis Otitis Abdominal pain Headache Pleuritic chest pain	Chronic debilitating conditions		Signs of pneumonia	Chest radiograph Sputum and blood cultures
Chronic or recurrent cough							
Postnasal drip	May not be aware of condition	Frequent throat clearing and hawking Cough worse in morning		Recumbency Allergic rhinitis Chronic sinusitis		Mucoid secretions in posterior pharynx Palpation, percussion, and transillumination of sinuses reveal sinusitis Mucosa of nose/oropharynx: cobblestone appearance	
Asthma	May have family history of allergies, atopy, or asthma	Recurrent cough Minimally or not productive (if productive, secretions clear and mucoid)	Shortness of breath	Exercise May be worse during seasonal allergies		Bilateral wheezing	Pulmonary function tests Response to isoproterenol and methacholine

Table continued on following page.

Differential Diagnosis of Cough *Continued*

CONDITION	NATURE OF PATIENT	NATURE OF SYMPTOMS	ASSOCIATED SYMPTOMS	PRECIPITATING AND AGGRAVATING FACTORS	AMELIORATING FACTORS	PHYSICAL FINDINGS	DIAGNOSTIC STUDIES
Chronic or recurrent cough *Continued*							
Chronic obstructive pulmonary disease (COPD)	Elderly patients		Shortness of breath			Lungs hyperresonant to percussion Auscultation reveals distant breath sounds, scattered rhonchi, wheezes, or prolonged expiration	Pulmonary function tests
Chronic bronchitis	Most common cause of chronic cough in adults (especially smokers)	May be minimally productive Often worse in morning			Smoking cessation	Scattered rhonchi	
Congestive heart failure	Elderly patients present differently May have only chronic, unexplained cough	Cough often nocturnal	Dyspnea on exertion Paroxysmal nocturnal dyspnea	Recumbency Exercise	Diuresis	Rales Pitting edema Tachycardia Gallop	Chest radiograph Potent diuretic for 2–3 days should improve symptoms
Gastroesophageal reflux	Usually adults	Irritative, nonproductive cough	Heartburn, eructation	Recumbency Ingestion of chocolate, caffeine, or alcohol Exercise	Antireflux measures, including diet, drugs, and elevating head of bed	Usually none	Upper gastrointestinal radiograph Esophagoscopy Esophageal pH monitoring

If an asthmatic cough is suspected and wheezing is absent, pulmonary function tests that measure response to isoproterenol should be performed. In rare instances, bronchial provocation with methacholine may be performed, but only with extreme care. If these tests are positive, asthma is the most likely cause of the cough.

A simple outpatient diagnostic test for a cough due to congestive heart failure is the administration of a potent oral diuretic for 2 to 3 days. If the patient diureses several pounds and demonstrates marked improvement of the cough, the cough probably is caused by pulmonary congestion secondary to heart failure.

Less Common Diagnostic Considerations

Most people who complain of cough do not have bronchogenic carcinoma. However, 70% to 90% of patients with bronchogenic carcinoma develop a cough at some time during the course of their disease. Various studies have documented that cough is the presenting symptom in 21% to 87% of patients with *bronchogenic carcinoma.* The possibility of bronchogenic carcinoma is especially strong in chronic cigarette smokers who develop a cough that lasts for months or who demonstrate a marked change in the character of their cough. Pulmonary tumors often are characterized by a change in the cough pattern, hemoptysis, chest pain, and enlarged supraclavicular nodes.

In patients with a *lung abscess,* cough is the dominant symptom more often than bloody sputum, pain, or dyspnea. The cough observed in patients with *bronchiectasis* usually is of long duration; productive of loose, moist, purulent sputum; and occasionally associated with hemoptysis. The cough of *tuberculosis* often is chronic (although it may be acute) and associated with hemoptysis, fever, night sweats, apical rales, and weight loss.

The physician should be particularly suspicious of disorders of the trachea or larynx in patients with inspiratory stridor or a dry, brassy, high-pitched, and unproductive cough. If the cough is associated with marked dyspnea, tachypnea, tachycardia, calf tenderness, prolonged immobility, atrial fibrillation, pleural friction, or hemoptysis, pulmonary embolism should be suspected.

Patients ranging in age from 3 months to 6 years may develop *croup* (laryngotracheobronchitis). This cough has a barking quality. Intercostal retraction with inspiration, inspiratory or expiratory wheezing, hoarseness, and difficulty with air movement all suggest this potentially critical condition. Hospitalization for intensive therapy may be necessary. In young children an inhaled foreign body also must be considered as the cause of coughing.

A rare and usually unrecognized cause of chronic cough is impaction of cerumen, a foreign body, or hair in the ear canal, which stimulates a cough through a reflex (ear-cough) mechanism. This cough is triggered by irritation of the external auditory canal or tympanic membrane.

Exposure to noxious gases, dusts, industrial pollutants, and smog can produce cough. This is particularly true in people who have underlying lung disease.

Angiotensin-converting enzyme inhibitors and beta blockers, including beta$_2$-blocker eyedrops, may cause a chronic nonproductive cough.

Reflux esophagitis does not usually present with cough, but patients with this condition may cough when recumbent. It should be considered in all instances of unexplained chronic cough.

Ornithosis, although rare, should be considered in patients who have a dry, hacking, unproductive cough with fever and who are in contact with fowl or pet birds. These patients often have a normal physical examination except for fever and cough. Coccidiodomycosis should be suspected if cough develops after the patient has visited an endemic area such as the San Joaquin Valley.

When complete history and thorough physical and laboratory examinations reveal no cause of cough, a *subdiaphragmatic process* (abscess or tumor) should be considered. If no organic cause for a chronic cough is found, a *psychogenic cause* may be strongly considered. Such patients do not cough at night and often can stop coughing if so instructed. This cough seldom is productive. In children it may be an attention-getting device; in adults it may be associated with other signs of hysterical behavior.

Selected References

Brashear RE: Cough: diagnostic considerations with normal chest roentgenograms. J Fam Pract 15:979–985, 1982.

Harding SM, Richter JE: The role of gastroesophageal reflux in chronic cough and asthma. Chest 111:1389–1402, 1997.

Kamei RK: Chronic cough in children. Pediatr Clin North Am 38:593–605, 1991.

Loudon RG: Cough: a symptom and a sign—basics of RD. Am Thorac Soc 9:1–6, 1981.

Mello CJ, Irwin RS, Curley FJ: Predictive values of the character, timing, and complications of chronic cough in diagnosing its cause. Arch Intern Med 156:997–1003, 1996.

Meyer AA, Aitken PV: Evaluation of persistent cough in children. Prim Care 23:883–892, 1996.

Parks DP, Ahrens RC, Humphries CT, Weinberger MM: Chronic cough in childhood: approach to diagnosis and treatment. J Pediatr 115:856–862, 1989.

Patrick H, Patrick F: Chronic cough. Med Clin North Am 79:361–372, 1995.

Philp EB: Chronic cough. Am Fam Physician 56:1395–1402, 1997.

CHAPTER 10

Diarrhea

In this chapter, *diarrhea* is defined as an increase in frequency, fluidity, or volume of bowel movements relative to the usual habit for a person. Acute diarrhea is second in frequency only to acute respiratory tract disease in American families. Diarrhea most frequently results from *acute gastroenteritis* caused by a virus or, less often, by bacteria or protozoa. Other common causes of diarrhea include *irritable bowel syndrome* (also called irritable colon, mucous colitis, or functional diarrhea) and ingestion of *antibiotics, antiinflammatory agents, magnesium-containing substances, alcohol,* and *excessive* (intolerable) *lactose.* Patients with *diabetes* also frequently have diarrhea.

When evaluating a patient's complaint of diarrhea, the physician must inquire about (1) the usual frequency and pattern of bowel movement, (2) the current pattern of bowel movements, (3) nocturnal diarrhea, (4) blood or mucus in the stool, (5) travel within the United States or abroad, (6) recent dietary changes, (7) exacerbation of diarrhea by particular foods such as dairy products, (8) recent drug ingestion, (9) change in the nature of food intake, and (10) any significant previous medical or surgical history.

Nature of Patient

In all age groups, *viral gastroenteritis* is the most common cause of acute diarrhea. This usually is a benign, self-limiting condition in adults but can result in severe dehydration in infants and children. In infants under age 3, *rotavirus* is responsible for about 50% of wintertime, nonbacterial gastroenteritis. This winter peak is even greater in temperate climates, such as found in the United States. *Salmonella* as a cause of gastroenteritis is more common in children ages 1 to 4 years. Epidemics of *Shigella* have been noted in children ages 1 to 4 years and in people living in closed environments, particularly those with substandard sanitation (e.g., in prisons and custodial institutions).

Giardiasis is not common in children, but infants are susceptible. Infants may be quite ill, in contrast to adults, who are often asymptomatic. However, acute or subacute diarrhea with marked symptomatology also may occur in some adults with giardiasis. Reports of symptomatic giardiasis have increased, primarily among hikers and campers, who are most likely to drink *Giardia*-infested water.

Whenever diarrhea in infants less than 1 year of age corresponds to increased ingestion of dairy products, *lactose intolerance* (lactase deficiency) should be suspected. This form of diarrhea is not limited to infants and young children. It is being reported with increasing frequency in adults, particularly those of Mediterranean extraction. Although these people may not have previously demonstrated lactose intolerance, lactase production normally decreases with age. This decrease is more pronounced in some people, and diarrhea seems to follow acute or chronic ingestion of large quantities of lactose, as found in milk, cheese, ice cream, and other dairy products. A transient lactase deficiency is common after infectious gastroenteritis.

Middle-aged women with chronic diarrhea are more likely to have functional diarrhea or an *irritable colon.* This condition seems to have a predilection for young women who are raising children, especially if they have the added responsibility of a job outside the home. It affects other stressed people as well. Another form of diarrhea reported to be more frequent among middle-aged women is the misuse or surreptitious use of purgatives. Patients who use laxatives surreptitiously often demonstrate other features of hysterical behavior. The addition of sodium hydroxide to the stool provides a simple test for some forms of laxative abuse. Ex-Lax, Feen-a-Mint, and Correctol contain phenolphthalein, which turns the stool red when alkali (sodium hydroxide) is added.

Patients with *diabetes* and associated neurologic dysfunction also may have chronic diarrhea. Some diabetic patients have gastric stasis and poor bowel motility. This permits bacterial overgrowth in the small bowel, which may produce an uncontrollable, explosive, postprandial diarrhea. Patients with this condition may refrain from eating before leaving their homes to avoid uncontrollable diarrhea at an inconvenient time. A therapeutic trial with tetracycline may effectively stop the diarrhea by combating the bacterial overgrowth.

Although acute diarrhea usually is benign and self-limiting, the following patients are particularly prone to serious complications from acute and chronic diarrhea: neonates, elderly people, patients with sickle cell disease, and those who are immunocompromised (by underlying disease or chemotherapy). Diarrhea due to enteric infections with protozoal, fungal, bacterial, and viral pathogens is common in patients with acquired immunodeficiency syndrome (AIDS).

Nature of Symptoms

A useful approach to the differential diagnosis of diarrhea is to separate *acute diarrhea* (which has an abrupt onset, lasts for less than 1 week, and may be associated with a viral prodrome, nausea, vomiting, or fever) from *chronic diarrhea* (in which the initial episode lasts longer than 2 weeks or symptoms recur over months or years). **The acute onset of diarrhea in a previously healthy patient, without signs or symptoms of other organ system involvement, suggests an infectious cause that most often is viral.** When vomiting and diarrhea begin suddenly and occur in many people at the same time, a preformed bacterial toxin (e.g., staphylococcal enterotoxin) is often the cause. Symptoms usually begin 2 to 8 hours after ingestion of contaminated food, most often in summer months when food may be inadequately refrigerated. With *Salmonella, Shigella,* or *Campylobac-*

ter, symptoms are delayed for 24 to 72 hours while the organisms multiply in the body. With *Giardia* this delay may be 1 to 2 weeks.

Chronic diarrhea most frequently is caused by the *irritable bowel syndrome, medications, dietary factors, chronic inflammatory bowel disease,* and *colon cancer.* Irritable bowel syndrome may present as chronic or intermittent diarrhea (which classically alternates with constipation) or as flare-ups of diarrhea that occur during stressful periods. Stools are looser and more frequent with onset of pain. A history of hard, often marblelike stools alternating with soft bowel movements, especially if associated with mucus in the toilet bowl or on the surface of the stool, suggests irritable bowel syndrome. Although a patient suffers from a chronic irritable colon, a superimposed case of viral gastroenteritis, salmonellosis, or giardiasis must still be considered. In such patients, a new cause of diarrhea should be sought if the usual diarrhea associated with their irritable colon changes or exacerbates.

Persistent diarrhea with frothy, foul-smelling stools that sometimes float suggests a *pancreatic* or *small-bowel* cause. Foul-smelling, watery, explosive diarrhea with mucus often is seen in *giardiasis.* The latency period may be 1 to 3 weeks. The onset of diarrhea due to giardiasis may be acute or gradual; it may persist for several weeks or up to 6 months.

Functional diarrhea almost never occurs at night and seldom awakens the patient. It is typically present in the morning. Copious amounts of mucus may be present, but blood seldom is in the stool, except that from hemorrhoidal bleeding. If questioned, the patient may admit to noticing undigested food in the stool and rectal urgency. Nocturnal diarrhea almost always has an organic cause.

Associated Symptoms

It often is diagnostically helpful to classify acute diarrhea into two types: *toxin-mediated diarrhea* (small bowel diarrhea) and *infectious diarrhea* (colonic diarrhea). Patients with a toxin-mediated diarrhea have an abrupt onset (often a few hours after eating potentially contaminated foods) of large-volume, watery diarrhea associated with variable nausea, vomiting, increased salivation, crampy abdominal pain, and general malaise, but little or no fever. The onset of neurologic symptoms in association with diarrhea suggests *Clostridia* toxin *(botulism).*

Diarrhea of an infectious cause should be suspected with a history of prior good health, acute onset of diarrhea, and no signs or symptoms of involvement of systems other than the gastrointestinal tract. This type of diarrhea is caused by *colonic mucosal invasion* and has also been referred to as *dysentery syndrome.* The presence of fever, vomiting, nausea, abdominal cramps, headache, general malaise, and myalgia along with a watery diarrhea suggests *viral gastroenteritis* and *Salmonella* or *Campylobacter.*

Diarrhea of *colonic origin* should be suspected if fever, early-morning rushes, hypogastric cramps, tenesmus, blood in the stools, or soft stools mixed with copious mucus are associated with diarrhea. Patients with fever and symptoms of small bowel or colonic diarrhea may have *shigellosis;* this is more common in summer. Diarrhea caused by *Salmonella* may have an acute or subacute onset or may present as chronic diarrhea. When a patient known to have intermittent chronic diarrhea due to an irritable colon has an increase in diarrhea, the cause may be additional stress or an infectious diarrhea (e.g., *Salmonella*) superimposed on an irritable colon. *Campylobacter jejuni* has been implicated in a large number of cases of food-borne diarrhea. It is usually associated with fever, bloody diarrhea, and abdominal pain.

When right lower quadrant pain is associated with diarrhea, *Yersinia* or *Campylobacter* infections may simulate *appendicitis.* The bacterial infections often cause diffuse abdominal tenderness and no rebound, thus militating against a diagnosis of appendicitis.

Blood on the surface of stools or on toilet paper suggests blood of anal origin, most often a bleeding hemorrhoid or small anal fissure, particularly if the bleeding occurs after hard stools are passed. Copious bleeding or blood mixed with the stools suggests a more serious cause, such as *ulcerative colitis.* Marked weight loss associated with persistent diarrhea and frothy, foul-smelling stools that sometimes float suggests a pancreatic or small bowel cause of *steatorrhea* and diarrhea. When acute diarrhea and severe vomiting (out of proportion to the diarrhea) begin 2 to 4 hours after eating potentially contaminated foods (especially milk products or meats), a *toxic staphylococcal gastroenteritis* should be suspected. The diagnosis is confirmed presumptively if these symptoms also developed in several other people who ate the same foods.

In addition to foul-smelling, watery, explosive mucoid stools, patients with giardiasis may have increased flatulence, nausea, and, in severe cases, anorexia and weight loss. Some patients complain of abdominal distention and occasional greasy stools.

Diarrhea associated with perianal excoriation (related to acidic stools), abdominal distention, occasional vomiting, fever, anorexia, and, in children, failure to thrive indicates *lactose intolerance.*

Muscle weakness, lassitude, and hypokalemia can be seen in all patients with protracted, copious diarrhea, but their presence should make the physician suspicious of surreptitious *laxative abuse,* particularly if other components of a hysteric personality are present.

Other associated findings that may suggest the etiology of the diarrhea include arthritis (inflammatory bowel disease), fever (inflammatory bowel disease, lymphoma, amebiasis, and tuberculosis), marked weight loss (malabsorption, cancer, and hyperthyroidism), lymphadenopathy (lymphoma and AIDS), neuropathy (diabetes), and peptic ulcer symptoms (antacid therapy and Zollinger-Ellison syndrome).

Precipitating and Aggravating Factors

Drug-induced diarrhea should be suspected if diarrhea develops after the administration of antibiotics or other drugs. The most commonly implicated antibiotics are ampicillin, tetracycline, lincomycin, clindamycin, and chloramphenicol. The diarrhea will range from mild and watery with nonspecific crampy abdominal pain and low-grade fever to a severe colitis with pseudomembrane formation. *Pseudomembranous enterocolitis* is life-threatening and is of the colonic or dysentery type. It is more common if several antibiotics have been administered but classically is caused by a clindamycin-associated *Clostridium difficile* superinfection. Symptoms may begin during or after the course of antibiotic therapy.

Magnesium-containing antacids, methyldopa, digitalis, beta blockers, systemic antiinflammatory agents, iron-containing compounds, laxatives, lactulose, colchicine, quinidine, phenothiazine, drugs, prokinetic agents such as metoclopramide or cisapride, and high doses of salicylates can also cause diarrhea.

If the onset of diarrhea is temporally related to acute stress, particularly *emotional stress,* a functional cause is probable. In these patients the onset of diarrhea may be gradual or acute and the duration protracted.

Ingestion of *contaminated water or food* may occur at any time, but especially during travel abroad or camping, thus producing "traveler's diarrhea." All patients with acute diarrhea should be asked about travel, medications, stress, food ingestion, exposure to others with similar symptoms, dairy product consumption, and recent illnesses.

Ameliorating Factors

The diarrhea of lactose intolerance abates with fasting or avoidance of foods that contain lactose. Functional diarrhea is alleviated with decreased stress. If diarrhea is relieved by antibiotics, bacterial overgrowth may have been the cause.

Physical Findings

Physical examination must include a careful abdominal examination and in some cases a rectal examination. Fever in association with acute diarrhea suggests an infectious cause. Thyroid enlargement and tremor suggest thyrotoxicosis; enlarged lymph nodes suggest lymphoma or AIDS. The colon may be tender to palpation in patients with irritable bowel syndrome, who also may have abdominal distention. Stools should be examined visually for blood or mucus and microscopically for fecal leukocytes, ova, and parasites.

Diagnostic Studies

Studies have shown that a specific causative agent cannot be isolated in about 60% of patients with acute gastroenteritis. Examination of patients with persistent,

Text continued on page 104.

Differential Diagnosis of Diarrhea

CONDITION	NATURE OF PATIENT	NATURE OF SYMPTOMS	ASSOCIATED SYMPTOMS	PRECIPITATING AND AGGRAVATING FACTORS	AMELIORATING FACTORS	PHYSICAL FINDINGS	DIAGNOSTIC STUDIES
Acute diarrhea Viral or bacterial gastroenteritis	All ages	Abrupt onset lasts <1 wk No symptoms of other organ involvement Most common cause of diarrhea *Adults:* benign, self-limiting *Children:* may lead to severe dehydration	Nausea and vomiting Fever Crampy abdominal pain			Hyperactive peristalsis Fever	Stool culture
Rotavirus	Most common in infants under age 3	Peak incidence in winter					
Salmonella *Shigella*	Peak incidence in children ages 1–4 years						Stool culture
Drug induced Laxatives	Mostly women	Diarrhea Muscle weakness Lassitude					Proctoscopy Stool sodium hydroxide test for phenolphthalein Barium enema Hypokalemia

Antibiotics	Taking antibiotics	Mild, watery diarrhea	Nonspecific crampy, abdominal pain Low-grade fever	Ampicillin Tetracycline Lincomycin Chloramphenicol Clindamycin
Pseudomembranous enterocolitis	Taking antibiotics, especially clindamycin	Severe colitis with pseudomembrane formation Life-threatening diarrhea of colonic or dysenteric type		Use of several antibiotics Classically, clindamycin-associated *Clostridium difficile* superinfection
Other drugs				Iron- or magnesium-containing compounds High doses of: Salicylates Quinidine Antiinflammatory agents Beta blockers Colchicine Methyldopa Digitalis Phenothiazines
Toxin-mediated (small bowel) diarrhea		Abrupt onset of large-volume, watery diarrhea	Nausea, vomiting Increased salivation Crampy abdominal pain General malaise Little or no fever	Contaminated food

Table continued on following page.

Differential Diagnosis of Diarrhea *Continued*

CONDITION	NATURE OF PATIENT	NATURE OF SYMPTOMS	ASSOCIATED SYMPTOMS	PRECIPITATING AND AGGRAVATING FACTORS	AMELIORATING FACTORS	PHYSICAL FINDINGS	DIAGNOSTIC STUDIES
Acute diarrhea *Continued*							
Clostridium toxin (botulism)			Neurologic symptoms	Contaminated food			
Staphylococcus toxin		Severe vomiting and diarrhea begins 2–4 hr after eating contaminated food (especially meat or dairy products)		Contaminated food			
Dysentery syndrome (infectious or colonic diarrhea)	History of prior good health	No symptoms other than gastrointestinal involvement Acute, watery diarrhea	Fever Nausea, vomiting Abdominal cramps Headache General malaise Myalgia				Microscopic stool examination for fecal leukocytes If leukocytes present, stool culture If high fever present, blood culture
Chronic diarrhea							
Inflammatory bowel disease	Adults	Initial episode >2 wk May recur over months or years	Weight loss Bloody stools Fever Arthralgia		Steroids	Fever Anemia	Proctoscopy Colonoscopy Gastrointestinal radiographs
	Children	Diarrhea must persist for >1 mo	Failure to gain weight	Enteritis Intestinal infections			

Irritable bowel syndrome (irritable colon, mucous colitis, functional diarrhea)	Most common in young women with children and in other stressed people	Chronic or intermittent diarrhea alternates with constipation More frequent and looser stools with onset of pain Hard, marblelike stools alternate with soft bowel movements Typical in morning; seldom at night Rectal urgency	Mucus in toilet bowl or on stool surface Sense of incomplete evacuation	Stress	Reduction in stress Pain relief with defecation	Colon tender to palpation Abdominal distention	
Lactase deficiency	Infants <1 yr Adults, especially African and Mediterranean descent	Diarrhea	Flatulence Perianal excoriation Abdominal distention Vomiting Fever Anorexia *Children:* failure to thrive	Lactose load Infectious gastroenteritis			Lactose tolerance test Mucosal biopsy
Diabetes	Diabetic	Uncontrolled, explosive postprandial diarrhea	Neurologic dysfunction	Meals	Antibiotics		Blood sugar Colony count of gastric contents
Giardiasis	Severe in children Adults may be asymptomatic Hikers and campers at higher risk	Foul-smelling, watery, explosive diarrhea Latency period of 1–3 wk Onset may be acute or gradual and may persist from weeks to 6 mo	Mucus in stool Increased flatuence Nausea Anorexia and weight loss Greasy stools Abdominal distention	Drinking water, infested with *Giardia lamblia*			Microscopic stool examination for *Giardia* Duodenal aspirate for *Giardia*

unexplained diarrhea should include colonoscopic examination with particular attention to the colonic mucosa. This frequently helps to establish the cause of diarrhea when radiographs and routine sigmoidoscopy are negative. Patients with invasive (so-called colonic) diarrhea have an erythematous colonic mucosa that may have ecchymoses, friability, excess mucus, and small ulcerations. These ulcerations must be differentiated from the ragged ulcers of *ulcerative colitis* and the discrete, punched-out ulcers that are almost pathognomonic of *amebic colitis.*

In addition to obtaining a precise history, the physician must examine the stool for fecal polymorphonuclear or mononuclear leukocytes. This is a simple test: a fleck of mucus or liquid stool is placed on a microscope slide, mixed with an equal volume of Löffler's methylene blue, and examined after 2 to 3 minutes with the "high, dry" objective. Because fecal leukocyte production is stimulated by bacteria that invade the colonic mucosa, these leukocytes are frequently seen in infections caused by *Salmonella, Shigella, Yersinia,* and invasive *Escherichia coli.* If fecal leukocytes are present, the stool should be cultured; blood should be cultured if high fever is present. Fecal leukocytes also are seen with disorders associated with colonic mucosa inflammation, such as *ulcerative colitis,* when blood and stool cultures are not remarkable.

Organisms that cause diarrhea by toxin production (*E. coli, Clostridium perfringens, Vibrio cholerae,* and *Staphylococcus*) or by induction of small bowel lesions (*Giardia* and viruses) may cause a watery stool without fecal leukocytes. Amebic dysentery usually is not associated with fecal leukocytes.

Microscopic examination of the stools reveals *Giardia* cysts in 50% of patients with giardiasis. If negative, a *Giardia* antigen test may be obtained. A jejunal biopsy and jejunal or duodenal aspiration also may reveal *Giardia* cysts.

In patients with diarrhea caused by laxative abuse, proctoscopic examination may reveal melanosis coli. Urine and stool tests may be positive for phenolphthalein. A barium enema may show increased haustral markings.

The stool pH is less than 6.0 and stool sugar is greater than 1 gram percent in patients with lactose intolerance.

Less Common Diagnostic Considerations

Less common causes of diarrhea include amebiasis, bacterial overgrowth after abdominal surgery, achlorhydria, gastric stasis (in diabetes), carcinoid syndrome, blind loop syndrome with bacterial overgrowth, inflammatory bowel disease, Crohn's disease, and ulcerative colitis.

Antidiarrheal drugs can result in obstipation. With obstipation and fecal impaction (which is more common in elderly patients), there may be frequent small, loose, and watery bowel movements without much solid stool. Fecal impactions usually can be diagnosed by rectal examination.

Patients with *inflammatory bowel disease* usually have frequent small stools or diarrhea with the passage of blood, mucus, and occasionally pus. They often have rectal leakage, nocturnal diarrhea, pain, urgency, and early-morning rushes. With the acute form, patients may appear toxic and have malaise, fever, dehydration, and tachycardia. Those with chronic inflammatory bowel disease may have weight loss, anemia, joint pains, and skin lesions (e.g., erythema nodosum).

Malabsorption conditions other than lactose intolerance include adult nontropical sprue (actually a gluten sensitivity); intolerance to carbohydrates, cow's milk, or protein; and loss of absorptive surface due to bowel resection, sprue, or pancreatic insufficiency.

Pancreatic islet cell tumors and colorectal carcinoma may present initially with diarrhea. *Colorectal cancer* is more common in middle-aged than elderly patients and may present with any change in bowel habits, most often diarrhea alternating with constipation. Diarrhea may be the only presenting symptom, particularly if the lesion is in the cecum or ascending colon.

Chronic Diarrhea in Children

The term *chronic* normally refers to prolonged diarrhea; the specific time that must elapse for diarrhea to be considered chronic is a matter of controversy. Although some agree that persistence for 2 weeks justifies diagnosing chronic diarrhea in adults, the prevalent belief is that diarrhea in a child must persist for 1 or more months to be considered chronic. In addition, the child must have either lost weight or failed to gain weight during that period for the situation to be considered clinically significant.

It is particularly important for the physician to have a concept of normal stool patterns in children. Under age 4 months, breast-fed infants pass two to four stools daily that are yellow to golden, soft, and have a pH near 5.0. Formula-fed infants under age 4 months have two to three stools daily that are firm and have a pH around 7.0. From ages 4 to 12 months, most children pass one to three stools per day. These stools are darker yellow and firmer. After age 1, children's stools are formed and resemble adult stools in odor and color.

One approach of the differential diagnosis of chronic diarrhea in children is to clarify them by type of stool: watery stools, fatty stools, or bloody stools. Watery stools are most often seen in the following situations: (1) *persistent postenteritis* diarrhea (with or without secondary carbohydrate intolerance); (2) *intestinal infections* from viruses, bacteria *(Shigella, Salmonella, E. coli, Yersinia),* and parasites (particularly *Giardia*); and (3) *disaccharidase deficiency.* A *lactose deficiency* secondary to an acute gastroenteritis is much more common than a primary lactase deficiency. A sucrase-isomaltase deficiency is rare.

Allergic gastroenteropathies, in which the child is allergic to cow's milk protein or soy protein, may also cause watery diarrhea in infants and children. Other, much less common causes include *Hirschsprung's disease, short bowel syndrome,* primary immune defects, and diarrhea associated with endocrine disorders.

Fatty stools suggest *cystic fibrosis, pancreatic insufficiency, celiac disease,* or *allergic gastroenteropathy.* Rarely, such drugs as neomycin may induce steatorrhea.

Chronic bloody diarrhea suggests *Shigella* or *Salmonella* infection, *dysentery, inflammatory bowel disease* (including ulcerative colitis and Crohn's disease), *amebic dysentery*, or less often antibiotic-induced pseudomembranous colitis.

Selected References

Agus SG: Approach to a patient with infectious diarrhea. Mt Sinai J Med 62:175–177, 1996.

Baldassano RN, Liacouras CA: Chronic diarrhea: a practical approach for the pediatrician. Pediatr Clin North Am 38:667–687, 1991.

Bramble MG, Record CO: Drug-induced gastrointestinal disease. Drugs 15:451–463, 1970.

Dupont HL: Guidelines on acute infectious diarrhea in adults: the Practice Parameters Committee of the American College of Gastroenterology. Am J Gastroenterol 92:1962–1975, 1997.

Kane JA, Blachlow NR: Infectious diarrhea. Prim Care 6:63–80, 1979.

Kroser JA, Metz DC: Evaluation of the adult patient with diarrhea. Prim Care 23:629–647, 1996.

Lipsky MS, Adelman M: Chronic diarrhea: evaluation and treatment. Am Fam Physician 48:1461–1466, 1993.

Matseshe JW, Phillips SF: Chronic diarrhea—practical approach. Med Clin North Am 62:141–154, 1978.

Talal AH, Murray JA: Acute and chronic diarrhea: how to keep laboratory testing to a minimum. Postgrad Med 96:30–32, 35–38, 43, 1996.

Talley NJ :Spectrum of chronic dyspepsia in the presence of the irritable bowel syndrome. Scand J Gastroenterol 26(suppl 182):7–10, 1991.

Yee J, Wall SD: Gastrointestinal manifestations of AIDS. Gastroenterol Clin North Am 24:413–435, 1995.

CHAPTER 11

Dizziness/Lightheadedness and Vertigo

Most patients who complain of dizziness do not have an ear problem. A careful history is particularly important for these patients. The physician must first determine whether the patient has true vertigo or dizziness/lightheadedness.

True vertigo is a hallucination of movement. *Objective vertigo* is the illusion that one's surroundings are moving. *Subjective vertigo* is the feeling that, with eyes closed, one's body or head is moving or turning in space.

In contrast, lightheadedness, dizziness, and giddiness represent a sensation of being about to faint *(near syncope);* this is not accompanied by true syncope or a feeling of rotation or movement. Some patients describe lightheadedness as a lack of strength or a generalized weakness and may feel that they will pass out if they do not lie down; this symptom usually improves rapidly with recumbency. Lightheadedness, dizziness, and near-syncope must be differentiated from true syncope (not discussed in this chapter), which has more serious implications, especially in elderly patients.

True Vertigo

Nature of Patient

Most vertiginous episodes in children are benign and self-limiting, except those associated with a seizure disorder. Although true vertigo is uncommon in children, they may complain of vertigo after an *upper respiratory tract infection* or an acute *viral infection* in which hearing was also disturbed. Vertigo may be secondary to an acute *viral labyrinthitis* or *benign paroxysmal positional vertigo,* often referred to as *benign positional vertigo* (BPV). Children with *serous otitis media* usually do not complain of dizziness or vertigo but may have nondescript balance disturbances. Vertigo or headaches may develop in children several weeks after a *head injury.* When paroxysmal vertigo occurs in children with a family history of migraine, it may represent a *migraine equivalent.* Vertigo seldom is the initial symptom of a seizure; when it is, it may be followed by transitory unconsciousness or amnesia of the event.

In adults, true vertigo frequently is caused by *BPV,* Meniere's syndrome (or disease), and *labyrinthitis.* Ototoxic and salt-retaining drugs, acoustic neuroma, and brain stem dysfunction are less common causes.

To facilitate diagnosis, vertigo can be separated into central and peripheral causes. *Central vertigo* is caused by brain stem or cerebellar lesions and is associated with diplopia, dysarthria, dysphagia, paresthesias, headache, or ataxia. *Peripheral vertigo* is caused by problems of the inner ear or vestibular nerve and often can be diagnosed by the duration of symptoms.

Nature of Symptoms

Although the clinical differential diagnosis of vertigo is best made on the basis of associated symptoms, physical findings, and diagnostic studies, vertigo has some distinguishing features. Recurrent attacks often are associated with *BPV,* and *Meniere's syndrome. Labyrinthitis* usually is not recurrent. The vertigo associated with *otitis media* has a gradual onset and may persist after the otitis subsides. If the vertigo has been continuous and progressive for several weeks or months, a *mass lesion* should be suspected.

Benign positional vertigo, Meniere's syndrome, and labyrinthitis have varying durations of symptoms. In positional vertigo, symptoms last from seconds to minutes; in *vertebrobasilar insufficiency,* minutes; in Meniere's syndrome, from minutes to hours; and in toxic labyrinthitis, vestibular neuronitis, or brain stem lesion, from days to weeks.

Prior episodes of vertigo may have been correctly diagnosed. If the previous physician did not obtain a precise history and perform an appropriate physical examination, however, prior episodes of vertigo may have been misdiagnosed as "nerves," "tension," or "low blood pressure." Lack of physician awareness of benign paroxysmal positional vertigo is a common cause of the misdiagnosis of dizziness in elderly people.

Associated Symptoms

Tinnitus, ear fullness, and other hearing disturbances usually are present with Meniere's syndrome, rare in labyrinthitis, and absent in BPV. Nausea and vomiting may be present in all. If vertigo is associated with an acute onset of unilateral weakness, uncoordination, diplopia, or numbness, the vertigo is caused by *brain stem disease,* such as vertebrobasilar insufficiency. These patients usually have normal hearing but may have other signs of brain stem dysfunction (e.g., vertical, lateral, or rotatory nystagmus).

Nystagmus is also observed in Meniere's syndrome and BPV. If the patient has a chronic, progressive, unilateral hearing deficit with tinnitus, facial numbness, or weakness, an *acoustic neuroma* should be suspected. Café au lait spots or neurofibromatosis also may be observed in patients with acoustic neuromas. Vertigo may be part of a *migraine* aura or may be a migraine equivalent, which is more common in adolescents.

Precipitating and Aggravating Factors

By definition, positional changes such as head turning, rolling over in bed, bending over and then standing erect, and looking up by extending the neck may precipitate or aggravate BPV. This is usually not true in Meniere's syndrome, which is thought to have its onset around *menstruation* and during times of *emotional stress. Ototoxic drugs* (e.g., streptomycin, aminoglycosides especially gentamicin, rarely furosemide) also may cause vertigo. Recurrent vertigo may be present when salt-retaining drugs (e.g., steroids, phenylbutazone) are ingested.

An acute onset of isolated vertigo suggests a *viral infection* or *middle or inner ear lesion.* Repeated vertigo episodes associated with nausea and vomiting of many years' duration suggest Meniere's syndrome or BPV.

Ameliorating Factors

During attacks of BPV, patients may be comfortable when they are still. Vertigo persists in patients with Meniere's syndrome, otitis, labyrinthitis, and acoustic neuroma even if they do not move.

Physical Findings

The symptoms caused by BPV can be replicated with caloric stimulation or certain postural maneuvers (e.g., Hallpike's). Nystagmus occurs in BPV, Meniere's syndrome, and labyrinthitis. Vertical nystagmus occurs only with central causes of nystagmus, and its presence excludes the previously mentioned (labyrinthine) causes of vertigo.

The typical lateral nystagmus of BPV occurs within a few seconds after the patient assumes a provocative posture or performs a provocative maneuver. The nystagmus abates after a few seconds and also fatigues (does not occur) with serial repetition of the maneuver.

No latency or fatigue exists when the nystagmus is caused by a central lesion.

Diagnostic Studies

The reader is referred to the references, particularly Drachman and Hart (1972) and Sloane (1996).

Less Common Diagnostic Considerations

Less common otologic causes of vertigo include tumors of the middle and inner ear, cholesteatoma, and impacted cerumen. Less common neurologic causes of vertigo include cerebellopontine angle tumors, brain stem tumors, multiple sclerosis, and vertebrobasilar insufficiency (more common in elderly patients). Ramsay Hunt syndrome, Lyme disease, and Wernicke's encephalopathy may cause vertigo in rare instances.

Lightheadedness/Dizziness and Giddiness

Many patients describe these symptoms as a sensation of dysequilibrium (worse while standing), nonspecific weakness, or faintness without actually fainting. This symptom may abate when they recline. The most common causes of lightheadedness include *psychological problems, circulatory problems* (sometimes related to *hypotensive drugs*), *arrhythmias,* and *hyperventilation.*

Nature of Patient

When lightheadedness occurs in children, especially those at or near puberty, a *psychological cause* (e.g., stressful home or school environments) should be suspected. Syncope and orthostatic lightheadedness occasionally occur during the adolescent growth spurt. Although much less common in children than in adults, *hyperventilation syndrome* may produce symptoms of lightheadedness.

When episodes of dizziness are associated with syncope or palpitations, the patient (child or adult) may have *sick sinus syndrome.* Some children and adults experience symptoms of lightheadedness during the tachycardia of *Wolff-Parkinson-White (WPW) syndrome* or *mitral valve prolapse.* Older children should be asked whether they are aware of any rapid or irregular heartbeat during the episode of lightheadedness.

An initial onset of lightheadedness in elderly patients suggests a *cardiovascular disturbance* or *cerebrovascular insufficiency;* vascular insufficiency secondary to cervical arthritis is less common. Postural dizziness related to *unstable vasomotor reflexes* is more common in elderly people but can be seen at any age. *Dysequilibrium,* a sense of imbalance or unsteadiness especially when standing, is more common in elderly patients. It can be caused by visual, proprioceptive, and cerebellar or motor defects, which occur in patients with stroke, vestibular disease, neuropathy, cerebellar disease, and particularly deconditioning. When a patient frequently complains of transient lightheadedness and no specific cause can be found, it probably is of psychogenic origin.

When a patient rarely complains of lightheadedness, a more thorough history and physical examination should be done. In this patient a psychogenic cause should be a diagnosis of exclusion. When lightheadedness occurs in a patient with a significant psychiatric disorder, *hyperventilation syndrome* or a *reaction to psychotropic agents* should be considered.

Nature of Symptoms

Psychogenic dizziness may be recurrent but often is persistent. Drug-induced giddiness also is persistent. Orthostatic hypotension, reactive hypoglycemia, and arrhythmias cause recurrent episodes of lightheadedness. Psychogenic dizziness and hypoglycemic dizziness are not necessarily related to position.

Associated Symptoms

Patients with *psychogenic dizziness* often have many "functional" complaints. If circumoral or digital paresthesias are present, the dizziness probably is caused by *hyperventilation.* An irregular or rapid heartbeat suggests an *arrhythmia* as the cause of the lightheadedness. Nervousness and sweating indicate *hypoglycemia.*

Precipitating and Aggravating Factors

If giddiness occurs while the patient is standing, *orthostatic hypotension* should be suspected. This most often is induced by antihypertensive drugs, vasodilators used for angina, and tricyclic antidepressants. Some patients who have significant systolic pressure reduction, especially elderly people, experience lightheadedness when they assume the erect posture, despite systolic levels greater than 120 mm Hg, particularly if the blood pressure has been reduced rapidly with antihypertensive agents. Orthostatic hypotension also may be secondary to severe diabetic or alcoholic neuropathy.

Patients may complain of lightheadedness or unsteadiness due to alcohol or *drug ingestion.* Antihypertensive agents of all types, particularly the more potent drugs, can produce *orthostatic hypotension,* the most common cause of recurrent dizziness and falls in elderly people. Vasodilators such as sildenafil (Viagra) and terazosin, used to treat erectile dysfunction and prostatic hypertrophy, respectively, may also cause lightheadedness. Phenytoin and psychotropic agents can produce feelings of unsteadiness. Ototoxic drugs (e.g., gentamicin, streptomycin, neomycin, quinine, salicylates in high doses) may cause lightheadedness without true vertigo. Dizziness occurs when selective serotonin reuptake inhibitors (SSRIs) are discontinued.

If dizziness has a temporal periodicity (middle to late morning, middle to late afternoon, or approximately 2 to 4 hours after eating), *reactive hypoglycemia* should be suspected. The dizziness can be caused by the hypoglycemia itself or hypoglycemia-induced paroxysmal tachycardia. Dizziness on arising in the morning should suggest orthostatic hypotension or hypoglycemia, particularly if the patient is receiving a long-acting insulin.

If transient episodes of lightheadedness (without syncope) have been occurring for many years and the history and physical examination do not suggest a specific cause, the patient should be reassured that most likely no serious illness exists. The symptom may be a manifestation of tension, and the patient should be instructed to record associated signs and symptoms as well as precipitating factors until the next visit.

Ameliorating Factors

If lightheadedness abates with recumbency, *orthostatic hypotension* should be suspected. If recurrent lightheadedness and dizziness abate when the patient is on vacation or removed from stressful situations, a *psychogenic cause* is indicated. If ingestion of carbohydrates or rebreathing in a paper bag alleviates the symptom, hypoglycemia or hyperventilation, respectively, should be considered.

Physical Findings

Usually, no abnormal physical findings are associated with psychogenic dizziness. Occasionally the patient can replicate the symptoms of hyperventilation syn-

Text continued on page 115.

Differential Diagnosis of Dizziness/Lightheadedness and Vertigo

CONDITION	NATURE OF PATIENT	NATURE OF SYMPTOMS	ASSOCIATED SYMPTOMS	PRECIPITATING AND AGGRAVATING FACTORS	AMELIORATING FACTORS	PHYSICAL FINDINGS	DIAGNOSTIC STUDIES
True vertigo							
Benign paroxysmal positional vertigo (benign positional vertigo, BPV)	Adults Uncommon in children	Recurrent over many years *Not* associated with tinnitus or hearing loss Episodes last seconds to minutes	Nausea and vomiting No neurologic defect	Positional changes (e.g., head turning, rolling over in bed)	Some relief if patient is motionless	Nystagmus and vertigo occur seconds after assuming a provocative posture Lateral or rotatory nystagmus	Symptoms can be replicated by caloric stimulation or certain postural maneuvers Electronystagmography
Otitis media	More common in children	Persistent vertigo	Earache	Upper respiratory infection		Those of otitis media (acute or chronic)	Audiometric testing Tympanogram
Meniere's syndrome (disease)	Adults	Sudden onset of vertigo Not precipitated by sudden movement Recurrent Duration minutes to hours	Tinnitus Hearing loss Ear fullness Nausea and vomiting	Menstruation Emotional stress		Lateral or rotatory nystagmus No nystagmus between attacks Hearing deficit	Audiometric testing
Labyrinthitis (peripheral vestibulopathy)	Any age	Sudden onset of vertigo Lasts days to weeks	Rarely associated with tinnitus Nausea and vomiting Hearing loss possible	May be precipitated by viral infection			Caloric test Postural maneuvers Electronystagmography

Acoustic neuroma	Adults	Gradual onset Persistent vertigo	Chronic, progressive unilateral hearing deficit Tinnitus Facial numbness Weakness Café au lait spots			May be café au lait spots Hearing loss Other neurologic problems	CT scan
Drugs							
Ototoxic		Persists days to weeks		Streptomycin Aminoglycosides Furosemide	Stop drug		
Salt retaining		Vertigo recurs when patient is taking drugs		Steroids Phenylbutazone Phenytoin			
Brain stem dysfunction (vertebrobasilar insufficiency, stroke, tumors)	Elderly	Acute onset of vertigo Normal hearing Recurrent Progressive with mass lesions	Blurred vision Diplopia Slurred speech Paresthesia Uncoordination Usually no nausea and vomiting			Vertical, lateral, or rotatory nystagmus	Electroencephalography CT scan
Dizziness/lightheadedness							
Psychogenic	Most common cause of dizziness in children	Recurrent Often persistent *Not* posture related	Many "functional" complaints	Emotional stress	Stress reduction		
Hyperventilation syndrome	More common in adults Anxious	Recurrent	Circumoral or digital paresthesias	Emotional stress	Rebreathing in paper bag	Hyperventilation infrequent Symptoms replicated by patient hyperventilating voluntarily	

Table continued on following page.

Differential Diagnosis of Dizziness/Lightheadedness and Vertigo *Continued*

CONDITION	NATURE OF PATIENT	NATURE OF SYMPTOMS	ASSOCIATED SYMPTOMS	PRECIPITATING AND AGGRAVATING FACTORS	AMELIORATING FACTORS	PHYSICAL FINDINGS	DIAGNOSTIC STUDIES
Dizziness/lightheadedness *Continued*							
Reactive hypoglycemia		Recurrent Dizziness has temporal periodicity Onset 2–4 hr after meals	Hypoglycemia-induced paroxysmal tachycardia Trembling Sweating	Carbohydrate ingestion	Temporary relief from carbohydrates Avoidance of excessive carbohydrate ingestion	Sweating Tachycardia	5-hr glucose tolerance test
Orthostatic hypotension	Elderly Hypertensive Diabetic	Recurrent Giddiness on standing	Occasional syncope	Erect posture Antihypertensive medication	Recumbency	Orthostatic hypotension	
Drugs or alcohol		Persistent light headedness or unsteadiness without true vertigo		Phenytoin Psychotropics Ototoxic drugs Vasodilators Discontinuation of SSRIs	Stop drugs		
Sick sinus syndrome	Adults Rare in children	Recurrent dizziness	Syncope Palpitations			Irregular pulse May be normal Bradycardia	Electrocardiography Holter monitoring His bundle study
Wolff-Parkinson-White (WPW) syndrome		Recurrent	Palpitations			May be normal between attacks	Electrocardiography Holter monitoring His bundle study

drome (dizziness, circumoral numbness) by hyperventilating voluntarily. Patients with reactive hypoglycemia may manifest excessive sweating and tachycardia. Intermittent tachycardia or bradycardia may be observed in patients with WPW syndrome or sick sinus syndrome, respectively. Orthostatic hypotension may be caused by drugs but also by a diabetic or alcoholic neuropathy.

Diagnostic Studies

Carotid Doppler studies, cerebral angiography, Holter monitoring, magnetic resonance imaging, and computed tomography (CT) scans may be helpful in selected patients.

Less Common Diagnostic Considerations

Less common diagnostic considerations include cardiac arrhythmias such as bradyarrhythmias, paroxysmal atrial fibrillation, complete heart block, paroxysmal atrial tachycardia, and WPW syndrome (especially in younger patients). Older patients with *subclavian steal syndrome* feel lightheaded after movement of their arms. These patients may have a decreased left carotid pulse, a bruit, or a decreased blood pressure in the left arm. Some patients with hemodynamically significant *aortic stenosis* or *idiopathic hypertrophic obstructive myocardiopathy* may experience lightheadedness, primarily after exertion.

Selected References

Baloh RW: Approach to the dizzy patient. Baillieres Clin Neurol 3:453–465, 1994.

Donaldson JA: Differential diagnosis of vertigo. AFP Family Practice Annual, 1982, pp 5–17.

Drachman DA, Hart CW: An approach to the dizzy patient. Neurology 22:323–334, 1972.

Edmeads J: Understanding dizziness: how to decipher this nonspecific symptom. Postgrad Med 88:255–268, 1990.

Gantz BJ: Differential diagnosis and management of the dizzy patient. Prim Care 9(2):413–427, 1982.

Hybels RL: History-taking in dizziness: the most important diagnostic item. Postgrad Med 75(3):41–46, 1984.

Jongkees LBW: The dizzy, the giddy, and the vertiginous. ORL J Otorhinolaryngol Relat Spec 40:293–302, 1978.

Kapoor WN: Syncope in older persons. J Am Geriatr Soc 42:426–436, 1994.

Lewis RF: Vertigo: some uncommon causes of a common problem. Semin Neurol 16:55–62, 1996.

Linstrom CJ: Office management of the dizzy patient. Otolaryngol Clin North Am 25:745–780, 1992.

Sloane PD: Evaluation and management of dizziness in the older patient. Clin Geriatr Med 12:785–801, 1996.

Smith JD: Evaluating vertigo. Emerg Med 12:45–51, 1980.

Towler HMA: Dizziness and vertigo. Br Med J 288:1739–1743, 1984.

Tusa RJ, Saada AA, Niparko JK: Dizziness in childhood. J Child Neurol 9:261–274, 1994.

Venna N: Dizziness, falling, and fainting: differential diagnosis in the aged. Geriatrics 41:30–36, 39, 42, 1986.

CHAPTER 12

Earache

Otalgia (earache) usually is a sign of an acute or chronic infection of the external auditory canal or mastoid or an acute infection of the middle ear. These infections can easily be identified with careful examination. **If otologic examination fails to show the source of the pain, referred pain should be considered.** Because the ear is innervated partially by sensory branches of the vagus nerve (Arnold's nerve), glossopharyngeal nerve (Jacobson's nerve), trigeminal nerve (auriculotemporal nerve), facial nerve, and branches of the cranial nerves (CN) II and III, pathologic conditions such as infection and malignant disease of the upper aerodigestive tract (carcinoma of larynx, hypopharynx, oropharynx, and base of tongue) and odontogenic disease also can cause otalgia (Fig. 12–1).

Most earaches are caused by an *acute infection of the middle ear or external ear canal.* Usually a careful examination will reveal the cause promptly; occasionally the differential diagnosis is more difficult. Other common causes of ear pain include *acute serous otitis media, eustachitis, acute otitic barotrauma, mastoiditis, traumatic perforation of the tympanic membrane, foreign bodies,* and *referred pain,* as with temporomandibular joint (TMJ) dysfunction, impacted third molars, periodontal abscess, and recent dental work. About 50% of referred ear pain is caused by a dental problem.

Nature of Patient

Otitis externa occurs more frequently in adults, particularly elderly diabetic patients, and in patients with seborrheic dermatitis or psoriasis of the scalp. "Swimmer's ear" is common in people who swim frequently but also occurs in those who clean their ears with cotton swabs, paper clips, towel tips, and so forth.

Otitis media is more common in children, particularly those younger than 8 years. Various studies suggest that 20% of all children have at least three episodes of otitis media in their first year of life and that two thirds of all children have at least one episode before age 2 years. After upper respiratory infection (URI) and tonsillopharyngitis, otitis media is the third leading reason for pediatric office visits. Premature children on respirators are at higher risk, as are those with cleft palate and Down syndrome.

Serous otitis also is more common in children. It usually is not associated with severe pain, except when an acute infection results in an acute otitis media. Serous otitis media often is asymptomatic but frequently is detected on routine audiometric testing of schoolchildren, since it is the most common cause of hearing deficiencies in children.

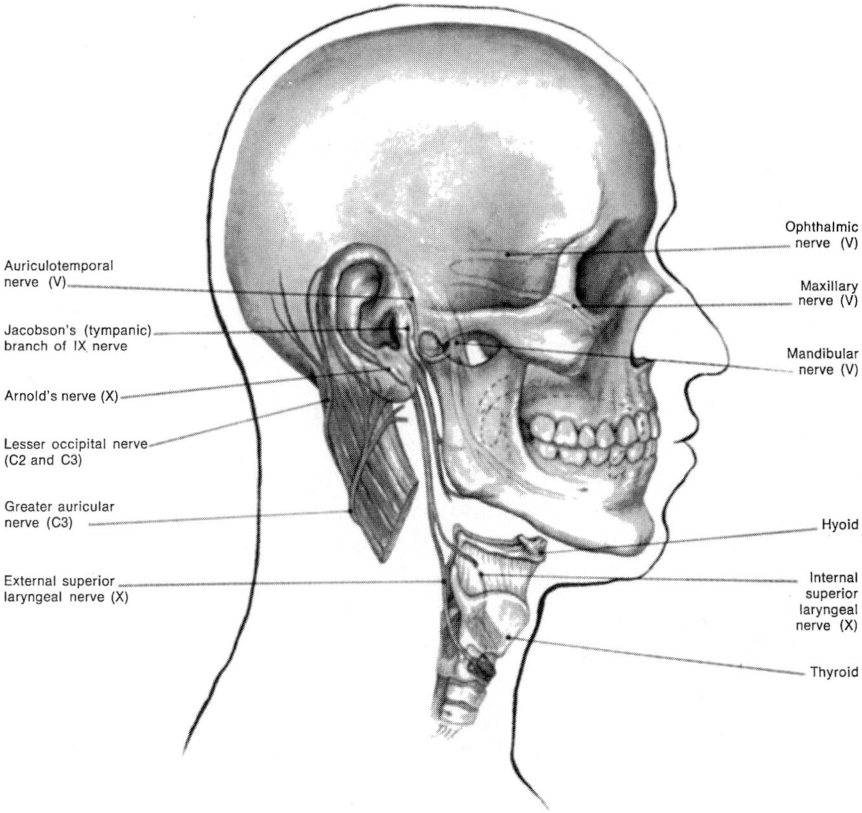

■ **Figure 12.1** Nerve supply to the ear. (From Beddoe GM: Otalgia. Am Fam Physician 11:108, 1975.)

Local causes of ear pain predominate in children, whereas the incidence of referred pain increases with age. One study showed that 60% of patients (mean age 36) referred to an ear, nose, and throat clinic had referred pain to their ears. In 80% the ear pain was caused by *cervical spine lesions, TMJ dysfunction,* or *dental pathology. Impacted third molars* are more common in women between ages 15 and 25 and may cause referred ear pain. In elderly patients, *malignant lesions* of the oropharynx and larynx can cause referred otalgia.

Referred pain to the ear does not rule out a local painful process. *Barotrauma* should be considered in patients who have recently traveled by air and in scuba-diving enthusiasts. Pain from direct trauma can result from a blast or a slap on the ear and in "ear pickers."

Nature of Symptoms

Otitis externa is easily differentiated from otitis media in that patients with otitis externa find movement or pressure on the pinna extremely painful. In addition, they may have tender swelling of the outer ear canal. *Bilateral pain* in the ears is more suggestive of otitis externa. Bilateral pain is unlikely in otitis media and virtually rules out a referred source of the pain. The pain of otitis media has been described as a deep-seated, severe pain that often prevents the patient from sleeping. Children who are too young to talk may present with irritability, restlessness, fever, poor feeding, or rubbing of the affected ear. Frequently the patient has a history of a recent URIs.

Serous otitis and *eustachitis* are not usually associated with a severe earache, but patients may have some intermittent discomfort and may state that they hear crackling or gurgling sounds. Severe pain in and especially behind the ear occurs with *acute mastoiditis.* These patients have exquisite tenderness on pressing over the mastoid process.

The pain of *barotrauma* may be severe and persistent, and a superimposed otitis media occasionally develops. The pain most frequently is experienced during descent in an airplane, especially if the patient has a concurrent URI with eustachian tube dysfunction. The pain may be excruciating.

Patients with *impacted cerumen* also may complain of severe pain in the ear, or they may have only a vague sensation of discomfort sometimes associated with impaired hearing. On questioning, the patients may admit to a longstanding problem with cerumen accumulation in the ears, with exacerbation leading to visits to the physician.

The pain of *TMJ dysfunction* usually is intermittent and often is worse in the morning if associated with night grinding. The pain also may occur toward the end of the day, especially if it is secondary to tension-induced bruxism (see Chapters 13 and 17).

Associated Symptoms

The usual sequence of symptoms in *otitis media* is a blocked feeling in the ear, pain, fever, discharge if the tympanic membrane perforates, and some relief of pain and fever with perforation. Patients with *serous otitis* usually are well and afebrile. They frequently present with impaired hearing as their only complaint, although they also may complain of a feeling of fullness in the ear, popping or crackling sounds, or tinnitus.

Symptoms typically associated with *TMJ dysfunction* include vertigo, tinnitus, headache, and a jaw click. The pain may be worse in the morning if the patient grinds the teeth during sleep ("night grinder").

Precipitating and Aggravating Factors

Otitic barotrauma is aggravated by URIs, hay fever, middle ear effusion, and stuffy nose. It often is precipitated by an increase in atmospheric pressure, as occurs with descent in an airplane. *Eustachitis* is often precipitated by pharyngitis or URI, which may cause mechanical or functional obstruction of the eustachian tube; air in the tube is reabsorbed, and the drum is retracted. *Acute otitis media* often precedes acute mastoiditis by 10 to 14 days. Pain in the ear that is referred from the second and third spinal nerve may be worse with flexion of the neck. Otalgia exacerbated by swallowing suggests *Eagle's syndrome,* an elongated styloid process.

Ameliorating Factors

The pain of *barotrauma* and *eustachitis* may be alleviated somewhat by chewing, Valsalva's maneuver, and nasal decongestants. *TMJ pain* may be eased by a dental bite appliance.

Physical Findings and Diagnostic Studies

The physical findings of otitis externa, otitis media, and serous otitis are well known (see references) and are not described here.

The physician must perform an accurate, complete examination of the eardrum to rule out otitis media. If an adequate view is obstructed because of wax accumulation or secondary external ear canal infection, otitis media cannot be ruled out; it can only be excluded if the entire drum is normal and there is no conductive hearing loss. In serous otitis a serous or glutinous fluid accumulates in the middle ear space. The drum may look abnormal because of the effusion, or it may be injected with noticeable radial vessels. With serous otitis and eustachitis the tympanic membrane may be retracted and may show decreased mobility on pneumatic otoscopy (Fig. 12–2). Impedance tympanometry (Fig. 12–3) helps to confirm the diagnosis.

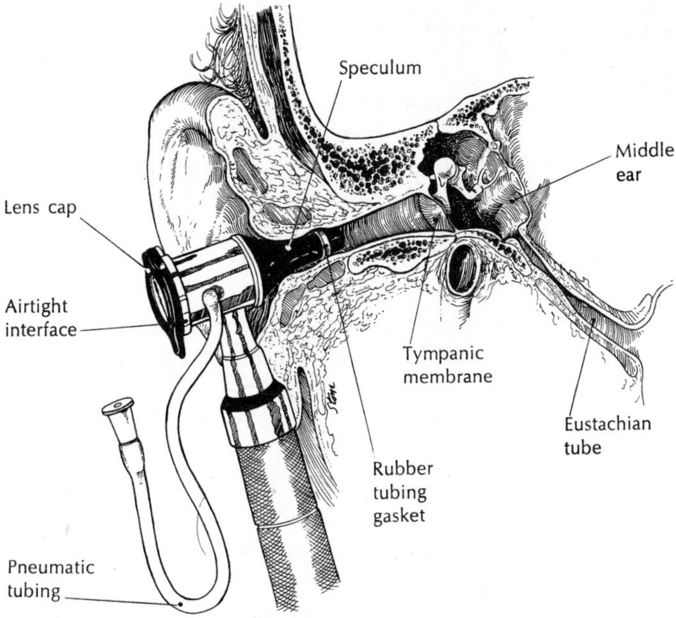

■ **Figure 12.2** Pneumatic otoscopy. (From Schwartz RH: New concepts in otitis media. Am Fam Physician 19[5]:91-98, 1979.)

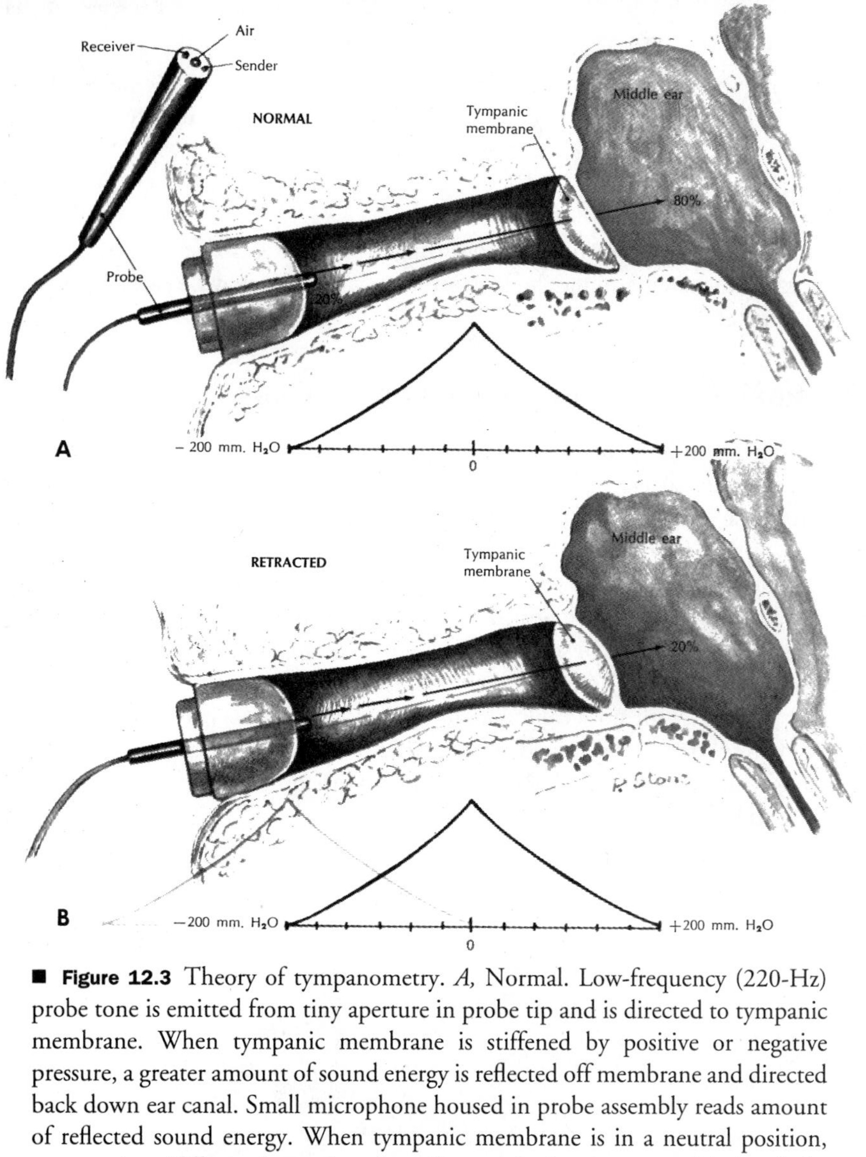

■ **Figure 12.3** Theory of tympanometry. *A,* Normal. Low-frequency (220-Hz) probe tone is emitted from tiny aperture in probe tip and is directed to tympanic membrane. When tympanic membrane is stiffened by positive or negative pressure, a greater amount of sound energy is reflected off membrane and directed back down ear canal. Small microphone housed in probe assembly reads amount of reflected sound energy. When tympanic membrane is in a neutral position, pressure in middle ear is equal to that of atmospheric pressure and is thus in its most mobile position. Here, most of sound energy from probe tone is absorbed by tympanic membrane into middle ear, and least amount is reflected back down ear canal. *B,* Retracted. Retracted tympanic membrane reflects negative pressure in middle ear relative to atmospheric pressure. Most compliant position of membrane (peak of tympanogram) is found when artificially induced negative pressure is introduced from manometer of instrument. Thus, pressure point at which peak of tympanogram occurs represents an indirect measure of middle ear pressure. Note that greater sound energy is reflected off tympanic membrane until pressure introduced down ear canal is equal to pressure in middle ear (in this case, –200 mm H_2O). (From Schwartz RH: New concepts in otitis media. Am Fam Physician 19[5]:91–98, 1979.)

When the patient complains of ear pain, has a fever and noticeable swelling behind the ear, or experiences tenderness to palpation over the mastoid process, *acute mastoiditis* is probable. The tympanic membrane often is red, bulging, and immobile because of an associated otitis media. It should be suspected whenever discharge from the middle ear is continuous for more than 10 days. Radiographs help to establish the diagnosis.

Whenever a patient complains of pain in the ear and examination of the ear canal and drum is normal, referred pain is most probable.

One common cause of referred pain to the ear is *TMJ dysfunction.* This may be either *acute,* resulting from opening the mouth extremely wide, or *chronic,* resulting from malocclusion or arthritis of the TMJ, which occurs more frequently in patients with *rheumatoid arthritis.* Malocclusion or enlarged masseter muscles caused by bruxism may be apparent on physical examination. In addition, the patient often has tenderness to palpation over the TMJ. Occasionally the examiner may hear clicking or palpate crepitus over the TMJ.

Patients with *impacted third molars* may have trismus and pain when pressure is applied above and behind the angle of the mandible. The diagnosis can be confirmed by dental radiographs.

Less Common Diagnostic Considerations

Pain in the ear can be caused by *infections* such as impetigo, insect bites, chondrodermatitis nodularis chronica helicis (an exquisitely tender nodule of the helix seen in older adults), perichondritis of the pinna, or gouty tophi (which usually are not painful). Rarely, *tumors* of the middle ear and meatus can produce nonremitting pain.

Patients with *herpes zoster oticus (Ramsay Hunt syndrome)* have severe pain in one ear for several days, after which vesicles appear on the auricle or in the meatus. These vesicles also may appear on the tympanic membrane and occasionally on the palate. Concurrent with the vesicles, a complete lower motor neuron lesion of CN VII usually occurs, associated with pyrexia, constitutional disturbances, deafness, tinnitus, vertigo, and nystagmus.

Drugs such as mesalamine and sulfasalazine may cause otalgia.

If otalgia develops in a child within 2 weeks of orthodontic treatment and otologic examination is normal, TMJ dysfunction should be considered, especially if otalgia recurs after orthodontic therapy. In infants and children, gastroesophageal reflux rarely may cause referred otalgia. Pain referred to the ear can occur from CN V lesions, dental caries, abscesses of lower molars, trigeminal neuralgia, sinusitis, and parotid pathology. Acute and subacute thyroiditis affecting one lobe may refer pain to the ear on the affected side. Ear pain can be referred from CN IX and X with lesions of the vallecula, posterior third of the tongue, tonsils, larynx, migraine, glossopharyngeal neuralgia, and carotidynia (persistent sore throat with normal pharynx, ear pain aggravated by swallowing, and tenderness over the carotid bulb).

Differential Diagnosis of Earache

CONDITION	NATURE OF PATIENT	NATURE OF SYMPTOMS	ASSOCIATED SYMPTOMS	PRECIPITATING AND AGGRAVATING FACTORS	PHYSICAL FINDINGS AND DIAGNOSTIC STUDIES
Otitis media	Children, especially <8 years	Pain is unilateral, deep, and severe	Irritability Restlessness Fever Poor feeding Ear feels full	URI	Tympanic membrane inflamed and bulging Decreased light reflex
Serous otitis media Eustachitis	Children and adults	Not usually painful Unilateral	Decreased hearing Crackling and gurgling sounds	URI	Fluid behind tympanic membrane Tympanic membrane shows decreased mobility Decreased conductive hearing Impedance tympanometry
Otitis externa	Adults Diabetic patients Patients with seborrhea "Ear pickers" Swimmers	Often bilateral			Pain on manipulation of pinna

Otitic barotrauma		Pain may be severe	URI Nasal stuffiness	Worse on airplane descent	Tympanic membrane retracted
Mastoiditis		Pain in and behind ear	Fever Drainage from middle ear >10 days	Otitis media 10–14 days previously	Exquisite pain with pressure on mastoid process Swelling behind ear Radiograph of mastoid
Foreign body Impacted cerumen	Children Adults	Pain or vague discomfort	May impair hearing Recurrent problem		Foreign body or cerumen in ear
Referred otalgia, as with TMJ dysfunction, dental problems, and tumors	Adults (increases with age)	Rarely bilateral TMJ dysfunction intermittent and often worse in morning	Resemble those of TMJ dysfunction: vertigo, tinnitus, jaw click Pain referred from infected tooth may be worse with hot or cold foods	TMJ arthritis Malocclusion or bruxism Impacted molar	Normal ear examination

Selected References

Clark JL: Otalgia: identifying the source. Postgrad Med 70(4):99–103, 1981.
Fletcher MM: The painful ear. Resident Staff Physician, July 1980, pp 45–51.
Ingvarsson L: Acute otalgia in children: findings and diagnosis. Acta Paediatr Scand 71(5):705–710, 1982.
Ludman H: Pain in the ear. Br Med J 281:1538–1541, 1980.
Murtagh J: The painful ear. Aust Fam Physician 20:1779–1783, 1991.
Schwartz RH: New concepts in otitis media. Am Fam Physician 19(5):91–98, 1979.
Thaller SR, DeSilva A: Otalgia with a normal ear. Am Fam Physician 36:129–136, 1987.
Thaller SR, Thaller JL: Head and neck symptoms. Postgrad Med 87:75–77, 80, 83–86, 1990.

CHAPTER 13

Facial Pain

Because the practitioner usually can differentiate headache from other causes of facial pain, the differential diagnosis of headache is discussed in Chapter 17. Typically, by the time patients consult a physician for facial pain, they already have visited a dentist several times. This illustrates the diagnostic difficulty.

The common causes of facial pain are diseases of local structures such as *dental disease, eye disease* (glaucoma), *nose or sinus disease* (sinusitis), and *temporomandibular joint (TMJ) dysfunction;* vascular pain such as *migraine* and *temporal arteritis;* neurologic pain such as *trigeminal neuralgia* and *sphenopalatine neuralgia;* referred pain, rarely from *angina pectoris* and occasionally from *muscle contraction headaches;* and psychogenic pain, as seen with *atypical facial pain, hysteria,* and *depression.*

Because pain is a symptom and cannot be seen or easily measured, the evaluation and diagnosis must depend on the patient's description; therefore, details that the clinician elicits are important. A patient's reaction to pain can be seen and may indicate the severity of the pain.

With chronic pain the initial symptoms may have been psychologically based, further complicating the diagnostic process. Despite that depressed, anxious, or neurotic people may seek help for organic causes of facial pain more frequently than do other people, chronic or recurrent episodes of facial pain can lead to depression and anxiety.

Nature of Patient

Trigeminal neuralgia is more common in patients over age 50. If facial pain occurs in a younger patient (less than age 40), trigeminal neuralgia is less likely, and other conditions that can mimic tic douloureux should be considered. These include *multiple sclerosis, acoustic neuroma,* and *trigeminal neuroma,* especially if the upper division (pain in the forehead or eye) is involved or if the symptoms are unilateral.

Glaucoma is more common in elderly persons; it affects 2% of those over age 40. It is more common in farsighted than in nearsighted people.

TMJ dysfunction is more common in patients over 40, particularly if they are edentulous or have worn posterior teeth or poorly fitting dentures, but it can accompany severe malocclusion or mandibular trauma at any age. Patients with rheumatoid arthritis appear to have a higher incidence of TMJ dysfunction.

Atypical facial pain is most common in women between ages 30 and 50; 60% of these patients have a similar family history. It tends to occur in people with a history of high stress, drug addiction, low self-esteem, impotence or frigidity, marital or family conflicts, or prior episodes of anxiety or depression. The typical patient is an edentulous, haggard-looking, middle-aged woman. She may have a history of concomitant psychiatric illness as well.

Facial pain from *sinusitis* can occur at any age but is less common in children and teenagers.

Nature of Symptoms

Dental pain is often severe, throbbing, and poorly localized. Excruciating, lancinating, stabbing, paroxysmal pain is characteristic of the *trigeminal, sphenopalatine,* and *glossopharyngeal* neuralgias. The pain of *glaucoma* is described as dull and frontally located. The pain of *acute narrow-angle glaucoma,* however, can cause severe pain of abrupt onset. Myofascial pain is often described as deep, continuous, and a dull ache.

Pain is relatively uncommon in patients with chronic or subacute sinusitis; it typically is seen with episodes of *acute sinusitis,* which may be superimposed on subacute sinusitis. Sinusitis pain usually is dull and relatively constant; occasionally it may be described as throbbing. This pain usually is located over the affected sinus or behind the orbit. With sphenoid sinusitis, however, pain may present at the vertex of the head and radiate to the neck and orbit. Sinusitis pain usually is unilateral but can be bilateral.

Neuralgia pains usually have a sudden onset. A typical attack may consist of two to three stabbing pains over 1 minute. Episodes may become more frequent with time, and several attacks may occur in a single day, with spontaneous remission for weeks or months. The pain may be recurrent, but it usually is paroxysmal and instantaneous. Although the actual pain may last only a few seconds and then disappear, some patients experience a gradual transition from lancinating pain to a vague ache or burning. Trigeminal neuralgia pains usually occur during the day, whereas glossopharyngeal pains often develop at night. Over time the episodes of trigeminal neuralgia may become more frequent and occur one or more times daily. These pains seldom awaken patients from their sleep.

The pain of *glaucoma* may be worse in dark rooms. It usually is gradual in onset, although the pain of acute narrow-angle glaucoma can begin suddenly and present as a dramatic emergency. The pain of sinusitis usually develops gradually and can last for days to weeks if not adequately treated.

Most causes of facial pain, including trigeminal neuralgia, sinusitis, glaucoma, and TMJ dysfunction, present with unilateral pain; occasionally, all can be bilateral or alternating. The pain of *trigeminal neuralgia* is located over the course of one of the three divisions of the fifth cranial nerve. It usually is unilateral but can be bilateral in 5% to 10% of patients. These bilateral attacks tend to be more common in certain families and possibly more common in women. Trigeminal neuralgia most often occurs along the distribution of the second (maxillary branch) or third (mandibular branch) division and seldom over the first division (ophthalmic branch). Most patients report that the pain is on the surface, not deep inside the head, which is more common with sphenopalatine ganglion neuralgia. **Both the lancinating nature of neuralgia pain and the tendency to be remittent and associated with trigger areas distinguish it from the more chronic pain of sinus infection, dental abscesses, and glaucoma.**

The anatomic distribution of the pain helps differentiate neuralgia from *atypical facial pain,* which is not confined to an anatomic distribution of any cranial or cervical nerve. The entire side of the head as well as the face, neck, or throat may be involved.

The pain of *subacute glaucoma* usually causes frontal headaches, whereas the pain of *acute glaucoma* often is described as pain in the eye or just behind the eye radiating to the head, ears, or teeth. The pain of *sinusitis* corresponds in location to the sinus involved. Patients with *maxillary* sinusitis usually complain of pain over the cheek or under the eye; the pain of *frontal* sinusitis is above the eyes or in the forehead; the pain of *ethmoid* sinusitis is most often supraorbital and may occasionally radiate to the vertex of the head. Sphenoid and ethmoid sinusitis seldom occur as isolated phenomena; they usually are associated with other forms of sinusitis.

Pain of *TMJ arthritis* or *dysfunction* normally is located in the TMJ area, although it may be referred to the ear or temples, thus simulating the pain of a tension headache. **Any time a patient complains of pain in the ear and physical examination of the ear is negative, the physician should palpate over the TMJ, question the patient for other signs and symptoms of TMJ dysfunction, and consider other causes of referred otalgia.** The pain of TMJ dysfunction may radiate to either the teeth or the ear.

Associated Symptoms

Involuntary facial contractions may occur with the severe pain of *trigeminal neuralgia.* A chronic painful syndrome causes sleeplessness, weight loss, anxiety, depression, and rarely a suicidal tendency. Patients with *sinusitis* often have or recently had symptoms of an upper respiratory infection. Patients with *atypical facial pain* frequently are depressed and emotional, with a large affectual component to their illness. Patients with *cluster headaches* (Horton's headache, histamine cephalalgia) may have ipsilateral lacrimation or rhinorrhea.

When patients see halos or rainbows around lights, have temporary obscuring of vision, and experience pain in and around the eye, *glaucoma* should be suspected. Occasionally these patients also complain of nausea and vomiting, which sometimes leads to the erroneous diagnosis of migraine headaches.

The associated symptoms of *TMJ dysfunction* include clicking, popping, crepitation, tinnitus, vertigo (rarely), pain in the ear, jaw clenching, bruxism, neckache, and headache. Patients may report that it is difficult to open their mouths widely because this elicits these symptoms.

Precipitating and Aggravating Factors

Dental pain may increase with ingestion of hot, sweet, or acidic foods. *Neuralgia* pains often are induced by touching of trigger points or by temperature extremes. *Sphenopalatine neuralgia* may be precipitated by sinusitis or a postnasal drip. Coughing and sneezing may exacerbate sinus pain. Erect posture may worsen pain caused by *maxillary sinusitis,* whereas recumbency exacerbates *frontal sinus* pain.

Darkness and drugs, which cause pupillary dilatation, often precipitate the pain of *glaucoma.* Bruxism and opening the mouth widely may aggravate *TMJ pain.* Mastication and temperature extremes may exacerbate dental pain. Acidic foods and mastication may precipitate pain from a sialolith. Pain in the jaw brought on by exertion suggests *angina pectoris,* especially in older patients.

Ameliorating Factors

Sinus pain often is relieved by postural changes; some sinuses drain better when the patient is erect, whereas others drain more effectively when recumbent. Because frontal sinuses drain better when erect, the pain of *frontal sinusitis* lessens as the day progresses. In contrast, the pain of *maxillary sinusitis* improves with recumbency, since the maxillary sinuses drain better in this position.

Effective relief of pain with carbamazepine (Tegretol) suggests that the pain is caused by *neuralgia.* Phenytoin also relieves neuralgic pain but seldom is effective in patients with migraine headaches. Patients with *atypical facial pain* rarely obtain relief from anything other than psychotherapy or antidepressants.

The pain of *TMJ dysfunction* occasionally is relieved by tranquilizers, antiinflammatory agents, and muscle relaxants. Depending on the cause, bite plates or correction of a malocclusion may be helpful. This may correct the malalignment of the TMJ but not necessarily the arthritic changes in the joint, whether primary changes or secondary to the malocclusion. Therefore, even extensive dental work does not always completely relieve TMJ pain.

Physical Findings

The physician must conduct a meticulous examination of eyes, ears, nose, nasopharynx, mouth, and hypopharynx to determine the source of facial pain. The physical examination usually is normal in patients with atypical facial pain and the various neuralgias. Rarely, patients with trigeminal neuralgia may have a sensory deficit over the division involved and pupillary inequality. If the trigeminal neuralgia is atypical or bilateral or occurs in patients under age 50, the physical examination should focus on findings that could be caused by a basilar artery aneurysm, multiple sclerosis, or cerebellar dysfunction. Patients with longstanding undiagnosed *neuralgia* may be partially or completely toothless; extractions may have been performed to relieve pain thought to be of dental origin.

The physical findings of *glaucoma* include increased intraocular pressure, as determined by tonometry, dilated pupil, and conjunctival injection. In the early stages of simple glaucoma, the patient usually does not notice any pain, obscuring of vision, halos, or visual field cuts. Patients with subacute glaucoma may have their vision temporarily obscured and see halos or rainbows around lights.

Patients with *acute glaucoma* may have marked conjunctival injection; therefore, acute glaucoma is part of the differential diagnosis of the patient with a "red eye." Other physical findings include edema of the eyelids, a hazy and "steamy" cornea, decreased corneal sensation, an injected discolored iris, and a pupil that is mildly dilated and occasionally vertically oval. The intraocular tension is raised, and the eye is hard to the touch and tender to gentle palpation.

Acute glaucoma can be differentiated from iritis (which may be painful) and conjunctivitis by the appearance of the cornea and the pupil. In conjunctivitis and iritis, the cornea is clear and sensitive (Table 13–1). In conjunctivitis the pupil is active, whereas in iritis it is small and fixed. In both conjunctivitis and iritis, intraocular tension is normal.

Patients with *acute sinusitis* have ipsilateral nasal fullness and pain over the affected sinus that is exacerbated by palpation or percussion. Transillumination over the affected sinus is impaired. Patients may complain of toothaches or tenderness on percussion of the upper teeth because the roots of these teeth are close to the floor of the maxillary sinus. Because maxillary sinusitis is so common, it occasionally is misdiagnosed as hay fever or chronic allergic rhinitis, and vice versa.

Fewer physical findings and symptoms are associated with *subacute* or *chronic sinusitis.* Patients with subacute sinusitis may complain of headache, postnasal drip, or purulent discharge from the nose or posterior pharynx when the sinus ostia permit drainage in this subacute phase. Patients with chronic sinusitis may have a mucopurulent discharge that is unresponsive to medical management. They may complain of vague ear pain or hearing loss that is secondary to a serous otitis. Often they have a sore throat secondary to a postnasal drip.

Patients with *TMJ dysfunction* may experience pain with palpation of the joint when they open and close the mouth. The TMJ can be palpated in the preauricular area or through the external auditory canal. The masseter muscles may be prominent in patients who grind their teeth. Auscultation over the joint may reveal a clicking sound with opening and closing of the mouth.

Tenderness on palpation of the temporal artery suggests *temporal arteritis.* Pain on palpation of the carotid bulb suggests *carotidynia.*

Cervical lymphadenopathy or neurologic deficits should suggest an intracranial or local *tumor.*

Diagnostic Studies

All patients with *unexplained* facial pain should be evaluated with dental, sinus, and skull radiographs or computed tomography (CT) scans, tonometry, studies of

TABLE 13.1 Points of Distinction Between Conjunctivitis, Iritis, and Acute Glaucoma

SITE	CONJUNCTIVITIS	IRITIS	ACUTE GLAUCOMA
Conjunctiva	Conjunctival vessels bright red and injected; movable over subjacent sclera; injection most marked away from corneoscleral margin; color fades on pressure	Ciliary vessels injected, deep red or bluish red; most marked at corneoscleral margin; color does not fade on pressure	Both conjunctival and ciliary vessels injected
Cornea	Clear, sensitive	Clear, sensitive	Steamy, hazy, insensitive
Anterior chamber	Clear; normal depth	Aqueous turbid; slightly shallow	Very shallow
Iris	Normal color	Injected, swollen, adherent to lens, muddy colored	Injected
Pupil	Black, active	May be filled with exudate Small, fixed	Dilated, fixed, oval
Intraocular tension	Normal	Normal	Raised

From Hart FD, editor: French's Index of Differential Diagnosis, 10th ed. Baltimore, Williams & Wilkins, 1973.

erythrocyte sedimentation rate (ESR), and thorough examination of the nose, nasopharynx, larynx, oropharynx, and hypopharynx.

The radiograph in *chronic sinusitis* may be negative or show haziness of the sinus cavity or thickening of the sinus mucosa. Generally, CT scans are preferred in the evaluation of the paranasal sinuses. Likewise, in *acute sinusitis,* radiographs can be negative in the earliest stage and become positive later. In other words, positive radiographic findings are confirmatory, although negative findings do not absolutely rule out acute or chronic sinusitis. Nasal endoscopy and modified CT scan of the sinuses may be abnormal and explain facial pain despite normal radiographs. The absence of radiographic changes significantly decreases the likelihood of chronic recurrent sinusitis.

Radiographic findings of *TMJ dysfunction* include the loss of the TMJ space, thinning or loss of lamina over the condylar head or glenoid fossa, flattening of the condylar head, and spur formation. Routine mandibular radiographs may be negative, but tomographic studies or magnetic resonance imaging (MRI) may show arthritic changes in the TMJ.

Less Common Diagnostic Considerations

Vague facial pain, neuralgia and headache, neck or throat pain radiating to the ipsilateral ear, and aching or sharp stabbing pain on swallowing, head movement, yawning, or coughing suggest *Eagle's syndrome.* This syndrome is related to an elongated styloid process or calcified stylohyoid ligament that is present in 4% of the population. Only 4% of those with an elongated styloid process have symptoms. The diagnosis may be confirmed radiographically.

Symptoms of burning, constant, and persistent pain affecting the upper division or any other division of the trigeminal nerve that begin after a recognized bout of herpes may signal a *postherpetic neuralgia.* This is most common in older patients who, after a bout of trigeminal neuralgia, continue to have local neuralgic pain with intermittent exacerbations.

Pain that usually occurs at night (in contrast to trigeminal neuralgia, which usually occurs during the day) should suggest the possibility of a *glossopharyngeal neuralgia.* Patients (usually older) describe the pain as stabbing, jolting, burning, or continuous. The pain may last seconds to minutes, and attacks tend to occur in clusters, lasting from days to months. The pain often is localized to the posterior half of the tongue, the tonsils, and the pharynx, although it may radiate to the ear, the neck, and the jaw. This diagnosis should be suspected when the pain begins at night or if it is triggered by swallowing, talking, yawning, or eating spicy, salty, or bitter foods. Its incidence is quite rare compared with that of trigeminal neuralgia.

When a patient complains of constant unilateral burning or aching in the region of the mandible, maxilla, or frontotemporal area, and if the pain is described as "deep" instead of "on the surface," the problem may be *sphenopalatine neuralgia (Sluder's syndrome).* It can be differentiated from trigeminal and glossopharyngeal neuralgia because it usually is a constant pain. It will last hours to

Text continued on page 135.

Differential Diagnosis of Facial Pain

CONDITION	NATURE OF PATIENT	NATURE OF PAIN	ASSOCIATED SYMPTOMS	PRECIPITATING AND AGGRAVATING FACTORS	AMELIORATING FACTORS	PHYSICAL FINDINGS	DIAGNOSTIC STUDIES
Neuralgia							
Trigeminal	> age 50	Lancinating Stabbing Sudden onset Usually occurs in daytime On surface Usually unilateral Maxillary or mandibular division more common		Touching of trigger points Extremes of temperature	Carbamazepine Phenytoin	Tenderness at trigger points	
Glossopharyngeal		Paroxysmal Recurrent Often nocturnal					
Sphenopalatine		Constant Pain "in deep"	Postnasal drip				
Sinusitis		Dull Constant Over affected sinus or behind orbit Recurrent or chronic Gradual onset or chronic	Nasal stuffiness Mucopurulent nasal discharge Upper respiratory infection	Upper respiratory infections Coughing and sneezing Frontal sinusitis pain worsens when recumbent Maxillary sinusitis pain may worsen when erect	Maxillary pain eases when recumbent Frontal pain lessens when erect	Tender to palpation or percussion Decreased transillumination Nasal congestion	Sinus radiographs Nasal endoscopy Sinus CT

Glaucoma	> age 40 Farsighted	Dull Severe with acute narrow-angle Usually unilateral	Nausea and vomiting			Increased ocular tension Pupil dilated	Tonometry
Acute		Orbital Severe Sudden onset	Halos or rainbows around light Temporary visual obscuration	Darkness Drugs that dilate pupils (e.g., sympathomimetics, psychotropics, anticholinergics)		Conjunctival injection Steamy cornea	
Subacute		Frontal Dull Gradual onset					
Temporomandibular joint (TMJ) dysfunction	> age 40 Those with rheumatic arthritis	Recurrent or chronic Usually unilateral over TMJ Felt in ear, temple, or teeth Worse in morning in night grinders	Tinnitus Clicking Crepitation of TMJ Bruxism	Bruxism Opening mouth widely	Bite plates Correction of malocclusion	Tender to palpation over TMJ Malocclusion Prominent masseter muscles	Radiographs, MRI, and tomograms of TMJ
Cluster headache (see Chapter 17)		Eye pain Frontal headaches	Ipsilateral lacrimation and rhinorrhea				

Table continued on following page.

Differential Diagnosis of Facial Pain *Continued*

CONDITION	NATURE OF PATIENT	NATURE OF PAIN	ASSOCIATED SYMPTOMS	PRECIPITATING AND AGGRAVATING FACTORS	AMELIORATING FACTORS	PHYSICAL FINDINGS	DIAGNOSTIC STUDIES
Temporal arteritis (see Chapter 17)			Headache Transient blindness			Temporal artery tender to palpation	Elevated ESR
Tumors of nasopharynx	Elderly	Constant pain in nose, ethmoid, midface					Skull radiographs and CT scans
Atypical facial pain	Women Anxious Similar family history Often depressed	Pain does not follow any cranial or cervical nerve Hemicrania	Large affectual component		Psychotherapy Antidepressants	Normal	
Dental abscess	Any age	Chronic pain in teeth, jaw, or maxillary region		Temperature extremes Mastication		Sensitive to hot or cold Tender to percussion over teeth	Dental radiographs

days, and nasal mucosa may be inflamed ipsilaterally. It often develops in patients who have sinusitis or postnasal drip. A diagnosis often may be made by anesthetization of the sphenopalatine ganglion. Cocaine or other topical anesthetics can be used on the tip of a nasal swab, which is inserted straight back through the nares after the nasal mucosa is shrunk.

The presentation and differential diagnosis of temporal arteritis are described in Chapter 17. If a patient complains of dull, aching pain in the lower jaw (either unilaterally or bilaterally) that occurs with physical exertion, it may be *atypical referred anginal pain.* The diagnosis is confirmed if the jaw pain is relieved by administration of sublingual nitroglycerin. Pain located in the nasal cavity, in the ethmoid region, or deep in the midface and that is not caused by one of the more common causes of facial pain should suggest the possibility of *nasal neoplasm,* particularly if the patient is elderly.

Pain in the eye most often is caused by trigeminal neuralgia, postherpetic neuralgia, sinus disease, or cluster headaches. Less common causes of referred pain to the eye can be observed in patients with hypertension, cranial arteritis, orbital tumors, and ophthalmoplegic migraine (pain with a third nerve palsy), which may be caused by an intracranial aneurysm. Direct causes of pain in the orbit include herpetic keratitis, herpes zoster of the ophthalmic branch, narrow-angle glaucoma, acute iritis, and keratoconjunctivitis sicca.

Sialolithiasis may be present if the patient complains of submandibular or parotid pain that is worse on chewing or swallowing, particularly with tenderness or swelling in the salivary glands. Exacerbation of the pain and swelling after instillation of lemon juice into the oropharynx or ingestion of lemon juice confirms the diagnosis.

Lyme disease may present with symptoms of TMJ and dental pain, facial pain, facial nerve palsy, or headache.

Selected References

Birt D: Headaches and head pains associated with disease of the ear, nose, and throat. Med Clin North Am 62:523–531, 1978.

Cooper BC, Cooper DL: Recognizing otolaryngologic symptoms in patients with temporomandibular disorders. J Craniomandib Pract 11:260–267, 1993.

Drinnan AJ: Differential diagnosis of orofacial pain. Dent Clin North Am 31:627–643, 1987.

Goodman BW: Temporal arteritis. Am J Med 67:839–852, 1979.

Gray G: Sinusitis—or is it? Aust Fam Physician 7:121–131, 1978.

Green DB: Orofacial and craniofacial pain: primary care concerns. Postgrad Med Spec, Aug 3, 1992, pp 57–64.

Kahn CH, Warfield CA: Orofacial pain. Hosp Pract 24:247–248, 253–254, 259, 1989.

Keith DA: Differential diagnosis of craniofacial pain. Cranio Clin Int 1:173–184, 1991.

Kennedy DW, Loury MC: Nasal and sinus pain: current diagnosis and treatment. Semin Neurol 8:303–314, 1988.

Pertes RA: A practical approach to the diagnosis of chronic orofacial pain. Part 1. Somatic Pain Compendium 9:554–555, 558–560, 562, 1988.

Schramm VL: A guide to diagnosing and treating facial pain and headache. Geriatrics 35:78–90, 1980.

Sluder G: The role of the sphenopalatine ganglion in nasal headaches. NY Med J 87:989, 1908.
Stohoe NL: Ocular pain in the elderly: simple symptom or hidden danger. Geriatrics 35:41–70, 1980.
Thaller SR, Thaller JL: Head and neck symptoms: is the problem in the ears, face, neck or oral cavity? Postgrad Med 87:75–77, 80, 83–86, 1990.

CHAPTER 14

Fatigue

Fatigue is the seventh most common complaint in primary care. It can be the presenting symptom of almost any disease. A thorough history and physical examination will establish a diagnosis in about 85% of patients. If, in addition to experiencing fatigue, the patient complains of localizing symptoms such as abdominal pain or hemoptysis, the diagnosis is easier. Specific attention then can be focused on abdominal or chest causes, respectively. If the patient's only complaint is fatigue, the diagnosis is more difficult.

Fatigue can be categorized as acute, chronic, or physiologic. *Acute fatigue* is most often a prodrome or sequela of an acute viral or bacterial infectious process. Heart failure and anemia also may present with a sudden onset of fatigue.

Chronic fatigue (of weeks' to months' duration) can be caused by *depression; chronic anxiety* or *stress; chronic infection,* especially *infectious mononucleosis, hepatitis,* or *tuberculosis; cancer; rheumatoid arthritis, fibromyalgia,* and other rheumatologic disorders; *heart failure; sleep apnea; serum electrolyte abnormalities* (hyponatremia, hypokalemia, hypercalcemia); *chronic lung disease;* or *anemia.* Prescribed and over-the-counter drugs are frequent, often unrecognized causes of chronic fatigue. These drugs include antihistamines, tranquilizers, psychotropics, hypnotics, and antihypertensives (particularly reserpine, methyldopa, clonidine, and beta blockers).

Patients with *physiologic fatigue* usually recognize the cause of their fatigue and usually do not consult a physician about this problem. Physiologic fatigue can result from overwork (either physical or mental) and insufficient or poor-quality sleep, which may be caused by depression, caffeine, drugs, alcohol, or chronic pain.

In about 50% of patients who present with fatigue, the cause is functional (*depression, anxiety,* or *somatoform disorder*); in the other 50% an organic cause exists. The physician must recognize that multiple causes of fatigue may be present. A patient who complains of fatigue, for example, may demonstrate signs and symptoms of depression and have hepatitis, infectious mononucleosis, or bronchogenic carcinoma.

Depression as a cause of fatigue is *not* a diagnosis of exclusion. Innumerable diagnostic tests to rule out all possible organic causes should not be performed before the diagnosis of depression is made. Rather, if a thorough history and physical examination do not reveal clues to an organic cause but do uncover symptoms of depression, depression is the probable cause of fatigue.

Nature of Patient

Fatigue is an uncommon complaint in children and young adults. When it is the presenting symptom, it usually is caused by a prodrome or sequela of an *acute infectious process.* Chronic fatigue in a young person most often is related to *infectious mononucleosis, hepatitis, substance abuse, depression,* or *chronic anxiety.*

Children seldom manifest depression by lowered mood or fatigue; rather, they present with somatic complaints such as headache or with "acting out." Often, depression is manifested in children by hyperactivity, withdrawal, eating problems, school troubles, sleep disturbances, or vague physical complaints. In adolescents, when fatigue is associated with "acting out" behavior (e.g., substance abuse, sexual misconduct), depression may be the underlying culprit. Illnesses such as cancer, chronic lung disease, heart disease, and leukemias are uncommon in children and adolescents.

As in younger patients, the most common cause of *acute* fatigue in adults is *infection.* The next most frequent causes of fatigue are *depression* and *anxiety.*

In adult patients, particularly the elderly, serious *organic illnesses,* such as circulatory and pulmonary disease, anemia, cancer, and endocrine abnormalities, are more likely to present with fatigue. In elderly patients, *masked hyperthyroidism* may present with a chief complaint of fatigue. Patients with this condition do not necessarily show the tachycardia, tremors, and other classic signs of hyperthyroidism. Weakness may be caused by diuretic-induced hypokalemia, psychotropic agents, alcoholism, and neuropathies.

Because fatigue is such a common symptom of depression in adults, the physician must recognize that the signs and symptoms of depression vary not only with age, but also with gender and socioeconomic status (Table 14–1). Men more often manifest depression by guilt, feelings of helplessness, pessimism, and

TABLE 14.1 Discriminators of Depression by Socioeconomic Class

	LOWER	MIDDLE	HIGHER
Affective	Hopelessness Self-accusation Crying Dissatisfaction Guilt Depressed mood	Loneliness Helplessness Guilt Crying Anxiety, tension Depressed mood	Decreased social life Pessimism Dissatisfaction Anxiety, tension
Somatic	Palpitation Headache Anorexia Waking early	Decreased libido Urinary complaints Trouble falling asleep Headache Anorexia Waking early	Fatigue Insomnia

Data from Rockwell DA, Burr BD: The tired patient. J Fam Pract 5(5):853–857, 1977; and Schwab J, Bralow M, Brown J: Diagnosing depression in medical patients. Ann Intern Med 67:695, 1967.

depressed moods. Early signs of depression in women include headache, insomnia, and withdrawal from social activities. Depressed patients of lower socioeconomic class are likely to have depressed moods, feelings of guilt, hopelessness, dissatisfaction, and crying spells. They may complain of palpitations, loss of appetite, early-morning waking, and headaches. Depressed middle-class patients state that they feel sad or blue, guilty, helpless, lonely, or anxious. They may complain of crying spells, initial insomnia, early waking, loss of appetite, headache, and decreased libido. Patients of the upper socioeconomic class more often complain of fatigue, insomnia, anxiety and tension, dissatisfaction, and decreased interest in work and social life.

About 90% of patients with *fibromyalgia* are women. They usually complain of fatigue, nonarticular rheumatism, and nonrestorative sleep.

Nature of Symptoms

The following historic clues suggest fatigue of *organic* origin: Fatigue is of shorter duration, related to exertion, *not* present in the morning but increasingly evident as the day goes on, relieved by rest, and progressive rather than fluctuating over time. Other obvious organic symptoms or signs may be present. The fatigue may be related to a specific muscle group (e.g., weakened arms or drooping eyelids, as in myasthenia gravis). Fatigue that increases over several months suggests a progressively deteriorating condition such as anemia or cancer.

Most cases of chronic fatigue in which an organic cause is not initially apparent are probably caused by psychosocial factors. Fatigue of *functional* origin usually is of longer duration than that of organic origin; it often is present and may be worse in the morning but improves gradually as the day progresses; it usually is not related to exertion. The cause of functional fatigue may become apparent during the history, especially if the onset of symptoms correlates with emotional stresses, including doubts about job security, major life changes, and significant loss (e.g., death of a spouse, loss of a job, or amputation of a limb). Fatigue that tends to be worse in the morning, even while the patient is in bed, and improves as the day progresses suggests *depression.* Fatigue that is constant over weeks or months, not aggravated by effort, associated with numerous somatic complaints, and shows no diurnal variation is probably caused by *chronic anxiety.*

Physiologic fatigue that does not represent a pathologic process should be expected in the following situations: prolonged physical activity without adequate rest; insufficient or poor-quality sleep; dieting; sedentary life-style; pregnancy and the postpartum period; and prolonged mental stress.

Associated Symptoms

Fatigue associated with dyspnea on exertion or shortness of breath suggests *chronic cardiorespiratory disease.* Fatigue associated with a low-grade fever suggests *infectious processes* such as hepatitis, tuberculosis, or subacute bacterial endocarditis

(SBE). *Inflammatory diseases* also may present with fatigue and a low-grade fever. Patients with these conditions also may present only with fatigue and no fever.

In adults complaining of fatigue who also have vague gastrointestinal (GI) symptoms (e.g., constipation, bloating, indigestion), skin disorders, and chronic pain syndromes, *depression* may be the cause. Fatigue associated with restlessness, irritability, sweating, palpitations, and paresthesias probably is caused by *chronic anxiety, stress,* or rarely *hyperthyroidism.*

When fatigue is associated with breathlessness, anorexia, weight loss, and pallor, *anemia* should be suspected. If these symptoms are accompanied by numbness in the legs or arms, *pernicious anemia* should be considered. If fatigue is associated with shortness of breath, swelling of ankles, or paroxysmal nocturnal dyspnea, *congestive heart failure* should be suspected. The presence of diffuse musculoskeletal pain and several tender points suggests *fibromyalgia.*

When chronic fatigue is associated with headache and upper respiratory complaints, *sick building syndrome* should be suspected. These patients usually work in modern office buildings with an impervious outer shell, inoperable windows, and inadequate ventilation.

Precipitating and Exacerbating Factors

Identifying a precipitating factor is often crucial in the diagnosis of fatigue. Initiation of medications, increased workload, insomnia, loss of job, and family problems all can be precipitating factors. If the onset of fatigue is associated with psychosocial problems, the cause may be chronic anxiety or stress; in such patients a minimal additional stress may exacerbate anxiety and result in a new complaint of fatigue. However, patients with organic disease may erroneously attribute their fatigue to a psychosocial problem.

Postpartum fatigue may be a symptom of medical or psychiatric illness, but it must be distinguished from severe tiredness, which typically occurs after delivery. Postpartum fatigue may be caused by thyroid disorders, anemia, infections, depression, and cardiomyopathy.

Ameliorating Factors

Fatigue reduced by rest is probably *physiologic.* If fatigue is improved on weekends and vacations, *chronic stress* related to employment may be underlying the fatigue. The symptoms of *sick building syndrome* (fatigue, headache, upper respiratory complaints) may also abate promptly when patients leave their workplace. *Drugs* are causal if fatigue disappears after they are stopped. If fatigue abates after a viral illness, the *viral infection* caused the fatigue.

Physical Findings

The most critical component in examining a patient complaining of fatigue is a thorough history that focuses on the onset of symptoms, relation to exertion, family and social history, a full systemic review, and questions about abuse of drugs or other substances.

Physical findings may provide clues about the cause of fatigue. Coarse hair, loss of the outer third of the eyebrows, hoarse voice, a doughy consistency to the skin, and myoclonic reflexes (particularly the "hung-up" ankle jerk) all suggest *hypothyroidism.* Tachycardia, tremors, fine hair, and warm, moist palms suggest *hyperthyroidism.* Conjunctival or skin pallor suggests *anemia.* Signs of avitaminosis, such as a smooth, glossy tongue and cheilosis, suggest a *nutritional deficiency.* Distended neck veins, rales at the lung bases, tachycardia, gallop, and edema suggest that *congestive heart failure* is the cause of fatigue. Auscultation of a midsystolic click or a late systolic murmur suggests *mitral valve prolapse.* This is a fairly common condition in which patients often complain of fatigue that is most often a manifestation of *anxiety.*

When associated with splenomegaly or hepatomegaly, adenopathy (particularly posterior cervical adenopathy) suggests *infectious mononucleosis.* Hepatomegaly (with or without jaundice) and pruritus suggest *hepatitis;* diffuse adenopathy suggests a *lymphoma,* such as *Hodgkin's disease,* or *acquired immunodeficiency syndrome* (AIDS). An enlarged liver with ascites and spider angiomata suggests *cirrhosis.* Increased bruising sometimes associated with pallor suggests a platelet deficiency, which may be part of some other *hematologic problem.*

Fever suggests an *infectious process.* Rales at the lung apices suggest *pulmonary tuberculosis.* Low blood pressure associated with increased skin pigmentation suggests *adrenal insufficiency.* Polyarticular arthritis suggests *rheumatoid arthritis,* whereas migratory arthritis suggests a *connective tissue disorder.*

Multiple (at least eight) hyperalgesic sites, usually in the neck, back, or trunk, suggest *fibromyalgia.* The tender points are in the midsupraspinatus muscle; midpoint of the upper trapezius; pectoralis insertion just lateral to the second costochondral junction; low cervical interspinous ligaments (C4–C6); low mid-lumbar interspinous ligaments (L4-S1); lateral epicondyle; upper outer quadrant of buttock (gluteus medius muscle); and medial fat pad of knee.

Diagnostic Studies

Laboratory tests seldom yield the cause of chronic fatigue. When the diagnosis is not readily apparent, however, the following laboratory tests should be performed: complete blood count (CBC) with differential, urinalysis, serum glucose, SMA-22, erythrocyte sedimentation rate (ESR), T-cell subsets; tests for human immunodeficiency virus (HIV); purified protein derivative (tuberculin, PPD); and chest radiograph. When the patient has a normal ESR, serious organic disease probably is not present. Depending on the diagnostic considerations, other laboratory tests may be indicated, such as a tuberculin test, a monospot test, thyroid function tests, and serum electrolyte evaluation. Sleep studies may be indicated if sleep apnea is suspected. In patients with chronic fatigue an abnormal laboratory finding does not necessarily indicate the cause.

Text continued on page 147.

Differential Diagnosis of Fatigue

TYPE	NATURE OF PATIENT	NATURE OF SYMPTOMS	ASSOCIATED SYMPTOMS	AMELIORATING FACTORS	PHYSICAL FINDINGS	DIAGNOSTIC STUDIES
Physiologic						
Prolonged physical activity Overwork Inadequate sleep Dieting Pregnancy and post-partum period	Usually recognizes cause of fatigue and does not complain to physician about it			Rest		Within normal limits
Sedentary life-style				Increased physical activity		
Functional	May appear depressed	Fatigue on arising; may diminish during day Onset with emotional stress (job insecurity, major life change, significant loss) Often chronic	Insomnia Vague GI symptoms Chronic pain			
Depression				Improvement in life situations	"Flat" affect	
Anxiety			Numerous somatic complaints Irritability Breathlessness	Removal of stress	No physical abnormalities	

Emotional stress		Of longer duration than that of organic origin Often present or worse in morning Improves during day Unrelated to exertion	Irritability Breathlessness	Removal of stress	No physical abnormalities	
Organic		Of shorter duration than that of functional origin Related to exertion Not present in morning but worsens during day Often related to onset of physical ailment	Symptoms of disease causing fatigue: dyspnea on exertion (cardiorespiratory disease), fever (infections), muscle weakness (myasthenia), cold intolerance (hypothyroidism)		Signs of organic pathology causing fatigue: pallor (anemia), rales (pulmonary congestion), weight loss (cancer), tachycardia (hyperthyroidism)	If diagnosis not clinically apparent: CBC with differential, urinalysis, serum glucose, SMA-22, ESR, chest x-ray, PPD, monospot test, thyroid function tests, serum electrolytes
Acute Viral or bacterial infections	Most common cause of acute fatigue in all age groups	Fatigue usually subsides in 2 weeks	Fever		Signs of particular infection	CBC with differential Cultures
Depression	Common cause of fatigue in adults		Sleep disturbances		No physical abnormalities	
Anxiety	Tense, nervous		Somatic complaints		May be signs of mitral valve prolapse	

Table continued on following page.

Differential Diagnosis of Fatigue *Continued*

TYPE	NATURE OF PATIENT	NATURE OF SYMPTOMS	ASSOCIATED SYMPTOMS	AMELIORATING FACTORS	PHYSICAL FINDINGS	DIAGNOSTIC STUDIES
Acute *Continued*						
Drugs and medications			Bizarre behavior Drowsiness		Bradycardia from methyldopa and beta blockers	
Organic illnesses						
Anemia		May have acute onset but increases progressively over time	Breathlessness Anorexia and weight loss Pallor Numbness of extremities (with pernicious anemia)		Conjunctival or skin pallor	Hemoglobin, hematocrit
Hypothyroidism			Weight gain		Coarse hair Loss of outer third of eyebrow Hoarse voice "Doughy" skin Myoclonic reflexes (especially "hung-up" ankle jerk)	Thyroid function tests
Serious organic illnesses (e.g., cancer, endocrine disorders)	Rare in children Most common in elderly		Depends on organic illness			

Chronic						
Depression (not a diagnosis of exclusion)	Does not present with fatigue in children Often overlooked in elderly Adolescents may present with somatic complaints and "acting out" behavior (e.g., abuse, sexual misconduct) Most common cause of chronic fatigue in adults	In adults, worse in the morning, improves as day progresses Signs and symptoms may vary with age, gender, and socioeconomic status	*Children:* Somatic complaints "Acting out" Hyperactivity School, eating, and sleeping problems Withdrawal *Adults:* Feelings of guilt, helplessness, pessimism, sadness, loneliness, anxiety, dissatisfaction Decreased libido Insomnia Early-morning awakening Weight loss and decreased appetite Social withdrawal Crying spells Headache Vague GI symptoms Skin disorders Chronic pain syndromes		"Flat" affect	Should *not* perform multiple diagnostic studies to rule out all possible organic causes before diagnosing depression
Medications	Users of antihistamines, psychotropics, tranquilizers, antihypertensives (reserpine, methyldopa, clonidine, beta blockers)	Onset correlates with beginning of drug ingestion		Cessation of drugs		

Table continued on following page.

■ Differential Diagnosis of Fatigue *Continued*

TYPE	NATURE OF PATIENT	NATURE OF SYMPTOMS	ASSOCIATED SYMPTOMS	AMELIORATING FACTORS	PHYSICAL FINDINGS	DIAGNOSTIC STUDIES
Chronic *Continued*						
Chronic anxiety or stress		Constant over weeks or months Shows no diurnal variation Is not aggravated by effort May be precipitated by psychosocial factors	Somatic complaints Restlessness Irritability Sweating Palpitations Paresthesias		With mitral valve prolapse, possible midsystolic click or late systolic murmur	
Organic illnesses						
Congestive heart failure Cancer Chronic infection	Adults		Vary with illness		Vary with illness	
Mononucleosis	Most common in adolescents and young adults				Posterior cervical adenopathy Hepatomegaly Splenomegaly	Monospot test
Hepatitis	Most common in alcoholics and IV drug users				Hepatomegaly with or without jaundice	Abnormal liver function tests and hepatitis antigens
Fibromyalgia	Adults, usually female	Fatigue may be severe; may occur after minimal exertion	Insomnia Nonrestorative sleep Nonarticular rheumatism	Often relieved by tricyclics or trazodone	Hyperalgesic tender sites: low cervical/lumbar spine, suboccipital muscles, lateral epicondyle, medial fat pad of knee	Abnormal sleep, electroencephalogram (EEG)

Less Common Diagnostic Considerations

The less common causes of fatigue include neoplasia, connective tissue diseases (e.g., disseminated lupus erythematosus, polymyalgia rheumatica, temporal arteritis), metabolic states (e.g., uremia, hypokalemia, hyponatremia), endocrine disorders (e.g., hypothyroidism, hyperthyroidism, hypoglycemia, Addison's disease, diabetes), malnutrition with or without malabsorption, chronic pain, chronic neurologic disorders (e.g., myasthenia gravis, post–polio syndrome, multiple sclerosis, Parkinson's disease), and chronic infections (e.g., AIDS, brucellosis, SBE, postviral fatigue syndrome). *Chronic fatigue syndrome* (CFS), also called *benign myalgic encephalomyelitis,* can be totally disabling.

Selected References

Bell DS, Bell KM, Cheney PR: Primary juvenile fibromyalgia syndrome and chronic fatigue syndrome in adolescents. Clin Infect Dis 18(suppl):21–23, 1994.

Bennett R: Fibromyalgia, chronic fatigue syndrome, and myofascial pain. Curr Opin Rheum 10:95–103, 1998.

Chester AC: Sick-building syndrome as a possible predation defense. Integr Physiol Behav Sci 30:68–83, 1995.

Doherty M, Jones A: Fibromyalgia syndrome. Br Med J 310:386–389, 1995.

Gordon M: Differential diagnosis of weakness—a common geriatric problem. Geriatrics 41:75–80, 1986.

Komaroff AL, Fagioli LR, Geiger AM, et al: An examination of the working case definition of chronic fatigue syndrome. Am J Med 100:56–64, 1996.

Lane TJ, Matthews DA, Manu P: The low yield of physical examinations and laboratory investigations of patients with chronic fatigue. Am J Med Sci 299:313–318, 1990.

Llewelyn MB: Assessing the fatigued patient. Br J Hosp Med 55:125–129, 1996.

Miller PM, Ingham JG, Davidson S: Life counts, symptoms and social support. J Psychosom Res 20(6):515–522, 1976.

Rockwell DA, Burr BD: The tired patient. J Fam Pract 5(5):853–857, 1977.

Ruffin MT, Cohen M: Evaluation and management of fatigue. Am Fam Physician 50:625–632, 1994.

Zala J: Diagnosing myalgic encephalomyelitis. Practitioner 283:916–919, 1989.

CHAPTER 15

Fever

This chapter emphasizes fever as the presenting problem rather than fever of unknown origin (FUO). **Classically, FUO is a temperature greater than 101°F that occurs on several occasions during a 3-week period in an ambulatory patient or during a 1-week period in a hospitalized patient.** Some suggest that the fever must persist only 10 to 14 days in an outpatient. The fever's cause should not be apparent, even after a complete history, physical examination, complete blood count (CBC) with differential, urinalysis, SMA-22, cardiogram, chest radiograph, monospot test, and intermediate-strength purified protein derivative (tuberculin, PPD) test.

In most febrile patients, a diagnosis is readily apparent or becomes evident within a few days. **FUO usually is caused by a common disorder that displays atypical manifestations or is a benign, self-limiting illness for which no specific cause is found.** Despite this, it is still important for the physician to search for occult sources of infection, especially if a response to antibiotics is possible.

Normal oral temperature is 98.6°F (37°C), plus or minus about 1°. Body temperature shows a normal diurnal variation; the lowest point is registered in the early-morning hours, and the highest is reached in the late afternoon.

Acute fevers most often are caused by *upper respiratory infections* (URIs), *tonsillitis, viral syndromes* (e.g., influenza, gastroenteritis), *drug reactions,* and *genitourinary* (GU) *tract infections* (e.g., cystitis, pyelonephritis, prostatitis). Less often, acute fevers accompany meningitis, intraabdominal abscess, and other forms of sepsis.

Chronic low-grade fevers most often are caused by *hepatitis, tuberculosis* (TB), *infectious mononucleosis* (especially in children and young adults), *lymphomas,* and *occult neoplasms* (especially in elderly patients). If the source of a fever is not readily apparent on the basis of history, symptoms, or physical examination, the possibility of *drug fever* (particularly from penicillins, cephalosporins, antituberculars, sulfonamides, macrolides, aminoglycosides, quinidine, methyldopa, procainamide, and phenytoin), *sinusitis, dental abscess, prostatitis, TB, infectious mononucleosis* (especially with associated fatigue), and *hepatitis* (both anicteric and icteric) should be considered. Cocaine, "Ecstasy," and amphetamine abuse may also cause fever.

Less common causes of fever without a readily apparent cause by presenting symptomatology include diverticulitis, subacute bacterial endocarditis (SBE), osteomyelitis, thrombophlebitis, and Crohn's disease.

Nature of Patient

The most common cause of fever in children is a viral URI. Young children usually have signs or symptoms of a respiratory infection but may show only fever. Common causes of fever in children who have no localizing signs or symptoms at the time of examination include *URIs, gastroenteritis, tonsillitis, otitis media, urinary tract infections* (UTIs), *measles,* and *roseola.* A true FUO in a child has serious implications. In one study, 41% of children with true FUO were found to have a chronic or fatal disease. Fever in children under age 3 months may be the only indication of a serious disease. Unexplained fever in adolescents may be a manifestation of *drug abuse* or *endocarditis.*

A history of UTI, sinusitis, prostatitis, and recurrent pneumonia on the same side increases the likelihood that the current febrile episode may be similar to those in the past.

In the absence of physical signs or symptoms suggesting the cause of fever, the physician should question specifically about occupational history (particularly exposure or contact with animals or chemicals), drug ingestion, and travel away from the patient's usual residence. Fever from unusual infections is more common in immunocompromised patients and those with human immunodeficiency virus (HIV) infection. In febrile, elderly patients who lack signs or symptoms that suggest a cause, *TB, occult neoplasm, cranial arteritis,* and *recurrent pulmonary emboli* must be considered. **Elderly patients often have a diminished or absent febrile response to infections.**

In the postoperative patient, fever may be caused by infection, atelectasis, or a reaction to anesthesia or medications.

Nature of Symptoms

Contrary to common belief, studies have shown that the fever pattern is not likely to be helpful diagnostically, although the magnitude may. Temperatures above 105°F (40.5°C) suggest *intracranial pathology, factitious fever, pancreatitis,* or *UTI,* especially with shaking chills. A mild fever suggests *URI* or *flulike syndrome.* Low-grade fever (especially when associated with fatigue) may be the initial manifestation of *TB, infectious mononucleosis,* or *hepatitis.* The fever range may also be helpful. A narrow range of fever, without spikes or chills, may be seen in lymphomas such as *Hodgkin's disease, lymphatic leukemia,* and *hypernephroma.*

A fever in an emotionally disturbed patient who is otherwise in good health and is employed in a health care–related position, has no weight loss, and demonstrates no related or proportional increase in pulse rate should make the physician suspect a factitious cause. Some investigators report that this is more likely in female patients. If a factitious cause is suspected, a simultaneous measurement of urine and rectal temperature should be obtained. **The temperature of the urine normally approximates rectal temperature, and a factitious cause should be suspected if the rectal temperature is significantly (usually more than 2.7°C)**

higher than the urine temperature. Other clues to a factitious cause include failure of temperature to follow a diurnal pattern, rapid defervescence without sweating, high temperature without prostration, and high temperature without weight loss or night sweats.

Drug fevers usually occur about 7 to 10 days after initial administration but reappear rapidly with subsequent administration.

Associated Symptoms

The following clues may help the physician differentiate viral from bacterial infections. **If the fever is high and there appears to be a sparsity of systemic symptoms (e.g., aches, pains, malaise, backache, fatigue), with the more specific findings limited to either the pharynx, abdomen, or chest, a *bacterial infection* is more likely. However, if there is a relatively low-grade fever of less than 101.5°F (38.5°C) associated with systemic complaints (e.g., aches, pains, backache, fatigue, and headache) and the localizing findings are sparse, a *viral infection* is more likely.** For example, the combined findings of a temperature of 103°F (39.4°C), a red sore throat, hoarseness, and possible dysphagia suggest a bacterial pharyngitis. A viral cause is more likely if the temperature is less than 101°F (38.3°C), the pharynx is injected and edematous but little evidence of follicular tonsillitis is present, and the patient complains of aches, pains, myalgia, and headache.

When rash is associated with fever, the rash may be a viral exanthem (e.g., rubella, rubeola, varicella) or a clue to a more serious illness (e.g., Rocky Mountain spotted fever, meningococcemia, thrombocytopenia, Lyme disease, infectious mononucleosis, erythema multiforme, vasculitis).

Shaking chills suggest a bacteremia frequently due to *pyelonephritis.* When fatigue is associated with a low-grade fever, *infectious mononucleosis* or *TB* is likely. Persistent fever after a URI, occasionally associated with a frontal headache, should suggest *sinusitis.*

When fever is associated with arthritis or endocarditis, the physician should suspect disseminated gonococcal infection, or *Lyme disease.* If fever is associated with generalized musculoskeletal pain, the physician must consider rheumatologic or autoimmune disorders.

Precipitating and Aggravating Factors

Contact with people with URI or influenza or a local endemic increases the likelihood of *URI* or *influenza.* These two conditions are particularly common in the winter and late summer.

In women a marked increase in sexual activity may precipitate *cystitis* or *urethritis,* referred to as "honeymoon cystitis." In men a sudden decrease in sexual activity, particularly after an increase in sexual relations (e.g., during a vacation), may precipitate *prostatitis.*

The pain of *sinusitis* may be exacerbated by bending forward, coughing, sneezing, or blowing the nose. Medications and over-the-counter drugs may also cause fever.

Physical Findings

In addition to conducting a careful, thorough physical examination, the physician should pay special attention to certain areas when evaluating a patient whose chief complaint is fever. Relative bradycardia, or a large dissociation between the fever and pulse rate, suggests a drug fever, factitious fever, or rarely typhoid. *Drug fever* should also be suspected if the patient looks "inappropriately well" for the severity of the fever. The sinuses should be percussed and transilluminated for evidence of *sinusitis.* The throat should be examined for signs of *bacterial* or *viral infection* as well as the enanthemas of *measles* or *infectious mononucleosis.* Carious teeth should be tapped for signs of *periapical abscess.* All lymph nodes should be palpated. Rectal examination must be performed for evidence of a *perirectal abscess* or *prostatitis.*

If an obvious source of fever is not made apparent by history or physical examination, attention should be focused on sources of fever that initially present without any clue other than fever. This is particularly true in children. Because significant physical findings and symptoms other than fever may be absent in young children, the physician may use the following clues to assess the severity of the illness: decreased playfulness, decreased alertness, reduced motor ability, respiratory distress, and dehydration. Fever may be seen as an early manifestation of many illnesses, ranging from *teething* to *roseola.* If the source of the fever in a child is not apparent, a urinalysis should be performed; pyuria and albuminuria may be the only manifestations of a UTI.

In teenagers and young adults, *infectious mononucleosis* should be suspected if the fever is associated with any one or more of the following: pharyngitis (either exudative or nonexudative), enanthema on the soft palate, posterior cervical or generalized adenopathy, hepatosplenomegaly, and exanthema. If these patients are given ampicillin, a rash similar to that seen after administration of penicillin may develop. If this occurs in patients with proven infectious mononucleosis, the likelihood of a true penicillin sensitivity is small.

Diagnostic Studies

Laboratory tests useful in determining the cause of a fever include CBC with differential (particular attention should be given to monocytes and atypical lymphocytes), urinalysis, monospot test, erythrocyte sedimentation rate (ESR), SMA-22, antistreptolysin titers, tuberculin test (PPD), antinuclear antibodies, febrile agglutinins, and cultures of blood, urine, pharynx, and stools. Computed tomography (CT) scans; sonograms; technetium, gallium, and indium-111 scans; and special radiographic studies may be helpful in some cases.

Less Common Diagnostic Considerations

The many uncommon illnesses that cause fever include SBE, acute bacterial endocarditis, bacteremia, meningitis, encephalitis, SLE, vasculitis, disseminated fungal infection, actinomycosis (including pelvic actinomycosis, often related to a retained intrauterine device), myocarditis, lung abscess, osteomyelitis, encephalitis, neoplasms in any location, retroperitoneal lesions, lymphomas, connective tissue disorders, inflammatory bowel disease, diverticulitis, periodic fever, metal fume fever, factitious fever, malaria, rat-bite fever, and pulmonary emboli (Table 15–1).

Neuroleptic malignant syndrome from antipsychotic medications (e.g., phenothiazines, haloperidol) may present with fever or even malignant hyperthermia.

TABLE 15.1 Causes of Fever of Unknown Origin in Adults*

CATEGORY	AUTHORS: PETERSDORF AND BEESON	SHEON AND VAN OMMEN	HOWARD ET AL	GLECKMAN ET AL	ESPOSITO AND GLECKMAN
Infection	36	21	37	18	36
Tuberculosis	11	5	4	6	8
Abdominal abscess	4	3	9	6	11
Hepatobiliary	7	0	7	0	6
Endocarditis	5	8	9	0	8
Pyelonephritis	3	0	4	0	0
Other	6	5	4	6	3
Neoplasm	19	17	31	9	24
Lymphoma	6	7	22	9	14
Carcinoma					
Renal	1	0	2	0	4
Pancreatic	2	0	0	0	1
Hepatobiliary	0	2	0	0	3
Unknown primary	2	2	2	0	2
Other	8	6	5	0	0
Connective tissue disorder	15	13	19	9	25
Giant cell arteritis	2	0	4	3	17
Systemic vasculitis	0	6	5	3	6
Lupus erythematosus	5	5	3	0	0
Still's disease	0	0	1	3	0
Rheumatic fever	6	2	0	0	1
Other	2	0	6	0	1
Miscellaneous	23	10	8	29	10
Pulmonary emboli	3	0	0	9	5
Factitious fever	3	0	0	0	0
Periodic disease	5	0	0	3	3
Drugs	1	0	2	0	2
Inflammatory bowel disease	0	4	4	3	0
Other	11	6	2	14	0
Undiagnosed	7	39	5	35	5

*All values are expressed as a percentage of total cases.

From Esposito AL, Gleckman RA: A diagnostic approach to the adult with fever of unknown origin. Arch Intern Med 139:575–579, 1979.

Differential Diagnosis of Fever

TYPE	NATURE OF PATIENT	NATURE OF SYMPTOMS	ASSOCIATED SYMPTOMS	PRECIPITATING AND AGGRAVATING FACTORS	PHYSICAL FINDINGS	DIAGNOSTIC STUDIES
Acute						
Upper respiratory infection (URI)						
Viral	Any age	Oral temperature usually $<101.5°F$	Signs of URI Possible systemic symptoms	Contact with people with URI Local endemic	Cough Oropharynx injected but not beefy red	
Bacterial	More common in children	Often high fever, $>101°F$	Marked signs of URI Few systemic symptoms Children restless		Pharyngotonsillar exudate Pulmonary findings	Positive culture
Other viral syndromes						
Influenza	Any age	Usually mild fever	Muscle aches Nausea Vomiting Cramps Diarrhea			
Gastroenteritis	Any age					
Drug reactions	Taking prescription, recreational, or over-the-counter drugs	Often high fever	Occasional rash		Fever abates when patient stops taking drug	
Urinary tract infection	More common in adults	Often high fever with chills	Backache Urinary frequency and urgency	Obstructive uropathy	Costovertebral angle tenderness	Urinalysis Urine culture
Prostatitis			Dysuria Backache	Marked change in sexual frequency	Prostate tenderness	Culture of prostate secretions
Bacterial sepsis		Often high fever with chills				Blood culture WBC with differential

Table continued on following page.

Differential Diagnosis of Fever *Continued*

TYPE	NATURE OF PATIENT	NATURE OF SYMPTOMS	ASSOCIATED SYMPTOMS	PRECIPITATING AND AGGRAVATING FACTORS	PHYSICAL FINDINGS	DIAGNOSTIC STUDIES
Chronic						
Hepatitis	More common in I.V. drug users	Usually low-grade fever	Fatigue Jaundice Anorexia		Hepatomegaly Liver tender to percussion Jaundice	Liver function tests Hepatitis antigens
Tuberculosis	More common in diabetics	Usually low-grade fever			Chest findings	Chest radiograph Tuberculin test
Infectious mononucleosis	Teenagers Young adults	Usually low-grade fever	Fatigue		Enanthema Pharyngitis Adenopathy (especially postcervical) Splenomegaly	Monospot test
Neoplasm	Elderly adults	Usually narrow fever range	Weight loss			
Occult infection (sinusitis, dental abscess, prostatitis, fungal infections, diverticulitis, SBE, osteomyelitis, inflammatory bowel disease)		Usually low-grade fever	Depends on cause		Depends on cause	Many, including radionuclide scanning
Drug reaction	Taking prescription, recreational, or over-the-counter drugs		Occasional rash		Fever abates when drug discontinued	CBC may show hematologic abnormality
Factitious fever	May be emotionally disturbed Associated with health care	Usually >105°F Can be low-grade	No weight loss Pulse rate not proportional to fever	Emotional stress	Disparity between rectal or oral temperature and urine temperature	

Patients (often of African, Eastern Mediterranean, or Southeast Asian descent) who have a *glucose-6-phosphate dehydrogenase deficiency* may develop fever after receiving sulfonamides, nitrofurantoins, phenacetin, antimalarials, or quinidine.

Cytomegalovirus disease, malignant histiocytosis, juvenile rheumatoid arthritis, Crohn's disease, and cryptic hematoma have been found to cause occult fevers.

Selected References

Carsons SE: Fever in rheumatic and autoimmune disease. Infect Dis Clin North Am 10:67–84, 1996.

Cunha BA: The clinical significance of fever patterns. Infect Dis Clin North Am 10:33–44, 1996.

Cunha BA: Fever of unknown origin. Infect Dis Clin North Am 10:111–127, 1996.

Esposito AL, Gleckman RA: A diagnostic approach to the adult with fever of unknown origin. Arch Intern Med 139:575–579, 1979.

Felton JM, Bryceson ADM: Fever in the returning traveller. Br J Hosp Med 55:705–711, 1996.

Froelich JW, Swanson D: Imaging of inflammatory processes with labeled cells. Semin Nucl Med 14:128–140, 1984.

Johnson DH, Cunha BA: Drug fever. Infect Dis Clin North Am 10:85–91, 1996.

Kimmel SR, Gemmill DW: The young child with fever. Am Fam Physician 37:196–206, 1988.

McCarthy PL, et al: History and observation variables in assessing febrile children. Pediatrics 65:1090–1095, 1980.

Nolan SM, Fitzgerald FT: Fever of unknown origin: the general internist's approach. Postgrad Med 81:190–198, 203–205, 1987.

Norman DC, Yoshikawa TT: Fever in the elderly. Infect Dis Clin North Am 10:93–99, 1996.

Schlossberg D: Fever and rash. Infect Dis Clin North Am 10:101–110, 1996.

Tabor PA: Drug-induced fever. Drug Intell Clin Pharm 20:413–420, 1986.

CHAPTER 16

Forgetfulness

Forgetfulness and loss of memory are common complaints, particularly in elderly patients. Often their families raise the issue. Gradual loss of memory in otherwise healthy, elderly individuals is so common that it was previously referred to as *benign senescent forgetfulness* (BSF). Despite this, patients are usually concerned that this might be an early sign of *Alzheimer's disease* (AD).

The most common causes of forgetfulness are *age-associated memory impairment* (AAMI, formerly referred to as BSF), depression, alcohol, substance abuse, medications, (particularly psychotropic drugs), *Parkinson's disease, primary degenerative dementia,* and *multiinfarct dementia.*

When patients complain of forgetfulness, particularly if they appear to be unreliable, it is essential to seek out someone more reliable, such as a friend or spouse, who can confirm the details of the patient's forgetfulness. **Although loss of memory and concentration may have a functional rather than organic origin, the clinician must not assume one or the other without an adequate assessment. This assessment must include an adequate history, physical examination, and especially a mental status examination.**

Nature of Patient

When adolescents or young adults complain of forgetfulness, memory impairment, or loss of concentration, the most likely causes are *severe anxiety, depression, alcohol abuse,* or *substance abuse.* In a middle-aged person who is not suffering from depression, a sudden onset of forgetfulness should suggest an organic cause such as *alcohol abuse, drug abuse,* administration of *psychotropic agents, brain tumor,* or the onset of a *dementing process.*

In a healthy patient older than 50 years, gradual impairment of memory is probably caused by *AAMI* when it is manifested in problems with everyday activities such as misplacing objects and forgetting the names of persons, multiple items to be purchased, or tasks to be done. In this age group a sudden loss of memory is more likely to reflect a serious etiology, including *stroke* (*cerebrovascular accident,* CVA), *intracranial hemorrhage,* and *brain lesions* (e.g., *tumor, normal pressure hydrocephalus* [NPH]).

Repeated *head trauma* (e.g., as experienced by boxers) may cause memory loss. If the patient is an alcoholic or substance abuser or has a history of treatment with psychotropic drugs, particularly tranquilizers and hypnotics, impaired memory and concentration can result.

Nature of Symptoms

It is particularly important to note whether the onset of memory impairment was sudden or gradual. A sudden onset may suggest administration of *psychotropic agents* (e.g., benzodiazepines, hypnotics), a *grieving process, stroke (CVA),* or *head trauma.* A gradual onset (or sudden onset less frequently) suggests *depression, progressive dementia, AD, Parkinson's disease,* or a *deteriorating medical disorder* (e.g., cardiac, respiratory, renal, or liver disease). **Loss of concentration, which may be confused with memory impairment, is a cardinal symptom of depression.**

Associated Symptoms

Feelings of sadness, impaired concentration, anhedonia, insomnia, and decreased libido suggest that the forgetfulness is probably caused by *depression,* although other major psychiatric disorders also can cause memory loss. Severe headaches, often worse with coughing and sometimes associated with vomiting, suggest the possibility of a *brain tumor.* Resting tremor, bradykinesia, festinating gait, and masked facies suggest that *Parkinson's disease* may be the cause of the memory loss. A progressive decrease in cognitive skills suggests a dementing process such as *AD* or *multiinfarct dementia.* If the patient has signs of infection, meningitis, or inflammatory brain disease, the sudden loss of memory may be caused by *viral, bacterial,* or *fungal brain disease,* especially in patients with *acquired immunodeficiency syndrome* (AIDS).

Precipitating and Aggravating Factors

Depression is probably the most common precipitating cause of forgetfulness and impaired concentration. This may come on spontaneously or be precipitated by bereavement or other severe loss. *Infectious, inflammatory,* or *neoplastic brain disease* may also precipitate memory loss. A single *head injury* resulting in a period of unconsciousness for more than 1 hour may cause a sudden memory loss. *Alcohol abuse, substance abuse,* and *psychotropic agents,* particularly hypnotics or benzodiazepines, may also precipitate a loss of memory. In some cases the administration of benzodiazepines to alleviate symptoms of bereavement may cause the continuation of forgetfulness after the normal grieving process has ended. *Multiple cerebral infarcts,* as seen in multiinfarct dementia, can present with a progressive loss of memory, as can the onset of other dementing diseases such as *AD* and *Parkinson's disease.*

Ameliorating Factors

Most often, simple reassurance by a physician that the symptoms do not represent a major debilitating condition such as AD or Parkinson's disease will alleviate

Differential Diagnosis of Forgetfulness

CONDITION	NATURE OF PATIENT	NATURE OF SYMPTOMS	ASSOCIATED SYMPTOMS	PRECIPITATING AND AGGRAVATING FACTORS	AMELIORATING FACTORS	PHYSICAL FINDINGS	DIAGNOSTIC STUDIES
Age-associated memory impairment	Older than 50 yr	Gradual onset	Difficulty remembering names and tasks to be done Misplacing objects		Reassurance Making lists Other memory-assisting techniques	Healthy	Mental status examination in all patients
Depression	All ages	Usually a gradual onset	Loss of concentration Anhedonia Decreased libido Low self-esteem	Grieving process Severe loss	Antidepressant medications	Depressed affect Weight loss	Serial 7s Gresham Ward questionnaire Wechsler Memory Scale
Alcohol and substance abuse	All ages, especially adolescents and young adults	Usually a sudden onset					Toxicology screen
Medications	All ages	Usually a sudden onset		Ingestion of psychotropic agents (e.g., benzodiazepines, hypnotics)	Stopping all medications, including OTC drugs		

Alzheimer's disease, multiinfarct dementia, other progressive dementing processes	Older patients	Gradual onset Progressive	Progressive decrease in cognitive skills		Disheveled appearance Abnormal behavior	CT scan MRI
Parkinson's disease	Older patients	Gradual onset Progressive	Resting tremor		Resting tremor Bradykinesia Festinating gait Masked facies	
Other intracranial pathology	All ages	Sudden onset	Severe headache Nausea Fever	Stroke (CVA) Infection AIDS Brain tumor Severe head trauma Repeated head trauma		CT scan Spinal tap

much of the patient's concern, even though minimal forgetfulness persists. In other patients, simple mnemonics, writing a list of items to be done, and other methods to diminish the effects of memory loss often help, particularly in individuals with *AAMI.* Treatment of depression with antidepressants usually alleviates the symptoms of forgetfulness and impaired concentration. Likewise, stopping any medications or over-the-counter (OTC) drugs that might interfere with memory or concentration may also be helpful.

Physical Findings

While taking a history and performing a physical examination, the physician should carefully observe the patient's general appearance and behavior, looking specifically for a depressed affect or abnormal behavior. In addition, the patient should be questioned carefully about mood, diurnal variations of mood, suicidal ideation, sleep disturbances, loss of weight, decreased libido, anorexia, and low self-esteem.

A physical examination must include a mental status examination. Memory and concentration can be examined by determining the patient's cognitive state. The physician asks patients to subtract serial 7s from 100, determines their digit span (ability to remember a series of numbers), and asks them to recite the months of the year in reverse. Recent memory can be tested by determining the patient's 5-minute recall of an address. Standardized tests for memory, orientation, and concentration include the Wechsler Memory Scale and the Gresham Ward questionnaire.

The physician also should look for signs of progressive medical disorders, such as *renal, cardiac, pulmonary,* or *hepatic disease.*

Diagnostic Studies

These studies should include standardized tests to determine mental status and memory capabilities. Certain psychological tests, such as the Mini–Mental State Examination (MMSE) and the Kendrick Cognitive Tests for the Elderly (KCTE), may help to discriminate dementia from functional illness, particularly depression. Computed tomography (CT) scanning may show ventricular and sulcal dilatation in AD, but 20% of normal elderly patients may demonstrate a similar picture. Magnetic resonance imaging (MRI) is often helpful in the early differentiation of patients with AD and multiinfarct dementia from those with AAMI. Serum electrolytes, thyroid function tests, and vitamin B_{12} and folate levels may be indicated.

In the early stages of memory loss, it may be impossible to determine whether the patient has early AD or AAMI. Serial examinations may be the most efficient way to make the correct diagnosis.

Less Common Diagnostic Considerations

Korsakoff's syndrome, herpes simplex encephalitis, NPH, and *multiinfarct dementia* can cause mild to severe memory impairment.

Selected References

Banford KA, Caine E: Does "benign senescent forgetfulness" exist? Clin Geriatric Med 4:897–916, 1988.

Blass JP: Age-associated memory impairment and Alzheimer's disease. J Am Geriatr Soc 44:209–211, 1996.

Bowen BC, Barker WW, Loewenstein DA, et al: MR signal abnormalities in mental disorder and dementia. Am J Neuroradiol 11(2):283–290, 1990.

Carlesimo GA, Fadda L, Boncia JJ, Caltagirone C: Differential rates of forgetting: long-term memory in Alzheimer's and multi-infarct dementia. Int J Neurosci 73(1–2):11, 1993.

Crook TH, Larrabee J, Youngjohn JR: Diagnosis and assessment of age-associated memory impairment. Clin Neuropharmacol 13(suppl 3):S81–S91, 1990.

Forno GD, Kawas CH: Cognitive problems in the elderly. Curr Opin Neurol 8:256–261, 1995.

Jacoby R: Loss of memory concentration. Br J Hosp Med 33:32–34, 1985.

Larrabee GJ, McEntee WJ: Age-associated memory impairment: sorting out the controversies. Neurology 45:741–747, 1995.

CHAPTER 17

Headache

About 80% of Americans experience some form of headache each year. Fifty percent of these patients have severe headaches, and 10% to 20% consult a physician with headache as the chief complaint. The most common type is the *muscle contraction,* or *tension-type,* headache. About 10% of the population have *vascular* headaches. Headaches caused by acute *sinusitis* also are fairly common. Less common causes of headaches include *glaucoma, medications, temporal arteritis* (more common in elderly patients), *cervical arthritis, temporomandibular joint* (TMJ) *dysfunction,* and *trigeminal neuralgia.*

Eye strain and hypertension are not common causes of headaches. Most patients with hypertension do not have headaches; most patients with headaches do not have hypertension. When headaches and hypertension coexist, the headaches usually are not related to the hypertension.

To establish a correct diagnosis, the physician must first differentiate acute headaches from recurrent and chronic headaches. Most common headaches are recurrent; a few are chronic. The physician should first elicit the "temporal profile" of the particular headache and a history of prior headaches. The examiner must ask any patient who complains of headaches about the number and types of headaches, age and circumstances at the time the headaches began, any family history of headaches, the character of pain (e.g., location of pain, frequency of attacks, duration of headache, time of onset of attack), any prodromal symptoms, associated symptoms, precipitating factors, emotional factors, previous medical history (especially past illnesses, concurrent disease, recent trauma or surgery), allergies, and responses to medication.

An organic disorder should be suspected if the patient has an isolated severe headache, consistently localized head pain that prevents sleep, headaches associated with straining, headaches accompanied by neurologic signs or symptoms, a change in usual headache pattern, or a chronic, progressively severe headache.

Nature of Patient

Tension headaches, *vascular* headaches (including migraine), and headaches due to *temporal arteritis* are significantly more common in women, whereas *cluster* headaches are much more common in men (male/female ratio, 9 : 1).

Muscle contraction (tension) headaches, the most common type in children and adults, usually are of psychogenic origin and often are induced by situational (home, family, school, or work) problems. Although most children with tension headaches may be suffering from simple anxiety or stress, the headache also may be a manifestation of depression, particularly if it is associated with mood change, withdrawal disturbances, aggressive behavior, loss of energy, self-deprecation, or weight loss. **If a headache has been present continuously for 4 weeks in the absence of neurologic signs, it is probably psychogenic in origin.** Migraine headaches are recurrent.

Studies of young children with *chronic* headaches have revealed that only a small fraction had an organic cause. In children and adolescents, organic headaches most often are caused by noncentral nervous system infections, fever, trauma, and migraine. In children, acute headaches may be the presenting symptom of a *febrile illness* such as pharyngitis or otitis media.

Children up to age 7 have a 1.4% incidence of *migraine;* among patients age 17, the incidence is 5%. Migraine headaches in young children are usually of short duration, and associated symptoms are infrequent. Population studies indicate a 12% incidence of migraine in postpubescent males and up to a 20% incidence in postpubescent females. Despite these studies, the physician must realize that 20% of all adults who experience migraine headaches have onset of symptoms before age 5, and 50% have onset of migraine symptoms before age 20. **Although combination headaches (tension and migraine) are common in adults, they are rare in children, and their frequency increases with adolescence.**

Sinus headaches are uncommon in children, but they may occur in young patients, particularly in association with persistent rhinorrhea, cough, otitis media, or allergies. The maxillary sinus is most frequently involved in children. Likewise, headaches of ocular origin are uncommon in children, although the possibility of *astigmatism, strabismus,* or *refractive error* must be considered. This is particularly true if the headaches appear to be related to reading or schoolwork or if they occur late in the afternoon or evening.

Increased intracranial pressure (ICP) should be suspected if a child who complains of headache has other signs of neurologic dysfunction or projectile vomiting without nausea or if the headache is precipitated or exacerbated by coughing or straining. Causes of increased ICP in children include tumors (headache usually progressive and chronic), *pseudotumor cerebri, hydrocephalus* (detected by serial head measurements), *subdural hematoma* (more common in battered children or after trauma), and *brain abscess* (which may be a complication of otitis media). *Malingering* can be the cause of headaches in children as well as in adults.

In *classic migraine (migraine with aura)* the aura and prodrome are prominent, and the headaches are throbbing and unilateral. The patient often goes to sleep and, on awakening, frequently finds that the headache has disappeared. *Common migraine (migraine without aura)* occurs more frequently than classic migraine. In common migraine the aura may be vague or not present. The prodrome may be vague and manifested only by personality change or malaise, nausea, and vomiting. Common migraine headaches are less often unilateral than classic migraine headaches.

Cluster headaches are extremely rare in children, although they may occur in teenagers. Cluster headaches have their highest frequency in the fourth to sixth decades of life. A family history of "vascular," "sinus," or "sick" headaches is present in most patients with migraine. A positive family history is not usually present in patients with cluster headaches. Most patients with vascular headaches have a history of headaches caused either by tension or by vascular problems. Prior diagnoses may be incorrect because of an inadequate or an incomplete history.

Because the incidence of significant disease causing the headaches increases with age, the onset of headaches in patients after age 50 requires careful evaluation and differential diagnosis. **Fewer than 2% of patients over age 55 experience new, severe headaches. If patients over age 55 have an acute onset of an unrelenting headache that lasts for hours or days, significant disease such as tumor, meningitis, encephalitis, or temporal arteritis should be suspected.** Headache may precede the onset of a neurologic deficit. A sudden new onset of headaches in elderly people occasionally strongly suggests *cerebral ischemia* and *impending stroke* as well as *arteritis.*

In patients over age 50, only a few conditions cause chronic severe headaches and include *temporal arteritis, cluster headaches, mass lesions, posttraumatic headaches, cervical arthritis, Parkinson's disease, medications,* and *depression.* **Depression is a common cause of chronic headache in patients over age 50, but these patients usually experienced chronic headaches before age 50 as well.** Temporal arteritis, although uncommon, occurs more frequently in elderly women; it should be suspected in elderly patients over age 60 who have unilateral chronic head pain, unexplained low-grade fever, proximal myalgia, greatly elevated erythrocyte sedimentation rate (ESR), or an unexplained decrease in visual acuity.

Other less common causes of headache in elderly patients include congestive heart failure, glaucoma, trigeminal neuralgia, and TMJ dysfunction. Iritis, cerebrovascular insufficiency, cerebral hemorrhage, subdural hematoma, and meningitis are even less common but are more serious causes of chronic headache.

Nature of Pain

The type, severity, and location of pain are important in the differentiation of the cause of headaches (Tables 17–1 to 17–3). *Tension (muscle contraction)* headaches usually are dull, not throbbing, steady, and of moderate but persistent intensity. If a patient with chronic tension headaches awakens with a headache, its severity may increase as the day progresses and then decrease toward evening. The pain of *migraine* headaches is severe, initially throbbing, and later boring. The severity of this pain increases rapidly and steadily. The pain of *cluster* headaches is much more severe and more stabbing and burning in quality than that of the usual vascular or tension headaches. Acute *sinus* headache pain usually is described as severe, throbbing, and pressurelike.

Common migraine headaches are usually unilateral but may be bilateral. Most often they are located in the frontotemporal or supraorbital region. *Classic*

TABLE 17.1 Causes of Headaches by Location

AREA OF PAIN	POSSIBLE CAUSE
Generalized	Muscle tension
	Hypertension
	Arteriosclerosis or anemia
	Central nervous system tumor
	Head trauma or chronic subdural hematoma
	Systemic: uremia, thyrotoxicosis
Frontal	
Upper	Muscle tension
	Frontal ethmoid sinusitis
	Rhinitis
Midfacial	Dental disease, maxillary sinusitis, nasal disease
	Ocular or vascular disease, tumor
	Neurologic (cranial nerve) or vascular degenerative disease
Lateral	
Temporal	Muscle tension
	Temporomandibular joint disorders, myofascial disease
	Vascular: arteritis, migraine, cluster headache
Facial or ear	Pharyngeal disease (referred pain)
	Otologic or dental disease; Ramsay Hunt syndrome
	Myofascial disease
Vertex	Sphenoid or ethmoid disease
	Hypertension
	Muscle tension
	Central nervous system, nasopharyngeal neoplasm
Occipital	Uremia
	Fibromyositis
	Subarachnoid hemorrhage
	Hypertension
	Muscle tension

From Schramm VL: A guide to diagnosing and treating facial pain and headache. Geriatrics 35:78-90, 1980.

migraine headaches are unilateral. Cluster headaches are unilateral and periorbital in any given cluster; the pain is described as in the eye and radiating to the front of the face or the temporal regions. Tension headaches are most often occipital, suboccipital, and bilateral, and patients describe the pain as similar to that caused by a constrictive band around the head or as tightness of the scalp. These headaches may radiate down the back of the head and neck. The pain of sinus headaches is usually over the involved sinus or sinuses: maxillary, ethmoid, or frontal. Some patients with *ethmoid sinusitis* present complaining of pain behind the eye that intensifies with coughing or sneezing.

Classic migraine headaches usually last for 2 to 8 days. Common migraine lasts from 4 hours to several days. The onset of most migraine headaches is gradual. Tension headaches usually persist all day for several days. Some patients state that these headaches are constant. Cluster headaches have a much shorter duration than tension headaches or migraines; most last from 20 to 60 minutes.

Patients with *trigeminal neuralgia* usually complain of facial pain, but occasionally their presenting symptom is headache (see Table 17–3). This pain is usually

TABLE 17.2 Diagnosis of Tension Headache Versus Migraine by History

	TENSION (MUSCLE CONTRACTION) HEADACHE			MIGRAINE* TYPE OF VASCULAR HEADACHE	
		PERCENTAGE OF PATIENTS			PERCENTAGE OF PATIENTS
CHARACTERISTICS	DESCRIPTION	1970s†	1950	DESCRIPTION	1950
Laterality	Bilateral	86	90	Unilateral	80
Locus	Occipital	25	–	Supraorbital frontal region	55
	Occipital and suboccipital	26	–		
	Frontal and occipital/ frontal	61	<50		
Quality of head pain	Nonthrobbing	73	70	Throbbing or pulsating	80
Onset of head pain	Severity increases gradually	81	–	Severity increases rapidly in classic, steadily in common	
Frequency	≤8 months	54	–	<1 week	60
	Constant or daily	–	50		
Duration	≤7 hours	50	–	<12 hours	50
	1-12 hours	–	33		
	1-3 hours	–	10		
Prodromes	None	88	90	Present	75
Autonomic symptoms	None	75	90	Present	50
Age at onset	15-24 years	52	–		55
	Before 20 years	–	30	Before 20 years	
Family history	No	54	60	Yes	65

*Percentages for common and classic combined.
†Percentages calculated from data of 1420 tension headache patients in three multicenter studies.
From Friedman AP: Characteristics of tension headache. Psychosomatics 20(7):451-457, 1979.

short, sharp, severe, and stabbing. Each episode lasts less than 90 seconds, but repeated pains persist for 2 to 3 minutes.

Headaches caused by *mass lesions* are persistent but intermittent, whereas headaches due to intracranial infections are usually constant.

Headache Patterns

The common varieties of headaches have a typical pattern for each patient. A change in the pattern should suggest the development of a new problem. If a patient who usually has tension headaches in the occipital region or in a bandlike region around the head develops unilateral headaches associated with nausea and vomiting, migraine headaches may have developed as an additional problem. *Migraine* headaches recur at irregular intervals and have no specific pattern; they may recur once or twice weekly or once a year. They often occur around the menstrual period.

The pattern of *tension* headaches varies with the cause of tension. They most often occur daily but may also occur several times a week. **A patient with chronic**

TABLE 17.3 Factors in Neuralgia and Vascular Pain

FACTOR	TYPICAL NEURALGIA	ATYPICAL NEURALGIA	MIGRAINE	CLUSTER HEADACHE	TEMPORAL ARTERITIS
Age	50–70 years	30–50 years	15–30 years	30–50 years	50–70 years
Gender	Equal	Predominantly female	About equal	Predominantly male	Predominantly female
Family history	Not significant	60%	Frequent	20%	Not significant
Pain location	Usually limited to one cranial nerve	Deep, diffuse, crosses sensory boundaries	Unilateral head and face	Unilateral face of orbit	Distribution of cranial artery, but multiple locations possible
Pain duration	Short, paroxysmal, seconds to minutes	Fluctuating, hours to days	Minutes to hours	Minutes to hours	Fluctuating, persistent
Pain type	Sharp, localized	Aching, drawing, pulling	Progressive, dull, boring; then throbbing	Repetitive burning or intense throbbing	Intense, deep boring, or throbbing
Precipitating factors	Touch, wind, others	Variable	None	None	None
Trigger zone	Usual	No	No	No	Artery tenderness only
Autonomic nervous system or other signs or symptoms	Unusual	Occasional lacrimation, flushing	Nausea, photophobia, scotomata, hemianopia, paresthesia	Common: lacrimation, rhinorrhea, flushing, congested nose, and conjunctiva Occasionally Horner's sign	Fever, malaise Anorexia Progressive decreased visual acuity
Effect of drugs					
Vasoconstrictors	None	Occasional relief	Relief	Relief	None
Analgesics	Inadequate	Relief with narcotic	Not adequate	Not adequate	Variable
Local anesthetics	Relief	Occasional relief	None	None	None
Steroids	None	None	None	None	Gradual relief
Effect of surgery					
Cranial nerve	Generally effective	Not effective	None	None	None
Biopsy	None	None	None	None	Diagnostic

From Schramm VL: A guide to diagnosing and treating facial pain and headache. Geriatrics 35:78–90, 1980.

tension headaches may awaken in the morning with a headache but rarely is awakened at night by it. A specific form of muscle contraction headaches is caused by *bruxism* (grinding of the teeth). Patients may present with a constant headache on awakening if they are "night grinders." Typically, *hypertensive* headaches also occur in the morning after nighttime recumbency and are usually throbbing in nature.

The frequency patterns of *cluster* headaches are diagnostic because these types of headaches usually occur in close succession. They often occur at approximately the same time of day for 3 to 8 weeks and may recur one to three times a day. They may have an inexplicable remission for months or years and an equally inexplicable recurrence. Although early-morning onset (1 to 5 AM) is typical of cluster headaches, some attacks occur during the day. If they happen at night, which is rare, they possibly are related to rapid eye movement during sleep. *Sinus* headaches also often begin in the morning, progressively worsen, but tend to improve toward evening.

Migraine headaches have prodromes, which are uncommon in cluster headaches; occasionally, some patients experience a burning sensation on the forehead before the onset of pain. The classic migraine prodrome occurs 15 to 30 minutes before the headache. It is abrupt in onset, lasts for 10 to 15 minutes, and is often contralateral to the headache. Visual auras include a variety of scotomata, transient blindness, blurred vision, and hemianopsia. Nonvisual auras may include weakness, aphasia, mood disturbances, and photophobia. In contrast to classic migraine, common migraine usually has no specific aura. When prodromes are present, they vary widely and may present as psychic disturbances, fatigue, gastrointestinal symptoms, or mood changes.

Associated Symptoms

With *classic migraine* the most common associated symptoms include anorexia, nausea, vomiting, sonophobia, photophobia, and irritability. Less common are dizziness, fluid retention, abdominal pain, and sleepiness. Symptoms associated with the *common migraine* include all those associated with classic migraine as well as fatigue, chills, diarrhea, and urticaria. Cyclic abdominal pain or vomiting in children and motion sickness in adults are typically seen in patients with migraine headaches.

Pain in the posterior cervical region that is exacerbated by neck extension often is seen in patients with *tension* headaches, who frequently are tense, anxious, significantly depressed, and fatigued. Patients with chronic tension headaches seem to be more emotionally involved in their headache symptoms; they seem to focus on their symptoms more than patients with migraines. In addition, the intensity of the affective disturbance is more marked in those with tension headaches than in those with migraine.

Patients with acute *sinus* headaches may complain of toothaches; this indicates a maxillary infection. Pain in the eye indicates an ethmoid sinusitis. Nasal discharge, percussion tenderness over the sinus area, and upper respiratory infection (URI) symptoms are often present. A *nasal* or *sinus neoplasm* may be present if the physician suspects a sinus headache that does not improve after approximately 2 weeks of appropriate therapy (including antibiotics and nasal decongestants) and if there is blood-tinged rhinorrhea. These symptoms recur despite therapy, and sinus radiographs may show evidence of bone destruction.

The symptoms associated with *cluster* headaches are significantly different and help the physician establish this diagnosis. Patients may complain of injection of the involved eye, a blocked nose with rhinorrhea, and marked ipsilateral lacrimation. They may have ipsilateral Horner's syndrome. About 25% of patients with cluster headaches have peptic ulcer disease.

Sick building syndrome should be suspected if fatigue and upper respiratory complaints are associated with the headache and the patient works in an inadequately ventilated building with an impervious outer shell.

Organic brain disease should be suspected if one or more of the following signs or symptoms are noted:

1. Intermittent or continuous headache that progressively increases in frequency and severity
2. Headache that is exacerbated by coughing or straining at stool
3. Headache that is worse in the morning (note that sinus and hypertensive headaches also may be worse in the morning)
4. Vomiting
5. Headache that disturbs sleep
6. Inequality of pupils
7. Fever
8. Seizures
9. Confusion
10. Recent onset of neurologic deficit
11. Papilledema
12. Onset of severe headaches after age 50

Precipitating and Aggravating Factors

Although migraine headaches may be precipitated by *menstruation,* their frequency increases as estrogen levels fall. Migraine headaches often are precipitated by emotional stress. Less frequently, they are precipitated by fatigue, bright lights, fasting, hypoglycemia, foods rich in tyramine (e.g., aged cheeses, sour cream, wines), odors, exercise, weather changes, and high altitude.

Patients may have a history of headaches that are caused by ingestion of certain foods and beverages (e.g., chocolate, yogurt, buttermilk). Headaches may be precipitated by foods that contain nitrites ("hot dog headache") or monosodium glutamate ("Chinese restaurant syndrome"). *Alcohol* and *caffeine* are frequent offenders, as is *caffeine withdrawal. Medications* such as reserpine, vasodilators, H_2-receptor blockers, indomethacin, angiotensin-converting enzyme (ACE) inhibitors, nitrates, beta blockers, calcium channel blockers, sildenafil, and oral contraceptives also may cause headaches. Some patients who have been heavy users of ergot drugs to control migraine may experience migraine headaches when these therapeutic agents are stopped.

Tension headaches can be precipitated by emotional or physical stress, extended periods of mental concentration, and prolonged, somewhat abnormal positions of the neck. Some muscle contraction headaches may occur with cessation of analgesics or tranquilizers used in their treatment. Dental malocclusion may stimulate contraction of the muscles of mastication, thus causing spasm of the muscles and headache. Poorly fitting dentures, particularly if they have been worn for 10 or more years, also may lead to tension headaches.

Cluster headaches may be precipitated by short naps, alcohol ingestion, nitroglycerin, tyramine, and emotional stress. *Sinus* headaches may be aggravated by coughing or sneezing, but this is also true of other types of headaches, especially vascular. Eye pain due to *glaucoma* often is precipitated by darkness or sympathomimetic drugs, which cause pupillary dilatation.

Ameliorating Factors

If the patient states that ergot-containing drugs improved the acute headaches, a vascular cause is probable. Likewise, relief with nasal decongestants and antibiotics suggests a sinus cause. A headache that is severe; associated with nausea, vomiting, scotomata, or aura; and relieved by sleep is probably migraine.

Physical Findings

In patients with *tension* or *migraine* headaches the physical findings seldom contribute to the differential diagnosis. Patients with *trigeminal neuralgia* may have a trigger point. During an attack of *cluster* headache, ipsilateral lacrimation and rhinorrhea may occur. Patients with acute *sinus* headaches may have a mucopurulent or blood-tinged nasal discharge. In addition, they may have tenderness to percussion or palpation over the involved sinus, which also may demonstrate impaired transillumination.

The presence of fever suggests an *infectious process* as the cause of the headache. Severe *hypertension* may suggest that the headaches are of hypertensive origin, although most patients with hypertension do not have headaches. Tenderness to palpation over the temporal artery suggests *temporal arteritis* as a cause.

When nuchal rigidity is found, *meningitis* or a *subarachnoid bleed* should be suspected. Nuchal rigidity must be differentiated from the stiff neck of patients with cervical arthritis (more common in elderly patients). In patients with true nuchal rigidity the neck is stiff throughout the arc as the examiner flexes it but not in extension or lateral rotation. In contrast, with *cervical arthritis* the early phase of flexion of the neck is supple; this is followed by a sudden, boardlike rigidity with resistance in other directions of movement as well.

Patients with *psychogenic* or *conversion* headaches may describe the pain in very vivid terms with much affect; the patient does not really appear to be in great pain.

Pain localized to one or both eyes with increased intraocular pressure indicates *glaucoma.* The presence of a jaw click or point tenderness to palpation over the temporomandibular joint suggests that the headache may be due to TMJ dysfunction.

Most patients with headaches do not exhibit any abnormalities on neurologic examination. However, a transient ipsilateral Horner's syndrome may be seen with some migraine headaches.

Diagnostic Studies

Only a few laboratory tests help in the differential diagnosis of headaches. Imaging studies are rarely useful in common tension or migraine headaches. Radiographs may confirm *acute sinusitis* if a typical fluid level exists in one or more of the sinuses. Patients may experience sinus headaches and still have normal sinus radiographs. The ESR is greatly elevated with *temporal arteritis.* A biopsy of the arterial wall showing giant cell infiltration is pathognomonic of arteritis.

If sudden onset of headache occurs in patients over age 50, the physician must make a difficult decision regarding whether to perform lumbar puncture. It is indicated in suspected cases of *cerebral hemorrhage* or *bacterial encephalitis,* but it is dangerous in patients with mass lesions or increased ICP. Noninvasive tests such as a computed tomography (CT) scan or magnetic resonance imaging (MRI) should be done first if intracranial disease is suspected. Arteriograms may show vascular abnormalities and mass lesions.

Less Common Diagnostic Considerations

Patients with *glaucoma* may complain of pain in one or both eyes and describe a visual halo around objects. Headaches often develop in a darkened environment. Intraocular pressure is increased, occasionally with tenderness to palpation over the globe.

Eye strain is a diagnosis that often is applied incorrectly. Headache from eye strain is unusual. It tends to occur in people who do work that requires close vision. In addition, the headaches tend to occur after a prolonged period of using the eyes.

Systemic causes of headaches include *uremia, occult carbon monoxide poisoning, sick building syndrome, thyrotoxicosis, severe anemia, brain tumors, chronic subdural hematoma, subarachnoid hemorrhage,* and *ocular disease.* Tumors of the eye, ear, nose, or throat also may present with headaches. Occult carbon monoxide poisoning may result from faulty furnaces, kitchen stoves, and propane space heaters at workplaces ("warehouse worker's headache").

SUNCT syndrome (**s**hort-lasting, **u**nilateral, **n**euralgiform headache with **c**onjunctival infection, **t**earing, and rhinorrhea) occurs more often in males. It shares

Text continued on page 177.

Differential Diagnosis of Headache

TYPE	NATURE OF PATIENT	NATURE OF SYMPTOMS	ASSOCIATED SYMPTOMS	PRECIPITATING AND AGGRAVATING FACTORS	AMELIORATING FACTORS	PHYSICAL FINDINGS	DIAGNOSTIC STUDIES
Tension (muscle contraction) headaches	Most common cause of headache at any age More common in females	Usually of psychogenic origin *Children:* may be manifestation of stress, anxiety, or depression *Adults:* Usually dull, nonthrobbing, with persistent, low intensity May last a few days Severity may increase as day progresses and then decrease toward evening Usually occipital, suboccipital, and bilateral Described as constrictive band around head or tightness of scalp Rarely wakes patient from sleep	Fatigue	Emotional or physical stress Abnormal neck positions (especially neck extension) Prolonged mental concentration Withdrawal of analgesics or tranquilizers Dental malocclusion or poorly fitting dentures Bruxism (nighttime grinding of teeth)	Stress reduction		

aches	population More common in women Family history of headaches			Sneezing	drugs Beta blockers
Common migraine: migraine headache without aura	More frequent in children	Vague or absent aura and prodrome Gradual onset Lasts up to 72 hours Not always unilateral Usually in frontotemporal or supraorbital region	Those of classic migraine General malaise Fatigue Chills Diarrhea Urticaria Motion sickness		Sleep
Classic migraine: migraine headache with aura	More common in women *Incidence:* 1.4% in children (under age 7 years) 5% in children at age 17 years 17% in postpubescent males 20% in postpubescent females 50% of adults with migraines have symptoms before age 20	Prominent aura *Prodrome:* Has abrupt onset Lasts 15–20 minutes Precedes headache by 15–30 minutes Often contralateral to headache *Headache:* Severe Throbbing Unilateral Gradual onset Intensity increases steadily and rapidly Lasts 2–8 days	Visual auras (scotomata, transient blindness, blurred vision, hemianopsia) Nonvisual auras (weakness, aphasia, mood disturbances, photophobia) Nausea and vomiting Anorexia Sonophobia Photophobia Irritability Dizziness Fluid retention Abdominal pain Sleepiness	Menstruation Emotional stress Fatigue Bright lights High altitude Weather changes Exercise Certain foods Fasting Hypoglycemia	Sleep

Table continued on following page.

Differential Diagnosis of Headache *Continued*

TYPE	NATURE OF PATIENT	NATURE OF SYMPTOMS	ASSOCIATED SYMPTOMS	PRECIPITATING AND AGGRAVATING FACTORS	AMELIORATING FACTORS	PHYSICAL FINDINGS	DIAGNOSTIC STUDIES
Cluster headaches	Highest incidence in fourth to sixth decade Rare in children Much more common in men than women (9 : 1) Family history of cluster headaches uncommon Recur at same time of day for 3–8 weeks, 1–3 times per day Typical early-morning onset	Pain more severe, stabbing, and burning than in vascular or tension headache Unilateral and periorbital in any given cluster May radiate to front of face or to temporal regions Duration: 20–60 minutes	25% of patients have peptic ulcer disease Injection of involved eye Rhinorrhea Marked ipsilateral lacrimation May be ipsilateral Horner's syndrome	Short naps Alcohol Nitroglycerin Tyramine Emotional stress			
Headaches due to febrile illnesses	Common cause of headache in children	Headache may be only presenting symptom in children	Fever	Pharyngitis, especially with otitis media		Fever	

Sinusitis (see Chap. 13)	Uncommon in children	*Children:* maxillary sinus most often involved *Pain:* Severe, throbbing, and intense pressure Usually over involved sinus Begins in morning, progressively worsens during day, improves toward evening	Persistent rhinorrhea Otitis media Allergies Symptoms of upper respiratory infection Toothache, with maxillary involvement Eye pain with ethmoid involvement	Coughing Sneezing		Mucopurulent or blood-tinged nasal discharge Percussion tenderness over involved sinuses	Transillumination of sinuses Sinus radiographs or CT scan
Depression	Common cause of headache in patients > age 50	Constant, chronic headache	Those of depression		Treat depression		
Temporomandibular joint (TMJ) dysfunction (see Chap. 13)	Adults	Usually pain in TMJ or ear, but may present with headache (temporoparietal)	Bruxism	Opening mouth too wide		Jaw clicks Point tenderness to palpation over TMJ Prominent masseter muscle	Radiograph of TMJ MRI of TMJ
Temporal arteritis	Most common in elderly women	Unilateral, chronic headache	Unexplained low-grade fever Proximal myalgia Decreased visual acuity			Tenderness to palpation over temporal artery	ESR greatly elevated

Table continued on following page.

Differential Diagnosis of Headache *Continued*

TYPE	NATURE OF PATIENT	NATURE OF SYMPTOMS	ASSOCIATED SYMPTOMS	PRECIPITATING AND AGGRAVATING FACTORS	AMELIORATING FACTORS	PHYSICAL FINDINGS	DIAGNOSTIC STUDIES
Cervical arthritis	Most common in elderly people	Occipital or nuchal headache				Stiff neck Early phase of flexion is supple but followed by sudden, board-like rigidity with resistance in other directions	Radiograph of cervical spine
Trigeminal neuralgia (see Chap. 13)	Adult	Pain is short, episodic, sharp, severe, and stabbing Each episode lasts <90 seconds but recurs for 2–3 minutes	Pain in face along distribution of one division of nerve	Trigger point Extremes of temperature		Possible trigger point	
Increased intracranial pressure		Progressive, chronic headache	*Children:* Neurologic dysfunction Projectile vomiting without nausea	Coughing Sneezing		Papilledema	CT scan Increased cerebrospinal fluid pressure
Glaucoma (see Chap. 13)		Frontal headache	Patient see halos Pain in eye	Darkened areas Drugs that dilate pupils		Increased intraocular pressure	Tonometry

features with cluster headaches and trigeminal neuralgia, but SUNCT appears to be rare.

The key to diagnosing headaches consists of a careful, detailed clinical history, headache diary, and neurologic examination. The physician usually has time to observe the patient and to evaluate the whole patient in relation to the family and environment, which is helpful in determining the underlying cause of headache. The physician should try to avoid the use of habituating drugs in the treatment of patients with chronic headaches.

Selected References

Couch JR: Headache to worry about. Med Clin North Am 77:141–167, 1993.

Coutin IB, Glass SF: Recognizing uncommon headache syndromes. Am Fam Physician 54:2247–2252, 1996.

Diamond S: Head pain: diagnosis and management. Clin Symp 46(3):1–34, 1994.

Edmeads JG: Headache as a symptom of organic disease. Curr Opin Neurol 8:233–236, 1995.

Evans RW: Diagnostic testing for the evaluation of headaches. Neurol Clin 14:1–25, 1996.

Hecherling PS, Leikin JB, Maturen A, Perkins JT: Predictors of occult carbon monoxide poisoning in patients with headache and dizziness. Ann Intern Med 107:174–176, 1987.

Lipton RB, Pfeffer D, Newman LC, Soloman S: Headaches in the elderly. J Pain Sympt Manage 8:87–97, 1993.

Marks DR, Rapoport AM: Practical evaluation and diagnosis of headache. Semin Neurol 17:307–313, 1997.

Rapoport AM: The diagnosis of migraine and tension-type headache, then and now. Neurology 42(2):11–15, 1992.

Rothner AD: Headaches in children and adolescents: classification and recommendations. Postgrad Med 81:223–230, 1987.

Schramm VL: A guide to diagnosing and treating facial pain and headache. Geriatrics 35:78–90, 1980.

Shankland WE: Differential diagnosis of headaches. Cranio 4:47–53, 1986.

Silberstein SD: Drug-induced headache. Neurol Clin 16:107–123, 1998.

Solomon S: Diagnosis of primary headache disorders: validity of the International Headache Society criteria in clinical practice. Neurol Clin 15:15–26, 1997.

Thompson JA: Diagnosis and treatment of headache in the pediatric patient. Curr Probl Pediatr 10:1–52, 1980.

CHAPTER 18

Heartburn and Indigestion

Heartburn and indigestion are common presenting complaints. Because these symptoms are often vague, it is difficult for the physician to determine a precise cause, and treatment is frequently ineffective.

Heartburn is a sensation of burning, warmth, or heat in the retrosternal region between the xiphoid and the manubrium that occasionally radiates toward the jaw or rarely the arms. Water brash (regurgitation of fluid) may be present.

Indigestion is a separate entity. *Dyspepsia,* which is similar to indigestion, is defined as episodic or persistent abdominal symptoms often related to feeding and thought to result from disorders of the proximal portion of the digestive tract. Dyspeptic symptoms include upper abdominal discomfort, postprandial fullness, early satiety, anorexia, belching, nausea, heartburn, vomiting, bloating, borborygmi, dysphagia, and abdominal burning. Usually these symptoms occur during the day and rarely at night.

The most common causes of heartburn and indigestion include *reflux esophagitis* (with or without hiatal hernia), ingestion of *drugs* (e.g., aspirin, nonsteroidal antiinflammatory drugs [NSAIDs], antibiotics, digitalis, potassium or iron supplements, theophylline derivatives), *gastritis, nonulcer dyspepsia,* excessive consumption of *food* or *alcohol, chronic active gastritis, gallbladder disease, pregnancy, aerophagia,* and *functional gastrointestinal* (GI) *disorder.* Although patients with tumors of the GI tract may complain of heartburn or indigestion, neoplasms are not a common cause of these symptoms.

This chapter focuses on indigestion and heartburn *not* associated with abdominal pain. Conditions associated with abdominal pain are discussed in Chapters 1 and 2.

Nature of Patient

Dyspeptic symptoms are a result of organic or, most often, functional causes. Younger patients are less likely to have organic causes of their indigestion, whereas older patients are more likely to have serious organic causes. Children rarely complain of indigestion or heartburn, although vague abdominal discomfort may affect children who experience *malabsorption* or *food intolerance.* With these conditions, certain foods may cause crampy abdominal pain or diarrhea. Weight loss may be noted with significant malabsorption. When children complain of distention or awareness of peristalsis and gurgling, they often have *functional GI disease.* If these complaints are intermittent and not disabling, if the patient is otherwise healthy, and if the results of the physical examination are normal, an emotional cause should be suspected. Questioning the child may reveal depression or other emotional problems. These problems frequently occur with external environmental stress such as divorce, birth of a sibling, illness in a family, starting school, and problems with a boyfriend or girlfriend.

In adults, heartburn is almost always caused by *reflux esophagitis.* This is more common in pregnant women, particularly during the later months. Patients with esophagitis may complain of severe heartburn that is relieved by alkali and aggravated by recumbency. Although *hiatal hernia* is three times more common in multiparous patients than in primigravid women, **symptoms of heartburn are caused by esophageal reflux and not by the hiatal hernia.** Pregnant patients have delayed gastric emptying, increased intraabdominal pressure, and increased estrogen levels, all of which facilitate esophageal reflux. From 30% to 50% of adults demonstrate hiatal hernias on radiographs; only 5% of this population report symptoms of heartburn.

Indigestion due to gastritis occurs frequently in patients who ingest large quantities of *alcohol* or *drugs* such as salicylates, corticosteroids, NSAIDs, theophylline, quinidine, and some antibiotics.

Travelers and campers who become infested with *Giardia* may experience just bloating, nausea, and upper abdominal discomfort. These dyspeptic symptoms may persist for months with only occasional episodes of diarrhea.

About 50% of all diabetic patients, whether or not insulin dependent, have delayed gastric emptying *(diabetic gastroparesis).* Many of these patients complain of pain, nausea, vomiting, or postprandial fullness *(diabetic dyspepsia).* In addition to these symptoms, the delayed gastric emptying may contribute to erratic absorption of oral hypoglycemic agents and thus poor blood glucose control.

Elderly patients are more likely to complain of vague feelings of indigestion, possibly related to bloating. Many of the symptoms of indigestion and abdominal bloating are caused by excessive *intestinal gas* and *disordered motility.* Virtually all intestinal gas is the result of bacterial fermentation, although the amount of discomfort is not necessarily proportional to the amount of gas in the intestines. The complaints of indigestion and bloating are more common in elderly patients because of relative gastric and intestinal stasis, hypomotility of the gut, altered intestinal bacteria, increased incidence of constipation, and lack of exercise, all of which tend to facilitate the production of intestinal gas. Elderly patients with *gastritis* or *duodenal ulcers* usually are infected with *Helicobacter pylori. H. pylori*–negative gastritis is usually caused by NSAID ingestion.

Tense and *anxious* patients are more likely to be aware of normal intestinal movement and are also more likely to complain about these feelings. Many patients with *gallbladder disease, irritable bowel syndrome,* and *ulcers* complain of vague abdominal discomfort and occasional distention.

Nature of Symptoms

Heartburn is a burning sensation that occurs in the xiphisternal region with occasional proximal radiation. It may vary in intensity from a mild feeling of warmth to extreme pain. Occasionally the pain may be indistinguishable from that of severe angina pectoris; it is therefore important for the physician to note that heartburn has *no relation to physical activity.* The pain is usually caused by esophageal spasm, is intermittent over several minutes, and recurs over long periods. Pain may radiate into the neck and occasionally into the arms, back, or jaw. According to one study, the pain radiated to the back in 40% of patients with proven *esophageal reflux* but radiated to the arms or neck in only 5%.

Initially, the pain of heartburn may be felt only after heavy meals or while the patient is lying down or bending over. In more advanced cases, the pain is more easily provoked, lasts longer, and is accompanied by *dysphagia.*

Patients with *gastritis* may have abdominal pain, vague indigestion, or heartburn as a presenting complaint. Epigastric discomfort that is worse after eating, loss of appetite, a sense of fullness, nausea, and occasional vomiting are also common complaints in patients with gastritis. These same symptoms may be seen in patients with nonulcer dyspepsia caused by *H. pylori.* Studies have shown that symptoms alone cannot differentiate nonulcer dyspeptic patients as positive or negative for *H. pylori.*

Heartburn is also a common complaint in patients with *bile gastritis,* which often occurs after gastric resection or pyloroplasty. Bile refluxes into the stomach and subsequently into the distal esophagus, causing heartburn. Some patients who have *peptic ulcer disease* do not complain of the classic symptoms but only of vague indigestion that is sometimes relieved by vomiting.

Symptoms in patients with *functional GI disorders* are often vague and nonspecific. Patients do not obtain consistent relief with any medication or therapeutic regimen. Other neurotic symptoms are often present, with no evidence of systemic disease or weight loss despite a long history of vague symptoms. Because various patients with an organic pathology (e.g., peptic ulcer, gallbladder disease, colonic tumors) may also have vague symptoms, a specific workup is required in some cases. When these vague symptoms occur in young adults, it is unlikely that a malignant process is present. Likewise, if the symptoms have been present for many years without any significant progression or evidence of systemic disease, a major disease process is also unlikely.

Other distinguishing characteristics often help the physician differentiate functional from organic pain. With *functional* illness, patients may have severe and continuous pain but no significant weight loss. The patients often give exaggerated descriptions of their pain and have a significant emotional investment; they may come into the office with a list of their symptoms. With *organic* disease, the pain, although severe, is often periodic and may be associated with weight loss.

Associated Symptoms

Patients with *peptic esophagitis* frequently have chest pain. They may complain of heartburn or chest pain when esophageal spasm occurs. Some patients complain only of substernal pain, which may radiate into the neck, jaw, or upper arms. When water brash is associated with heartburn, *gastroesophageal reflux* is most likely. When nocturnal pain is associated with abdominal pain and dyspepsia, *peptic ulcer* is likely. **If dyspepsia is continuous, exacerbated by food, and especially with associated anorexia and weight loss, gastric cancer is more likely.**

Belching secondary to *aerophagia* is often seen in patients with reflux esophagitis and in patients with functional GI disease. If indigestion is associated with nausea, right upper quadrant (RUQ) pain, or pain in the right shoulder (particularly the inferior angle of the right scapula), *duodenal loop distention* or *cholelithiasis* should be considered. Hematemesis suggests *peptic ulcer disease* or *variceal bleeding,* regardless of how vague the other symptoms are.

Precipitating and Aggravating Factors

In many patients with symptoms caused by *reflux esophagitis,* coronary artery disease (CAD) or hysteria has been previously diagnosed. **Clues to the correct diagnosis of esophagitis are that the pain is not usually brought on by exercise, frequently occurs in the recumbent position, and is often relieved by antacids.** Despite these clues, chest pain caused by reflux esophagitis may be induced by exercise. Anything that distends the lower third of the esophagus, irritates its mucosa, or reduces lower esophageal pressure can precipitate reflux esophagitis. This includes recumbency, acidic foods, gastric stasis, large meals, and fatty foods, which delay gastric emptying. Several studies show that in addition to gastric juices, bile and other duodenal juices may play a role in the pain of reflux esophagitis.

Conditions that increase intraabdominal pressure (e.g., pregnancy, marked ascites) can facilitate regurgitation of gastric or duodenal contents into the distal esophagus. Caffeine frequently causes heartburn in susceptible people. Certain spices, carminatives (e.g., oil of spearmint and peppermint), garlic, onions, chocolate, fatty foods, alcohol, and carbonated beverages may reduce lower esophageal pressure and thus facilitate reflux. Cigarette smoking also reduces lower esophageal pressure and stimulates gastric acidity. Certain drugs, particularly theophylline derivatives, isoproterenol, and anticholinergics, lower esophageal pressure and may precipitate reflux and heartburn. Other precipitating factors include straining, recumbency, lifting, and ingestion of orange juice, tomato juice, and spicy foods and drinks.

In some patients who swallow air, chew gum, or eat rapidly, heartburn develops as a result of belching and subsequent regurgitation of gastric juices into the distal esophagus. Although some patients with hiatal hernia have heartburn or chest pain, a hiatal hernia does not establish the presence of esophagitis.

Ameliorating Factors

In general, avoidance of precipitating factors reduces and may eliminate the discomfort. In addition, raising the head of the bed (by tilting the entire bed, not by merely using another pillow), retiring with an empty stomach, sucking on antacid tablets, eating small frequent meals, following a low-fat diet, and avoiding tight garments may help.

The pain of *peptic esophagitis* is frequently relieved by antacids, which reduce gastric acidity and reestablish more normal lower esophageal sphincter pressure, thus reducing reflux. The physician must remember that the pain of peptic esophagitis may be relieved by nitrates, typically thought to relieve only the pain of angina pectoris. **Relief of substernal pain by nitroglycerin does not necessarily establish the diagnosis of angina pectoris, since this drug can also relieve the pain of lower esophageal spasm.** Patients with peptic esophagitis who obtain inadequate relief from the usual therapeutic measures (antacids, bethanechol, cimetidine, metoclopramide) may receive additional relief from nitroglycerin. **If the pain is relieved by ingesting viscous lidocaine (Xylocaine Viscous), it is probably caused by peptic esophagitis.** Some suggest using this procedure as a diagnostic tool, although false-positive results may occur among patients with chest pain of coronary origin. Therefore, this test is useful but will not rule out CAD with absolute certainty.

Once the diagnosis of serious disease is excluded, patients with vague symptoms of indigestion and functional GI complaints should be treated with reassurance and occasionally tranquilizers. If the symptoms of the dyspepsia are relieved by ingestion of bismuth salts (e.g., Pepto-Bismol), antibiotics, or both, an *H. pylori* infection should be suspected.

Physical Findings

Most patients who complain of indigestion or heartburn demonstrate no abnormal physical findings. Auscultation of peristalsis in the chest should suggest a large diaphragmatic *hernia.* Mild, diffuse, abdominal tenderness associated with abdominal distention sometimes is observed with *pancreatitis* or *excessive swallowed air* in the intestinal tract. A succussion splash can often be elicited in patients with *gastric dilatation,* whether reflex or secondary to pyloric obstruction.

Some patients with *gastritis* have tenderness on abdominal palpation, whereas others may have no physical findings other than midepigastric tenderness to percussion. The same is true for patients with *peptic ulcer disease.* Patients with *cholelithiasis* may have no symptoms but occasionally have RUQ tenderness to palpation or percussion. In some patients with *gallbladder hydrops* a dilated gallbladder is palpable or ballotable.

Diagnostic Studies

Endoscopy is the most reliable diagnostic technique for establishing the cause of upper GI symptoms, although most patients with vague symptoms do not require this invasive procedure. Early endoscopy should be recommended if the dyspeptic patient (1) has onset of symptoms or change in dyspeptic symptoms after age 45; (2) is *H. pylori* positive or taking NSAIDs if less than age 45; (3) has had dyspepsia more than 1 year; (4) has anorexia, weight loss, anemia, or blood in the stools, and colonic pathology has been excluded; or (5) is immunocompromised.

Esophageal reflux can be observed on upper GI radiographs. Esophagitis can be detected by esophagoscopy, and its symptoms can be produced by instillation of dilute hydrochloric acid in the distal esophagus (Bernstein test). Esophageal pH monitoring is the most sensitive test.

Gastritis is best diagnosed by gastroscopy. Gallbladder disease can be diagnosed by sonography, cholecystography, and isotopic studies.

Less Common Diagnostic Considerations

When the patient finds that abdominal discomfort is intensified by bending over or wearing a tight garment, *gas entrapment* (e.g., hepatic or splenic flexure syndrome) should be suspected. Sometimes this discomfort is relieved by the passage of flatus. Gas entrapment can be confirmed if flexion of the right or left thigh on the abdomen replicates the pain or if an abdominal radiograph shows a large bubble of trapped gas in the hepatic or splenic flexure. The pain of gas entrapment in the hepatic or splenic flexure is often referred to the chest, and the patient may complain of chest pain.

Heartburn may be caused by viral *esophagitis* and *esophageal candidiasis. Disseminated sclerosis* that invades the esophagus may also cause severe heartburn. Indigestion may be the presenting symptom in *uremia, pulmonary tuberculosis, migraine, gastric dilatation, glaucoma, hypercalcemia, diabetes,* and *CAD. Barrett's esophagus* and *gastric cancer,* although often asymptomatic, may cause symptoms of indigestion.

Selected References

Barbara L, Camilleri M, Corinaldesi GP, et al: Definition and investigation of dyspepsia: consensus of an international ad hoc working party. Dig Dis Sci 34:1272–1276, 1989.

Chamberlain CE, Peura DA: *Campylobacter (Helicobacter) pylori:* is peptic disease a bacterial infection? Arch Intern Med 150:951–955, 1990.

Collins JSA, Knill-Jones RP, Sloan JM, et al: A comparison of symptoms between non-ulcer dyspepsia patients positive and negative for *Helicobacter pylori.* Ulster Med J 60:21–27, 1991.

De Luca VA: Gastroduodenal dyspepsia: a personal view integrating clinical, endoscopic, histological and management criteria. Dig Dis 14:27–42, 1996.

Gremse DA, Sacks AI: Evaluation of dyspepsia. Pediatr Ann 26:251–259, 1997.

Long WB, Cohen S: The digestive tract as a cause of chest pain. Am Heart J 100:567–572, 1980.

Differential Diagnosis of Heartburn and Indigestion

CAUSE	NATURE OF PATIENT	NATURE OF SYMPTOMS	ASSOCIATED SYMPTOMS	PRECIPITATING AND AGGRAVATING FACTORS	AMELIORATING FACTORS	PHYSICAL FINDINGS	DIAGNOSTIC STUDIES
Reflux esophagitis	Adults More common in pregnant women in later months	Severe heartburn Water brash with and without recumbency Recurrent pain radiates to back (40%), arms, or neck (5%)	Chest pain Dysphagia Belching (from aerophagia) Cough Asthma, especially nocturnal	Recumbency Straining or lifting Drinking alcoholic, caffeinated, or carbonated beverages Eating heavy meals or fatty, spicy, or acidic foods Smoking Pregnancy Exercise	Raising head of bed Antacids Small, frequent, low-fat meals Avoidance of tight garments		Pain often relieved by viscous lidocaine Esophagoscopy Upper GI radiograph Esophageal pH monitoring
Gastritis	Especially alcoholics	Abdominal pain Vague indigestion Heartburn	Decreased appetite Sense of fullness Nausea and vomiting	Alcohol Meals Drugs (aspirin, NSAIDs, corticosteroids, antibiotics, antiasthma agents)	Bile gastritis may be relieved by vomiting	Tenderness to abdominal palpation or epigastric percussion	Endoscopy Upper GI radiograph Gastric biopsy
Active chronic gastritis	Especially older adults	Indigestion			Bismuth compounds (Pepto-Bismol) Antimicrobials		Gastric mucosal biopsy Urea breath test Serologic test for *H. pylori*

Nonulcer dyspepsia		Diffuse abdominal pain or discomfort	Nocturnal pain uncommon		Pain not usually relieved by antacids		Endoscopy
Functional GI disorder	Children and adults	Distention Awareness of peristalsis and gurgling Intermittent symptoms Vague, nonspecific symptoms No weight loss Continuous pain	Significant emotional investment Other neurotic symptoms Belching (from aerophagia)	Social/environmental stresses		No signs of systemic disease	Studies normal
Excessive intestinal gas	Common in elderly	Vague feelings of indigestion	Abdominal bloating Belching Passing flatus	Increased ingestion of flatulogenic foods (e.g., bagels, legumes, high-fiber foods) GI stasis Gut hypomotility Bacterial change Constipation Lack of exercise	Belching Passing flatus		
Gas entrapment (hepatic or splenic flexure syndrome)		Abdominal discomfort Pain often referred to chest	Chest pain	Bending over Wearing tight garments	Passing flatus	Flexion of thigh on abdomen replicates symptoms	Abdominal radiograph shows trapped gas in hepatic or splenic flexure
Gallbladder disease		Vague abdominal discomfort Occasional distention Indigestion	Nausea Pain in right shoulder	Fatty foods			Cholecystograms Sonograms

Pound SE, Heading RC: Diagnosis and treatment of dyspepsia in the elderly. Drugs Aging 7:347–354, 1995.

Richter JE: Dyspepsia: organic causes and differential characteristics from functional dyspepsia. Scand J Gastroenterol 26 (suppl 182):11–16, 1991.

Talley NJ: Nonulcer dyspepsia: current approaches to diagnosis and management. Am Fam Physician 47:1407–1416, 1993.

Talley NJ, Silverstein MD, Agreus L, et al: AGA technical review: evaluation of dyspepsia. Gastroenterology 114:582–595, 1998.

Thompson WG, Heaton KW: Functional bowel disorders in apparently healthy people. Gastroenterology 79:283–288, 1980.

CHAPTER 19

Insomnia

Of all the sleep problems, disorders of initiating and maintaining sleep (insomnias) are the most common. Studies have shown that hypnotics are used regularly by about 20% of the adult population. Insomnia includes the following problems: delay in falling asleep, poor quality of sleep (deficiency of deep and rapid eye movement [REM] sleep), frequent awakening, and early-morning wakefulness.

Insomnia can be caused by *physical disorders* (e.g., congestive heart failure, pregnancy, hyperthyroidism, nocturnal asthma, nocturnal seizures); *painful* or *uncomfortable syndromes* (e.g., toothache, arthritis, restless legs syndrome), *psychiatric illnesses* (e.g., depression, anxiety, schizophrenia, mania), use or withdrawal of *drugs* (e.g., caffeine, alcohol, antidepressants, sympathomimetics, beta blockers, hypnotics); and *situational stressors.* **The most common causes are ingestion of caffeine, alcohol consumption, anxiety, and depression.** Insomnia may be transient or chronic.

Nature of Patient

Nocturnal enuresis (bedwetting), *sleepwalking, talking while asleep,* and *night terrors* are thought to be arousal disorders because they usually occur with emergence from deep non-REM sleep. Children who experience nocturnal enuresis and sleepwalking often have difficulty sleeping. Bedwetting is the most common sleep-arousal disorder in children between ages 3 and 15. It is more prevalent in males than in females. When no obvious organic or psychological cause exists, bedwetting usually occurs in the first part of the night as the child emerges from delta sleep and before the first REM sleep. The change of sleep state often is accompanied by body movements and increased muscle tone; urination occurs during this period. Although most of these problems have a psychological cause, many investigators believe that such disorders have a psychophysiologic rather than strictly psychological basis.

Nightmares and night terrors often disturb sleep. Nightmares, in both children and adults, occur during REM sleep. Night terrors, characterized by sudden screams and arousal, occur during deep sleep. **Insomnia in children is most often caused by psychological stress but occasionally results from organic disease** (e.g., hip disorder).

Some patients who snore have *sleep-induced apnea,* which causes nocturnal wakefulness and daytime drowsiness. These patients typically are obese males and loud snorers. They may have as many as 100 episodes of sleep apnea each night; many episodes lead to brief arousal.

Sleep patterns often change with aging; many elderly people require less sleep than they did in their younger years. Elderly patients often complain of both delay in falling asleep and poor sleep quality. They also sleep less efficiently in that the time spent asleep while lying in bed decreases 70% to 80%. They are more likely to awaken from environmental stimuli such as noise and temperature.

Many patients who ingest products that contain *caffeine* (e.g., coffee, tea, cola) complain of insomnia. Even those patients who previously tolerated caffeine well may develop sleeping problems. Because the half-life of caffeine may range from 2 to more than 6 hours in different people, the ingestion of caffeine, especially after 6 PM, may contribute significantly to insomnia. Patients may or may not be aware that caffeine is the cause of their insomnia. People who drink *alcohol,* even in moderate amounts (i.e., two drinks at night), as well as recovering alcoholics, often experience poor sleep quality with frequent awakening.

Poor sleep at night may be related to napping or dozing during the day, which is more common in elderly people. Elderly patients with *dementia* are often restless and wakeful at night. *Depression,* a common cause of sleep disturbances, is frequently undiagnosed in elderly patients.

Depressed (unipolar affective disorder) patients of all ages frequently experience insomnia characterized by delayed sleep onset (prolonged latency), frequent awakening, and classically, early-morning wakefulness. Patients with *manic depression (bipolar affective disorder)* may experience marked insomnia, especially just before and during the manic phase. Patients who suffer from *anxiety* may have trouble falling asleep but seldom experience early-morning wakefulness.

Nature of Symptoms

Patients usually describe insomnia rather loosely as "trouble sleeping." The physician must determine whether they have difficulty with falling asleep (prolonged sleep latency), staying asleep (poor quality), early-morning wakefulness, or a combination of these problems. Because a patient may have one or more types of insomnia, the physician must question specifically for each type of insomnia to diagnose the cause correctly and to provide effective, specific therapy. *Short-term* (less than 2 weeks) insomnia is most often caused by a life stress, such as emotion, noise, pain, stimulation, grief, anxiety, jet lag, or a change in working hours. *Chronic* insomnia may result from psychiatric disorders (e.g., depression, dysthymic disorder), conditioned insomnia, drugs, caffeine, or alcohol.

Asking patients what they are thinking about before they fall asleep and when they awaken often provides significant clues to the cause of their insomnia. It is also important to interview the sleep partner of an insomniac about snoring, apnea, leg twitches, seizures, and unusual sleep postures. Bedside tape recorders may also help to document snoring.

Prolonged sleep latency (the time from turning the lights out until stage 1 sleep) is most common in anxious patients, caffeine and alcohol users, and elderly patients, especially those who sleep during the day. Most patients overestimate the latency period. Some complain of poor-quality sleep when they do not feel rested despite adequate sleep; this is usually caused by a deficiency of deep REM sleep and is particularly common in patients with painful syndromes, pregnant women, people who consume alcohol, and recovering alcoholics.

Some patients, particularly alcoholics, complain of frequent awakening; this is usually from stage 2 sleep. **Early-morning awakening from which a patient cannot return to sleep is most common and particularly characteristic of depressed patients.** Some studies show depressed patients to have prolonged sleep latency, decreased total sleep, increased intermittent awakening, and less deep sleep than other patients.

Associated Symptoms

Painful and *uncomfortable conditions* such as pleurisy, peptic esophagitis, toothaches, pregnancy, and even severe itching can interfere with normal sleep. *Restless legs* while awake, especially in the evenings, may be associated with *periodic limb movements* while asleep, thus disturbing sleep or even causing full awakening. Paroxysmal nocturnal dyspnea, nocturnal asthma, hyperthyroidism, alcoholism, use of caffeine or other drugs, recent cessation of hypnotics or antidepressants, and severe snoring may also contribute to sleeping problems.

Although anxiety and depression often cause insomnia, patients with these conditions usually have additional symptoms. *Anxious patients* often have somatic complaints such as headaches, chest pain, palpitations, dizziness, gastrointestinal distress, nervousness, and feelings of foreboding. *Depressed patients* frequently complain of decreased appetite, weight loss, lack of energy, lack of interest in activities, decreased libido, constipation, and vague aches and pains. Patients with fibrositis *(fibromyalgia)* and insomnia (which some investigators attribute to depression) may obtain excellent relief of their aches, pains, and insomnia with antidepressant medication.

The daytime consequences of insomnia may provide diagnostic clues. Fatigue, poor performance, impaired concentration, and irritability are common to both insomnia and depressive disorders.

Precipitating and Aggravating Factors

Patients who complain of insomnia should be questioned about whether certain situations (e.g., death in the family, financial concerns, family crises, school examinations, changes in life patterns, alterations in work schedules, changes in drug habits) coincided with the onset of insomnia. So-called rebound insomnia often occurs with cessation of benzodiazepine drugs, especially at higher dosage levels. Paradoxically, these drugs may have originally been used as hypnotics. The patient should also be questioned about prior episodes of insomnia and what may

Differential Diagnosis of Insomnia

CAUSE	NATURE OF PATIENT	NATURE OF SYMPTOMS	ASSOCIATED SYMPTOMS	PRECIPITATING AND AGGRAVATING FACTORS
Bedwetting (nocturnal enuresis) Nightmares and night terrors	Children (especially ages 3–15) More common in males More common in children	Arousal after deep sleep Arousal during REM sleep	Sleepwalking	Environmental or psychological stresses and fears
Painful or uncomfortable conditions Physical disorders	Any age	Delayed latency Poor sleep quality	Symptoms related to physical disorder or painful or uncomfortable condition	Toothache Pleurisy Arthritis Pregnancy Esophagitis Nocturnal asthma or seizures Congenital hip lesions Hyperthyroidism Nocturia
Change in sleep habits	Elderly people	Delayed sleep latency Poor sleep quality	Daytime naps or dozing	
Unipolar depression	Depressed	Delayed sleep latency Early-morning wakefulness	Anorexia Fatigue Lack of interest in activities Decreased libido Constipation Vague aches and pains	Conditions, medications, and situations that produce depression
Bipolar depression	Manic Manic-depressive	May not sleep at all during manic phases	Agitation Hyperactivity Flight of ideas	Worse just before and during manic phase

Anxiety	Any age	Delayed sleep latency	Somatic complaints Headaches Chest pain Palpitations Dizziness Gastrointestinal symptoms Nervousness Feelings of foreboding	Situations that produce anxiety
Sleep apnea	Adults Often obese males	Frequent awakening Poor sleep quality	Snoring Excess daytime sleepiness	Sleep apnea Obstruction Central apnea
Caffeine	Any age	Delayed sleep latency Poor sleep quality	May have previously tolerated caffeine well	Use of caffeine (especially after 6 PM)
Alcohol	Teenagers Adults Elderly	Delayed latency Frequent awakening	Nervousness Signs of alcoholism	Alcohol Alcoholic withdrawal Recovering alcoholics
Withdrawal of antidepressants or hypnotics	Any age	Similar to prior symptoms	May redevelop symptoms of anxiety, depression	
Medications and drugs	Any age	Poor sleep quality Prolonged sleep latency	Depends on drug responsible	Psychotropics Beta blockers Bronchodilators Sympathomimetics Diuretics Hypnotics Appetite suppressants Amphetamines Cocaine

have precipitated them. Transient insomnia may occur in anticipation of a joyous event or during periods of excitement.

According to one study of patients referred to a sleep center, the most common cause of insomnia is ingestion of *caffeine* in any form. Many of these patients previously tolerated caffeine well. The second most common cause is *alcohol.* Although small amounts of alcohol may facilitate sleep onset for some patients, it may also cause early awakening or nightmares, contrary to common belief. These patients often note poor quality of sleep and frequent awakening.

In evaluating sleep disturbances, physicians should have patients keep a sleep diary for 1 week. Patients should note the time they retire, their latency period, number of awakenings, time of last awakening, any sleep events (e.g., dreams, nightmares, need to urinate), and any comments made by the sleep partner. It is particularly important for patients to note their thoughts during latency and on awakening, since these may help establish the cause of their insomnia.

Other precipitating and aggravating factors in insomnia include fear of illness and even pruritus. Although these factors may be tolerated during the day when the patient is active, they may be distracting enough to cause insomnia when the patient is at rest.

Ameliorating Factors

Hypnotics, including over-the-counter preparations, are occasionally helpful for short periods of insomnia. However, their continued use (for more than 1 week) may exacerbate insomnia, particularly if REM sleep has been suppressed. Hypnotics are *rarely* indicated to treat the symptom insomnia. **Insomnia is treated by dealing with its cause.**

Daytime naps or pain can be identified as the probable cause of insomnia if cessation of the former or relief of the latter results in improved sleep. If avoidance of caffeine (in all forms) after noon permits the return of normal sleep patterns, caffeine was probably responsible for the insomnia. When changes in work shifts are associated with insomnia, patients should be advised to try to return to their original sleep schedule to determine whether this eliminates their insomnia. Avoidance of noisy or extremely warm environments and strenuous exercise at night also may facilitate a return to normal sleep patterns.

Physical Findings

The physical examination is usually not helpful in determining the cause of insomnia. Occasionally, medical conditions that contribute to insomnia may yield abnormal physical findings; this occurs in hyperthyroidism, congestive heart failure, peptic esophagitis, pulmonary disease, ulcer disease, seizure disorders, and prostatism. Any condition that causes frequent nocturia may interfere with normal sleep patterns.

Diagnostic Studies

When the cause of insomnia cannot be determined and the patient cannot find relief, he or she should be referred to a sleep center for polysomnographic studies.

Less Common Diagnostic Considerations

Conditions that occur less frequently include nocturnal *myoclonus,* painful erections, central *sleep apnea,* and *restless legs syndrome.* The last two conditions are more common in elderly people. Sleep apnea often is exacerbated by hypnotics and alcohol.

Recently, physicians are increasingly recognizing *primary* sleep disorders rather than assuming that insomnia is a symptom of other disorders.

Selected References

Folks DG, Fuller WC: Anxiety disorders and insomnia in geriatric patients. Psychiatr Clin North Am 20:137–164, 1997.

Gillen JC, Byerly WF: The diagnosis and management of insomnia. N Engl J Med 322:239–248, 1990.

Hauri PJ, Esther MS: Insomnia. Mayo Clin Proc 65:869–882, 1990.

Kales A, Soldatos CR, Kales JD: Sleep disorders: insomnia, sleepwalking, night terrors, nightmares and enuresis. Ann Intern Med 106:582–592, 1987.

Kogeorgos J, Scott DF: Sleep and sleep disorders. Practitioner 224:717–721, 1980.

Pring PN, Vitiello MV, Raskind MH, Thorpy MJ: Geriatrics: sleep disorders and aging. N Engl J Med 323:520–526, 1990.

Reite M, Buyase D, Reynolds C, Mendelson W: The use of polysomnography in the evaluation of insomnia. Sleep 18:58–70, 1995.

Spielman AJ, Nunes J, Glovinsky PB: Insomnia. Neurol Clin 14:513–543, 1996.

Walsh JK, Mahowold MW: Avoiding the blanket approach to insomnia: targeted therapy for specific causes. Postgrad Med 90:211–224, 1991.

Ware JC, Morewitz J: Diagnosis and treatment of insomnia and depression. J Clin Psychiatry 52(6):55–61, 1991.

Yousaf F, Sedgwick P: Sleep disorders. Br J Hosp Med 55:353–358, 1996.

CHAPTER 20

Menstrual Irregularities

Abnormal Bleeding

Menstrual irregularity is especially common in the perimenarchal and perimenopausal years. Bleeding from the vagina is considered *abnormal* when it occurs at an unexpected time of life (before menarche or after menopause) or when it varies from the norm in amount or pattern. *Spontaneous abortions, pregnancy complications,* and *bleeding from polyps* or other pathologic processes account for approximately 25% of the cases of abnormal vaginal bleeding.

Dysfunctional uterine bleeding is a confusing nonspecific diagnostic term. It has been defined as abnormal uterine bleeding not due to structural or systemic disease. Therefore, this diagnosis may be reached only by a process of exclusion. It is almost always associated with anovulatory cycles. With advances in the understanding of the neuroendocrinologic basis of the menstrual cycle, diagnosis and therapy have become more specific (see references).

To understand and diagnose the various causes of menstrual irregularities, the examiner must have a thorough knowledge of normal physiology (Fig. 20–1). **Although the history is important, it seldom is diagnostic and serves only as a guide to the origin of the bleeding. In most patients, hormonal or cytologic studies are necessary to establish the correct diagnosis.**

Anovulatory Bleeding

Hormonal mechanisms of endometrial bleeding include *estrogen-withdrawal bleeding, estrogen-breakthrough bleeding, progesterone-withdrawal bleeding,* and *progesterone-breakthrough bleeding.* **Anovulatory, hormone-related bleeding is most common.** This form of dysfunctional uterine bleeding is caused by estrogen-withdrawal or estrogen-breakthrough bleeding.

Estrogen-withdrawal bleeding. In estrogen-withdrawal bleeding the endometrium proliferates and remains stable as long as the estrogen level remains above the threshold. When the estrogen falls below the threshold, bleeding occurs. In the absence of progesterone, the endometrium is not in the secretory phase, and bleeding is often prolonged and profuse. This type of bleeding often occurs during adolescence and the climacteric.

Estrogen-breakthrough bleeding. This type of bleeding has been divided into two categories. The first is associated with low but constant levels of estrogen (near the threshold). This causes portions of the endometrium to degenerate and results in spotting. **This type of threshold-breakthrough bleeding occurs with the use of low-dose oral contraceptives.**

The second type of estrogen-breakthrough bleeding occurs when estrogen

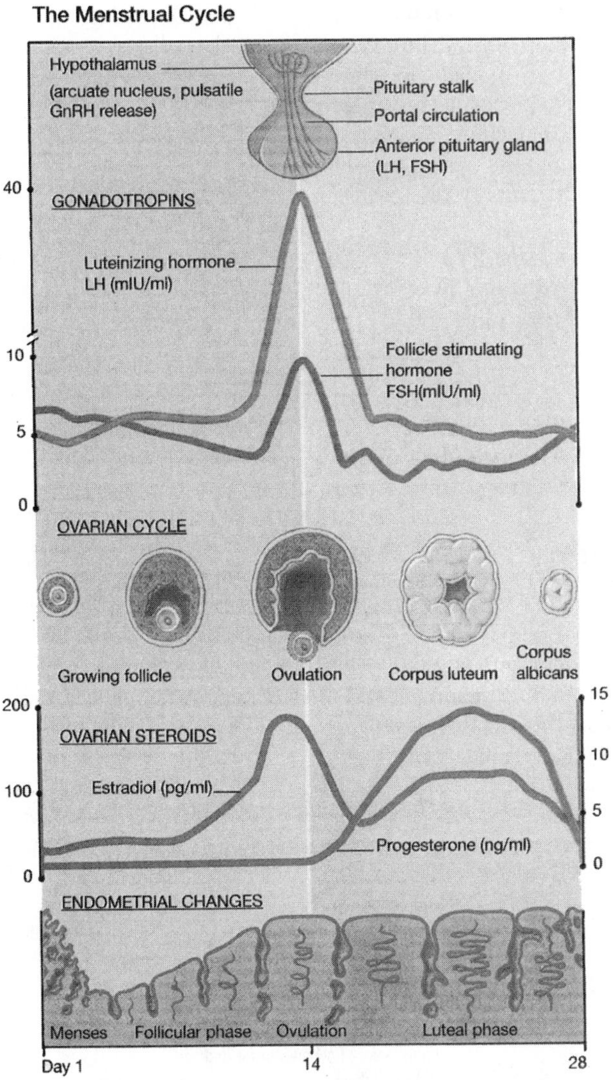

■ **Figure 20.1** Normal menstrual cycle, with pituitary anatomy and levels of gonadotropins, ovarian activity and levels of ovarian steroids, and changes in endometrium. *GnRH,* Gonadotropin-releasing hormone. (From Braverman PK, Sondheimer SJ: Menstrual disorders. Pediatr Rev 18:18, 1997; Illustration by Marcia Smith.)

levels are initially well above the threshold. This causes the endometrium to proliferate and become hyperplastic. Areas of endometrium outgrow their blood-borne hormone supply, resulting in degeneration and irregular, prolonged bleeding.

Progesterone-withdrawal bleeding. As in polycystic ovarian syndrome, this type of bleeding occurs only with an estrogen-primed endometrium. When estrogen therapy is continued as progesterone is withdrawn, progesterone-withdrawal bleeding occurs. This type of bleeding is observed when intramuscular progesterone or oral medroxyprogesterone acetate (Provera) is administered as a test for the presence of endogenous estrogen.

Progesterone-breakthrough bleeding. This form of estrogen-breakthrough bleeding occurs when a high dose of progestational drug is given.

Dysfunctional Ovulatory Bleeding

Dysfunctional ovulatory bleeding may be suspected by history and confirmed with simple investigations (Table 20–1). Ovulatory bleeding is usually associated with a regular cycle length, occasional ovulation pain (mittelschmerz), premenstrual symptoms (e.g., breast soreness, bloating, weight gain, mood changes), and a biphasic basal body temperature. *Anovulatory bleeding* causes an irregular cycle in which bleeding is not preceded by or associated with subjective symptoms. The basal body temperature pattern is monophasic.

Bleeding Patterns

Recognition of particular bleeding patterns is another way of considering cases of abnormal vaginal bleeding (Table 20–2). *Menorrhagia,* or *hypermenorrhea* (excessive menstrual bleeding), is often caused by local gynecologic disease (e.g., polyps, cancer, salpingitis, uterine fibroids). It also occurs in association with intrauterine contraceptive devices (IUDs).

TABLE 20.1 Differentiation of Ovulatory and Anovulatory Bleeding

CRITERIA	OVULATORY BLEEDING	ANOVULATORY BLEEDING
History	Regular cycle length Ovulation pain (mittelschmerz) Premenstrual molimina (breast soreness, bloating, weight gain, mood change) Dysmenorrhea (cramps up to 12 hours before flow and/or for first 2 days of flow)	Irregular cycles in which bleeding is not preceded by or associated with subjective symptoms
Basal body temperature record	Biphasic pattern	Monophasic pattern
Cervical mucus	Preovulatory: thin, clear, watery mucus with stretchability (spinnbarkeit) and ferning	Always dominated by estrogen
Maturation index	Preovulatory: dominated by superficial cells Postovulatory: shift to high percentage of intermediate cells	Always a marked right shift due to high estrogen level
Premenstrual endometrial biopsy	Secretory endometrium	Proliferative and possibly hyperplastic changes
Serum progesterone level	Preovulatory: <1 ng/mL Postovulatory: >5 ng/mL	Never exceeds 5 ng/mL; usually preovulatory values

From Strickler RC: Dysfunctional uterine bleeding: diagnosis and treatment. Postgrad Med 66:135–146, 1979.

TABLE 20.2 Nomenclature to Describe Menstrual Disturbances

TERM	BLEEDING PATTERN
Menorrhagia	Excessive flow (amount and/or duration) with normal cycle (21-35 days)
Polymenorrhea	Normal flow with cycle less than 21 days
Polymenorrhagia	Excessive flow with cycle less than 21 days
Metrorrhagia	Excessive flow that is acyclic
Metrostaxis	Continuous bleeding
Ovulation bleeding (pseudopolymenorrhea)	Spotting or light flow at time of midcycle estrogen nadir
Premenstrual staining	Spotting or light flow up to 7 days before menstruation in ovulatory cycle

From Strickler RC: Dysfunctional uterine bleeding: diagnosis and treatment. Postgrad Med 66:135-146, 1979.

Metrorrhagia (intermenstrual spotting between otherwise normal periods) is also often caused by local disease. It frequently is associated with exogenous estrogen therapy. *Menometrorrhagia* is bleeding that is unpredictable with regard to amount and frequency. It can be caused by local lesions, complications of early gestation, or endocrine dysfunction (e.g., dysfunctional bleeding).

Polymenorrhagia is excessive cyclic hemorrhage occurring at intervals of 21 days or less. This type of bleeding is most often the result of anovulatory cycles.

Nature of Patient

Before menarche, a characteristic sequence of events begins at about age 8 (Fig. 20–2). Breast buds develop, pubic hairs appear, breasts enlarge, axillary hairs appear, and finally a height spurt occurs. Menstrual function usually begins after the height spurt. About 6 months before menarche, a physiologic leukorrhea occurs. In the first year after menarche, 55% of menses are anovulatory, with a sharp decline to about 7% by 8 years after menarche. Usually 15 months are required for completion of the first 10 menstrual cycles. This means that when menses begin, it is unusual for them to occur at regular monthly intervals.

The average age at which girls begin to menstruate is 12 years. Table 20–3 shows the characteristics of normal menstruation. Bleeding that occurs before 9 to 10 years of age is abnormal, and local pathology as well as adrenal and ovarian tumors must be suspected. Because some teenage girls are reluctant to volunteer information about their menstrual periods, it is essential that physicians routinely ask a series of questions:

1. When did your menses begin?
2. How often do your menstrual periods occur?
3. On what date did your last period occur?
4. Is there any pain associated with menstruation?
5. Are you sexually active?
6. Are you practicing any form of birth control?

These questions must be asked in a nonthreatening way so that the patient feels at ease and understands that the physician is willing to listen. Likewise, when asking

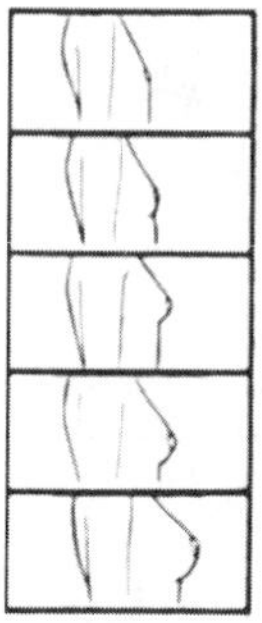

Stage	Description
Breast development	
B1	Preadolescent: elevation of nipple only
B2	Breast-bud stage: elevation of breast and nipple as a small mound
B3	Further enlargement of breast and areola with no separation of contours
B4	Projection of areola so as to form a secondary mound
B5	Mature stage: nipple projects from general contour of breast

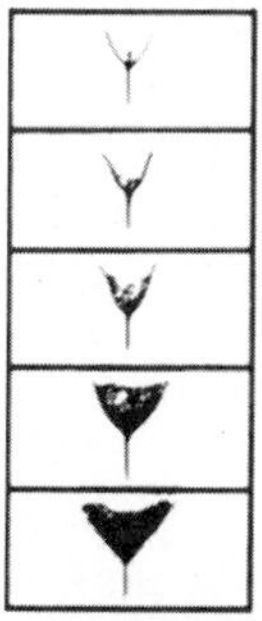

Stage	Description
Pubic hair development	
PH1	None
PH2	Sparse growth of long straight hair along labia; no hair on mons pubis
PH3	Thicker, coarse, curled hair on mons pubis
PH4	Adult-type hair on mons pubis but not reaching the medial aspect of thighs
PH5	Hair reaches the medial surface of thighs

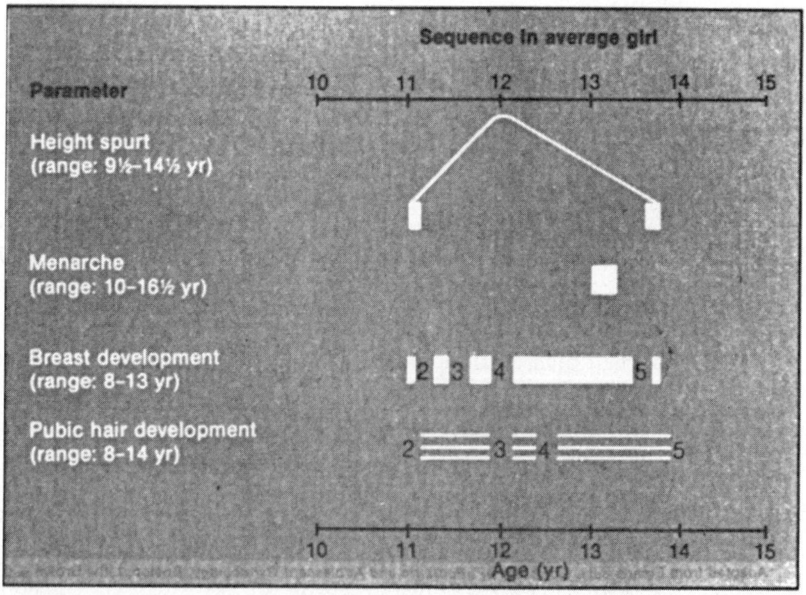

■ **Figure 20.2** Relationship of pubertal events in adolescent girls. (From Lopez RI: Menstrual irregularities in teenage girls. Drug Therapy, April 1981, p 49.)

TABLE 20.3 Characteristics of Menstruation*

CHARACTERISTICS	RANGE	AVERAGE
Menarche (age of onset)	9-17 years	12.5 years
Cycle length (interval)	21-35 days	28 days
Duration of flow	1-8 days	3-5 days
Amount of flow	10-80 mL	35 mL
Onset of menopause	45-55 years	47-50 years

*Range and averages for American women.
From Hamilton C: Vaginal bleeding: evaluation and management. Resident Staff Physician, November 1981, pp 62-64.

questions about sexual activities, the physician must remain nonjudgmental. The teenager should be reassured that any discussion of this nature will remain a private matter between patient and physician.

The adolescent typically has cycles of variable length. Anovulation may be associated with both short and long cycles together with short follicular and luteal cycles. Menarche may be delayed in underweight adolescents, as well as in some teenage girls who are on strict diets to remain fashionably thin and in athletes with normal body weight but low body fat. Menarche often has a familial pattern; girls often start menstruating at about the same age as their mothers and sisters did.

Several significant age-associated conditions can cause abnormal vaginal bleeding. In children, insertion of *foreign bodies* into the vagina may cause bleeding. During the reproductive years, *dysfunctional uterine bleeding* and bleeding from *pregnancy complications, tumors,* and *fibroids* may occur (Table 20–4). **A menstruating woman of any age can bleed from complications of pregnancy.** Anovulatory *estrogen-withdrawal bleeding* is the most common cause of irregular menses during the reproductive and perimenopausal years and accounts for 40% of menstrual disturbances in the perimenopausal years.

Other less common causes of abnormal vaginal bleeding in perimenopausal women include *organic lesions* (neoplasm or inflammatory diseases of the cervix, vagina, and endometrium), *constitutional diseases* (hypothyroidism, hyperthyroidism, Cushing's disease, cirrhosis, thrombocytopenia), and certain *drugs* (Table 20–5). In postmenopausal women, bleeding may result from *endometrial* and *cervical cancers.*

Nature of Symptoms

Prolonged irregular and profuse bleeding may occur with either estrogen-breakthrough or estrogen-withdrawal bleeding. The bleeding may be spotty (threshold-breakthrough bleeding). Anovulatory bleeding is usually unexpected and painless. Anovulatory cycles may result in *polymenorrhagia.* With ovulatory menstrual abnormalities, there may be a short luteal phase, in which case menstrual cycles may be variable in length with excessive flow. Patients with these problems may also complain of premenstrual bleeding or staining. When *menor-*

TABLE 20.4 Causes of Vaginal Bleeding in the Reproductive Years

Menstruation and variations	**Exogenous hormones**
Ovulation spotting (midcycle)	Estrogen
	Estrogen-progestin oral contraceptives
Pregnancy complications	**Trauma**
Early (<20 weeks)	**Anticoagulant drugs**
Implantation bleeding	**Organic gynecologic disease**
Abortion	Pelvic infections
Ectopic pregnancy	Neoplastic diseases
Trophoblastic disease	Benign
Late (>20 weeks)	Malignant
Placenta previa, vasa previa, other	Adenomyosis
Postpartum	**Systemic disease**
Uterine atony	Generalized bleeding disorders
Retained products	Thyroid disease
Normal delivery	
Disorders of central nervous system–hypothalamic-ovarian-pituitary axis	
Dysfunctional uterine bleeding	
Anovulatory (80%–90%)	
Ovulatory	
Functioning ovarian cysts or tumors	
Emotional stress	
Anticholinergic drugs	

From Hamilton C: Vaginal bleeding: evaluation and management. Resident Staff Physician, November 1981, pp 62–64.

rhagia is present, *tumors, fibroids, cancer, polyps, salpingitis,* or *IUDs* may be the cause. *Endometriosis* (see Chapter 21), *salpingitis,* and *cancer* may also cause minimal bleeding and should be suspected if purulent discharge is present.

During the reproductive years, abnormal vaginal bleeding often represents *pregnancy complications.* The patient may have a history of sexual activity without adequate contraceptive measures. In addition, symptoms of pregnancy, such as missed periods, morning sickness, and breast tenderness, may be present. In these patients the uterine bleeding initially results from endometrial sloughing, and therefore spotting rather than amenorrhea may occur before gross hemorrhage.

Gross hemorrhage may be concealed or visible. *Ectopic pregnancy* is strongly suggested by an adnexal or cul-de-sac mass in a pregnant woman who has a normal or only slightly enlarged uterus. Concealed pelvic hemorrhage from a ruptured ectopic pregnancy can occur either with or without vaginal bleeding. This diagnosis should be suspected when the patient has amenorrhea, pelvic or abdominal fullness, abdominal pain (particularly if unilateral or referred to the shoulder), tenesmus, and urinary frequency or urgency. Fever, signs of peritoneal irritation, purulent vaginal discharge, and pain can be seen in patients with ectopic pregnancy or salpingitis.

Copious vaginal bleeding most often results from pregnancy complications and less often from local gynecologic disease or dysfunctional bleeding. Bright-red hemorrhage with clots suggests a brisk nonmenstrual flow. A darker tint of blood implies slower hemorrhage acted on by cervical or vaginal secretions. Irregular bleeding during pregnancy may result from separation of the placenta or the embryo from its attachment, but malignant cervical erosions, polyps, and local vaginal lesions must be excluded.

Menorrhagia during puberty is usually caused by anovulation. This gradually abates within several months of the onset of the menarche. Menorrhagia during the reproductive years can also result from anovulation, as can *polymenorrhagia.* Menorrhagia that occurs during the reproductive years may be caused by *fibromyomas.* **The chief characteristic of a uterine fibroid is an asymmetrically enlarged uterus.** More than one fibroid may be present in the uterus, and the shape can be extremely irregular. As a rule, the consistency of the fibroid is hard and unyielding. Usually the cervix and uterine fibroid move together.

It may be difficult for the physician to distinguish a fibromyoma from an *ovarian cyst.* **A helpful point in the differentiation of fibroids from ovarian**

TABLE 20.5 Common Drugs That May Alter Menstrual Bleeding

GROUP AND GENERIC NAMES	TRADE AND COMMON NAMES
*Amphetamines	*Desoxyn, Obetrol
Anticoagulants	Coumadin, heparin
*Benzodiazepines	
Diazepam, oxazepam	*Valium, Serax
Benzomide derivatives	
Procainamide, procarbazine	Pronestyl, Matulane
*Butyrophenones	*Haldol, Inapsine
Cannabis	Marijuana
Chlordiazepoxide	Librium
*Cimetidine	Tagamet
Ethyl alcohol	Whiskey, wine, beer
*Isoniazid	*INH
*Methyldopa	*Aldomet
Monoamine oxidase inhibitors	Eutonyl, Nardil
*Opiates	*Morphine, heroin, methadone
*Phenothiazines	*Compazine, Thorazine, Phenergan
Prostaglandin inhibitors	Motrin, Indocin
Rauwolfia	Raudixin
*Reserpine	*Serpasil
*Spironolactone	*Aldactone
Steroids	
Gonadal	
*Estrogens	*Premarin, oral contraceptives
*Progesterones	*Provera, oral contraceptives
*Testosterone	*Android
Thyroid hormones	Synthroid, Cytomel
*Thioxanthenes	*Navane
*Tricyclic antidepressants	*Elavil

*May also produce galactorrhea.

Modified from Murata JN: Abnormal genital bleeding and secondary amenorrhea: common gynecological problems. J Obstet Gynecol Neonatal Nurs 19:26–36, 1990.

cysts is that ovarian cysts almost never cause menorrhagia. Ovarian tumors usually create no menstrual disturbances. *Adenomyoma* of the uterus usually causes symmetric uterine enlargement, but absolute differentiation must be accomplished by pathologic examination.

Chronic salpingo-oophoritis (hydrosalpinx, tubo-ovarian abscess, or *chronic salpingitis*) and *ovarian endometriosis* can cause menorrhagia, and congestive (premenstrual) dysmenorrhea is usually present as a prominent symptom. Menorrhagia can also be caused by IUDs, thrombocytopenia, and other coagulation defects.

Irregular menstrual bleeding may be divided into three groups: (1) irregular bleeding during menstrual life, (2) bleeding before puberty and after menopause, and (3) bleeding during pregnancy.

Irregular Bleeding During Menstrual Life (see Table 20–4)

Metrorrhagia. The most common cause of bleeding or spotting between regular menses is breakthrough bleeding associated with oral contraceptives, but complications of pregnancy must always be considered. The lesions of the reproductive organs that cause metrorrhagia include *cervical carcinoma, benign* and *malignant uterine tumors, endometritis,* and rarely *tuberculous endometritis. Fibromyomas* usually cause menorrhagia but occasionally can cause metrorrhagia. Fibroids tend to produce irregular bleeding when they are submucosal or in the process of extrusion. A carcinoma can develop in a patient known to have uterine fibroids, and a fibroid occasionally can undergo sarcomatous degeneration. Rapid enlargement of the uterus associated with irregular bleeding is very suggestive of a *sarcoma.* However, several fibroids can be present in the same uterus and are a common cause of rapid uterine enlargement. *Choriocarcinoma* is a rare cause of uterine enlargement that follows a *hydatidiform mole* in about 50% of the recorded cases. It should be suspected during early pregnancy when abortion is a threat and the uterus is extremely enlarged. Choriocarcinoma is also likely in women who have persistent uterine enlargement.

Cervical erosions usually do not bleed. If irregular bleeding occurs from the erosion or if the cervix bleeds during an examination, cancer should be excluded.

Menorrhagia. *Polyps* and *fibroids* are common causes of menorrhagia, which has been defined as blood loss of greater than 80 mL per period or as menses lasting longer than 7 days. Typical menstrual blood loss is 30 to 40 mL. *Dysfunctional uterine bleeding* can occur at any age. Half of cases occur in women between ages 40 and 50, about 10% develop at puberty, and the remaining 40% occur between puberty and age 40. Dysfunctional uterine bleeding, most frequently due to an anovulatory cycle, usually is in the form of menorrhagia, although the interval between periods may be shortened.

Women using *estrogen preparations* to control menstrual symptoms or to prevent conception may develop menorrhagia while the drugs are being taken or following their withdrawal. The menorrhagia is often related to the dosage of estrogen.

Coagulopathies and hypothyroidism may present as menorrhagia.

Bleeding associated with *ovulation* is uncommon; when it occurs, it is midway between the periods (approximately at the time of ovulation). Midmenstrual cycle bleeding accompanied by lower abdominal pain is termed *mittelschmerz.*

Bleeding Before Puberty and After Menopause

Vaginal bleeding in neonates is usually caused by a temporarily *high fetal estrogen concentration.* Postmenopausal bleeding may result from *malignant growths, polyps, senile endometritis,* or *cervicitis. Carcinoma of the uterine body* seldom causes much uterine enlargement, and any increase in size usually occurs slowly. Because the postmenopausal uterus shrinks considerably, a uterine size that would be regarded as normal in a younger woman indicates abnormal enlargement in a postmenopausal woman.

Bleeding During Pregnancy

It is important for the physician to differentiate the uterine hemorrhage of extrauterine gestation from that due to threatened abortion. Bleeding can be caused by *placenta previa* and *abruptio placentae.*

Associated Symptoms

Ovulatory irregular bleeding is often associated with midcycle ovulation pain (mittelschmerz), premenstrual symptoms, and dysmenorrhea. Fever, purulent vaginal discharge, and pain may be clues to *pregnancy complications,* including spontaneous and induced *abortion.* These same signs and symptoms may be observed in cases of *ectopic pregnancy* and *salpingitis.* Irregular menses associated with galactorrhea suggests a *prolactinoma.* Anovulatory irregular bleeding associated with hirsutism and occasionally hypertension suggests *polycystic ovarian syndrome.*

Precipitating and Aggravating Factors

Anovulatory irregular menstrual bleeding often occurs during the first 12 to 18 months after menarche. It is seen most often in obese patients; in women who have adrenal disease, pituitary tumors, polycystic ovary syndrome, Cushing's disease, diabetes, malnutrition, chronic illness, or hypothyroidism; and in patients who use phenothiazines or opiates (see Table 20–5).

Physical Findings

Physical examination should include thorough pelvic, vaginal, and abdominal evaluations. It should be directed at detection of systemic diseases such as *endocrinopathies,* including adult-onset adrenal hyperplasia, Cushing's disease, thyroid dysfunction, polycystic ovaries, and obesity.

Diagnostic Studies

Diagnostic tests useful in the differential diagnosis of patients with abnormal vaginal bleeding include a complete blood count (CBC), reticulocyte count, platelet count, and coagulation studies; pregnancy tests; thyroid-stimulating hormone (TSH), follicle-stimulating hormone (FSH), and luteinizing hormone (LH) tests; plasma glucose; and urinalysis. Other diagnostic tests that help the physician evaluate the cause of abnormal vaginal bleeding include uterine curettage; endometrial, vaginal, and cervical biopsies; a Papanicolaou test for detection of cancer; and Gram's stain and culture for determination of infections. Transvaginal ultrasonography is useful in diagnosing the cause of menometrorrhagia.

Pelvic ultrasonography helps the physician diagnose ectopic pregnancies, ovarian cysts, and tumors. **Because most patients of reproductive age who have severe uterine bleeding are pregnant, human chorionic gonadotropin (HCG) levels should be determined.** HCG is produced during uterine or ectopic pregnancy, development of hydatidiform moles, and formation of choriocarcinoma. The most sensitive test for detecting early pregnancy is radioimmunoassay (RIA) for the beta subunit of HCG. This test often allows the physician to detect pregnancy as early as 1 week after fertilization, whereas less sensitive urine tests may not confirm a normal pregnancy until the seventh week. **This test is particularly important, since the physician cannot exclude the possibility of an ectopic pregnancy on the basis of a negative urine test.** However, a negative serum RIA almost always excludes an ectopic pregnancy.

Although ectopic pregnancy accounts for only 0.5% of all pregnancies, it is the cause of 10% to 15% of maternal deaths. More than 90% of ectopic pregnancies are caused by tubal implants that rupture during the first trimester. Major risk factors for ectopic pregnancy include history of a previous ectopic pregnancy, salpingitis, previous tubal procedure, and pregnancy that occurs when an IUD is in place.

The physician is unlikely to miss a catastrophic rupture; however, some ectopic pregnancies leak slowly over several days, so they may go unrecognized until the patient's second or third visit. Ultrasonography helps rule out an ectopic pregnancy by confirming the presence of a uterine gestational sac with an intrauterine pregnancy. With a positive culdocentesis or a suspicious sonogram, laparoscopy must be performed, followed by surgical exploration if an ectopic pregnancy is seen. A negative RIA for the beta subunit of HCG essentially excludes any pregnancy complication.

Less Common Diagnostic Considerations

Patients with *endometriosis* may have abnormal vaginal bleeding but usually have dull backaches and dyspareunia associated with congestive dysmenorrhea. *Cervical erosions* can be detected on physical examination. *Bleeding disorders,* including idiopathic thrombocytopenic purpura, may present with menometrorrhagia. *Thrombocytopenia* is often seen in patients with disseminated lupus.

Because *clear cell adenocarcinoma* of the vagina or cervix can be fatal, the possibility of this tumor must always be considered. It is most common in daughters of the 2 to 3 million women who took diethylstilbestrol (DES) as a fertility drug. These "DES daughters" also may have congenital abnormalities of the cervix, uterus, and upper vagina. In addition, they demonstrate an increased risk of pregnancy complications (e.g., threatened, spontaneous, or induced incomplete abortion and ectopic gestation).

Abnormal vaginal bleeding may also be a sign of a *coagulation defect,* especially platelet deficiency, von Willebrand's disease, or leukemia.

Amenorrhea

The average age of menarche in the United States is 12.7 years, and the age range for menarche is 11 to 15 years (99% of women reach menarche by 16 years). *Primary amenorrhea* refers to the condition in women who fail to menstruate at all. Most young patients simply have delayed menarche. Because weight loss, excessive exercise training, and eating disorders can result in delayed menarche, it is particularly important for the physician to determine the patient's diet. In addition, substances such as amphetamines, cannabis, estrogens, and phenothiazines may interfere with the onset of menstruation (Table 20–6).

TABLE 20.6 Common Drugs That May Cause Amenorrhea

GENERIC NAME	TRADE AND COMMON NAMES
Amphetamines	Desoxyn, Obetrol
Benzodiazepines	
Diazepam, oxazepam	Valium, Serax
Benzomide derivatives	Pronestyl, Matulane
Butyrophenones	Haldol, Inapsine
Calcium channel blockers	
Nifedipine, verapamil, diltiazem	Adalat, Cardizem, Calan
Cannabis	Marijuana
Chemotherapeutics	Cytoxan, Myleran, Leukeran, Platinol
Cimetidine	Tagamet
Isoniazid	INH
Methyldopa	Aldomet
Monoamine oxidase inhibitors	Eutonyl, Nardil
Opiates	Morphine, heroin
Phenothiazines	Compazine, Thorazine, Phenergan
Rauwolfia	Harmonyl, Raudixin
Reserpine	Serpasil
Spironolactone	Aldactone
Steroids	
Gonadal	Ingredients of oral contraceptives
Estrogens	
Progesterones	
Thyroid hormones	Synthroid, Cytomel
Thioxanthenes	Navane
Tricyclic antidepressants	Elavil

Modified from Murata JN: Primary amenorrhea. Pediatr Nurs 15:125–129, 1989.

Primary amenorrhea is rare; it usually is associated with an endocrine imbalance or congenital abnormalities. In patients with this condition, the physician must rule out chromosomal aberrations and genital malformations. In all cases, chromatin analysis of a buccal smear should be performed (Table 20-–7).

Short stature and a webbed neck should suggest *Turner's syndrome.* Age is a significant factor in the diagnosis. For example, a 15-year-old girl who has not yet menstruated usually has a delayed menarche, whereas a 17-year-old girl who has not begun to menstruate is considered to have primary amenorrhea (Fig. 20–3).

Patients with *secondary amenorrhea* have menstruated but then stop. **During the reproductive years the most common cause of secondary amenorrhea is pregnancy.** An endocrine imbalance may be an associated factor, but tumors seldom cause secondary amenorrhea. A vaginal smear and evaluation of the cervical mucus will help in determining whether there is ovarian estrogen production. Various endocrinologic tests help determine whether ovarian progesterone production is normal and whether levels of ovarian androgen are normal or elevated. If a patient with secondary amenorrhea has galactorrhea, a *prolactinoma* is probable.

Table 20–8 lists the various causes of secondary amenorrhea.

Diagnostic studies that are useful in the evaluation of amenorrhea include buccal chromatin analysis, blood and urine hormone estimation, chromosomal analysis, basal body temperature, vaginal smear, tomographs of the pituitary fossa, computed tomography (CT) scans, and a progesterone withdrawal test for determination of whether estrogen is being manufactured.

Less common causes of amenorrhea include *nutritional disorders* and strict *dieting; systemic disorders* such as tuberculosis, diabetes, prolactinoma, hypothy-

Text continued on page 213.

■ **TABLE 20.7 Diagnostic Scheme for Evaluation of Primary Amenorrhea**

Anamnesis — Physical examination

Positive — *Chromatin analysis* (buccal smear) — Negative

Hypogonadotropic amenorrhea Primary ovarian failure	Gonadal dysgenesis ⟶ Testicular feminization XY	Turner's syndrome (XO) Mosaicisms (XO/XY, XO/XX)
Central nervous system tumor or trauma Congenital adrenogenital hyperplasia Congenital absence of uterus and/or vagina Endocrine active ovarian tumors Psychogenic amenorrhea	Pure gonadal dysgenesis (Swyer syndrome XY)	
	Quinacrine staining for Y chromosomes	
	Positive	Negative
Endocrine diagnostic	Testicular feminization Pure gonadal dysgenesis Mosaicisms (XX/XY)	Gonadal dysgenesis (Turner's syndrome) Mosaicisms (XO/XX)

From Lehmann F: Diagnostic approach to ovarian dysfunction. Hormone Res 9:319-338, 1978.

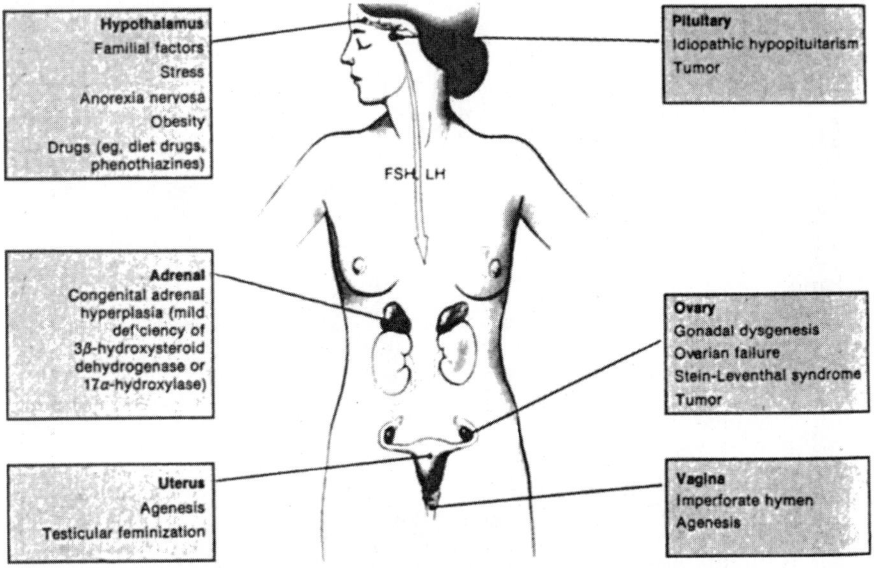

■ **Figure 20.3** Possible causes of primary amenorrhea and delayed menarche. *FSH,* Follicle-stimulating hormone; *LH,* luteinizing hormone. (From Lopez RI: Menstrual irregularities in young girls. Drug Therapy, April 1981, p 42.)

■ **TABLE 20.8 Possible Causes of Secondary Amenorrhea**

	OVARIAN HORMONE PRODUCTION		
NORMAL (CYCLIC)	DECREASED (ACYCLIC)		INCREASED (ACYCLIC)
Asherman's syndrome Endometrial destruction Infective tuberculosis, schistosomiasis) Iatrogenic (curettage, irradiation)	*High gonadotropin levels:* Premature ovarian failure Castration (surgical or radiation)	*Low or normal gonadotropin levels:* Functional aberrations of hypothalamic-pituitary axis Psychogenic factors Nutritional factors Nongonadal endocrine disorders (thyroid, adrenals, pancreas) Systemic infections and chronic diseases Pharmacologic factors (psychotropic drugs, post-pill oversuppression, drug addiction) Central nervous system disease (tumor or trauma)	Polycystic ovary syndrome Virilizing ovarian tumors (arrhenoblastoma, hilus cell tumor) Feminizing ovarian tumors (granulosa cell, thecal cell)

From Lehmann F: Diagnostic approach to ovarian dysfunction. Hormone Res 9:319–338, 1978.

Differential Diagnosis of Menstrual Irregularities

CAUSE	NATURE OF PATIENT	NATURE OF SYMPTOMS	ASSOCIATED SYMPTOMS	PRECIPITATING AND AGGRAVATING FACTORS	PHYSICAL FINDINGS	DIAGNOSTIC STUDIES
Dysfunctional uterine bleeding (hormonal causes)	Can occur at any age 10% of cases occur at puberty 50% of cases occur between ages 40 and 50	Usually due to anovulatory cycles Menorrhagia Interval between periods may be decreased				Diagnosis only by process of exclusion
Anovulatory cycles	Normal occurrence in 55% of girls within first year of menarche	Irregular cycle length Polymenorrhagia Bleeding not preceded by or associated with subjective symptoms		Obesity Adrenal or pituitary disease Polycystic ovaries Diabetes Malnutrition Chronic illness Hypothyroidism Phenothiazines or opiates		Monophasic basal body temperature Serum progesterone level never exceeds 5 ng/mL
Estrogen-withdrawal bleeding	Most common cause of irregular menses in reproductive years, especially adolescence and climacteric	Prolonged, irregular, profuse bleeding	Painless			Endometrial biopsy Serum FSH and LH Pregnancy test
Estrogen-breakthrough bleeding						
Threshold bleeding		Spotty bleeding		Low-dose oral contraceptives		

With estrogen levels above threshold		Prolonged, irregular, profuse bleeding				
Progesterone-breakthrough bleeding Progesterone-withdrawal bleeding				High-dose progestational drugs Intramuscular progesterone or oral medroxyprogesterone acetate (Provera) as test for endogenous estrogen		
Ovulatory cycles		Cycle length is usually regular Premenstrual staining or bleeding Dysmenorrhea	Mittelschmerz Premenstrual syndrome (PMS)			Biophasic basal body temperature Serum progesterone level >3 ng/mL
Complications of pregnancy	Reproductive age	Spotting precedes gross hemorrhage (visible or concealed)	Missed periods Morning sickness Breast tenderness			Serum HCG

Table continued on following page.

Differential Diagnosis of Menstrual Irregularities *Continued*

CAUSE	NATURE OF PATIENT	NATURE OF SYMPTOMS	ASSOCIATED SYMPTOMS	PRECIPITATING AND AGGRAVATING FACTORS	PHYSICAL FINDINGS	DIAGNOSTIC STUDIES
Ectopic pregnancy	Increased risk with previous ectopic pregnancy, salpingitis, previous tubal procedure, or pregnancy with IUD	Amenorrhea Pelvic or abdominal fullness Abdominal pain (usually unilateral) May refer to shoulder May or may not be vaginal bleeding Purulent vaginal discharge	Tenesmus Increased urinary frequency or urgency		Adnexal or cul-de-sac mass Normal or slightly enlarged uterus Peritoneal irritation	
During uterine pregnancy		Irregular bleeding due to separation of placenta or embryo from its attachment				
Spontaneous abortion		Hemorrhage (sometimes with clots)	Fever Purulent vaginal discharge or pain			
Endometriosis (see Chap. 21)		Slight bleeding	Dysmenorrhea Purulent vaginal discharge Dull backache		Implants may be palpable	Pelvic ultrasonography

Endometrial and cervical cancer	Postmenopausal women	Extent of bleeding may vary	Purulent vaginal discharge			Dilatation and curettage Biopsy Pap test
Fibroids	Women of reproductive age	Menorrhagia, occasionally metrorrhagia Irregular bleeding			Uterus is asymmetrically enlarged Fibroids are hard and unyielding Cervix and fibroids usually move together	Pelvic sonogram
Intrauterine device		Menorrhagia	Cervical discharge		IUD	
Salpingitis	Usually occurs in reproductive years	Menorrhagia or slight bleeding	Purulent discharge Fever Abdominal pain Dysmenorrhea		Signs of peritoneal irritation	
Insertion of foreign body into vagina	Most common cause of abnormal vaginal bleeding in children				Foreign body	

Table continued on following page.

Differential Diagnosis of Menstrual Irregularities *Continued*

CAUSE	NATURE OF PATIENT	NATURE OF SYMPTOMS	ASSOCIATED SYMPTOMS	PRECIPITATING AND AGGRAVATING FACTORS	PHYSICAL FINDINGS	DIAGNOSTIC STUDIES
Amenorrhea						
Primary	In girls up to age 17; delayed menarche most common cause Girls age 18 or older who have not yet menstruated (rare)			Severe malnutrition Weight loss Vigorous exercise Amphetamines Phenothiazines Cannabis Endocrine and congenital abnormalities Chromosomal aberrations	Abnormal pubertal development Abnormal external or internal genitalia Short stature	Chromatin analysis
Secondary	Patients have menstruated and then stopped menstruating			Pregnancy Endocrine imbalance Tumors Breast-feeding Oral contraceptives "Postpill" amenorrhea		Vaginal smear and evaluation of cervical mucus to determine ovarian estrogen production and other hormone levels Serum HCG
Prolactinoma			Galactorrhea			Serum prolactin levels CT scan of sella

roidism, and hyperthyroidism; and *psychogenic disturbances,* including severe stress and anorexia nervosa.

Hyperandrogenic chronic anovulation, which includes polycystic ovarian syndrome, should be suspected in obese young women who have normal sexual development, hypertension, and hirsutism. They may have secondary amenorrhea or oligomenorrhea. Early polycystic ovarian syndrome may include severe dysfunctional bleeding and elevated serum gonadotropin levels. The patient also may have severe acne. *Congenital adrenal hyperplasia* (virilizing tumor) is also manifested by hirsutism and severe acne.

Secondary amenorrhea has been reported in female marathon runners, a finding that probably is related to the marked decrease in total body fat in these women. It also has been reported in competitive swimmers and ballet dancers for the same reason.

Asherman's syndrome is amenorrhea due to destruction of the basal layer of the endometrium and adhesions following "overenthusiastic" uterine curettage.

Selected References

Braverman PK, Sondheimer SJ: Menstrual disorders. Pediatr Rev 18:17–27, 1997.

Burnett RG: Diagnostic strategies for amenorrhea. Postgrad Med 87:241–247, 250, 1990.

Dewhurst J: Secondary amenorrhea. Pediatr Ann 10(12):38–42, 1981.

Dodson MG: Use of transvaginal ultrasound in diagnosing the etiology of menometrorrhagia. J Reprod Med 39:362–372, 1994.

Higham JM, O'Brien PM, Shaw RW: Assessment of menstrual blood loss using a pictorial chart. Br J Obstet Gynaecol 97:734–739, 1990.

Kiningham RB, Apgar BS, Schwenk TL: Evaluation of amenorrhea. Am Fam Physician 53:1185–1194, 1996.

Kustin J, Rebar RW: Menstrual disorders in the adolescent age groups. Prim Care 14:139–166, 1987.

Marul EL, Dawood MY: Amenorrhea. Clin Obstet Gynecol 26(3):749–761, 1983.

Neinstein LS: Menstrual problems in adolescents. Med Clin North Am 74:1181–1203, 1991.

Nesse RE: Managing abnormal vaginal bleeding. Postgrad Med 89:205–214, 1991.

Powell LL: Evaluation of abnormal genital bleeding. Clin Issues Perinatal Womens Health Nurs 2:328–338, 1991.

Reindollar RH, Novack M, Tho SPT, McDonnough PG: Adult onset amenorrhea: a study of 262 patients. Am J Obstet Gynecol 155:531–543, 1986.

Soules MR: Adolescent amenorrhea. Pediatr Clin North Am 34:1083–1103, 1987.

Spellacy WN: Abnormal bleeding. Clin Obstet Gynecol 26(3):702–709, 1983.

Strickler RC: Dysfunctional uterine bleeding: diagnosis and treatment. Postgrad Med 66:135–146, 1979.

Wathen PI, Henderson MC, Witz CA: Abnormal uterine bleeding. Med Clin North Am 79:329–343, 1995.

CHAPTER 21

Menstrual Pain

Dysmenorrhea is the term used to describe painful menstruation. It also may occur before menstruation. Approximately 50% of postpubescent women experience dysmenorrhea; 10% of these women are incapacitated by pain for 1 to 3 days per month. As the greatest single cause of lost working hours and school days among young women, dysmenorrhea has been found to be associated with substantial economic losses to the entire community as well as to the patient. In some patients, anticipatory fear of the next menstrual period can cause anxiety during the intermenstrual period.

In evaluating a patient with pelvic pain at menstruation, the physician must first decide whether the patient has *premenstrual syndrome* (PMS) or dysmenorrhea. **PMS usually begins 2 to 12 days before the menstrual period and subsides at the onset or early in the course of menstruation.** The major symptoms of PMS are a diffuse, dull pelvic ache, mood changes (irritability, nervousness, headaches, depression), swelling of the breasts and extremities, occasional weight gain, and a sensation of abdominal bloating. The diagnostic process is sometimes more difficult when, as typically occurs, the symptoms of PMS overlap or are followed by those of dysmenorrhea. PMS is quite common and causes minor mood changes, whereas *premenstrual dysphoric disorder* affects only 3% to 8% of women and is characterized by severe irritability, tension, dysphoria, and lability of mood that seriously interferes with life-style.

It is helpful to classify dysmenorrhea as primary or secondary. *Primary dysmenorrhea* is the most common menstrual disorder and occurs in 30% to 50% of young women. Dysmenorrhea is classified as primary (intrinsic, essential, or idiopathic) if it occurs in a woman who has no pelvic abnormality. About 95% of female adolescents have primary dysmenorrhea, and this problem is a major cause of school absenteeism.

Secondary dysmenorrhea (extrinsic or acquired) results from organic pelvic diseases such as *endometriosis, fibroids, adenomyosis, bacterial infections,* and infections caused by *intrauterine contraceptive devices* (IUDs). Because effective therapy is now available for primary and secondary dysmenorrhea, it is not sufficient merely to diagnose "dysmenorrhea." The physician must distinguish among PMS, primary dysmenorrhea, and secondary dysmenorrhea.

Some women will not initiate a discussion of dysmenorrhea with their physician. They may have been taught that it is normal or that relief cannot be obtained. It is therefore essential that the practitioner ask the patient whether dysmenorrhea is a problem.

Nature of Patient

Severe primary dysmenorrhea is common in young women, with the greatest incidence in the late teens and early 20s. **When dysmenorrhea begins within the first 2 to 3 years of menarche, primary dysmenorrhea is the most likely diagnosis.** Primary dysmenorrhea usually occurs with ovulatory cycles; these normally begin 3 to 12 months after menarche, when ovulation occurs regularly. Primary dysmenorrhea usually begins a few months after menarche and becomes progressively more severe.

If a patient has gradually increasing monthly pain without menstruation, a *congenital abnormality* obstructing menstrual flow must be considered. These rare abnormalities may lead to hematocolpos, hematometra, and eventually intraperitoneal bleeding.

Secondary dysmenorrhea usually begins many years after menarche. Dysmenorrhea that develops after age 20 is usually of the secondary type. A history of pelvic infection, menorrhagia, or intermenstrual bleeding suggests underlying pelvic pathology. Dysmenorrhea often can be caused by an *IUD.* If dysmenorrhea develops after cervical conization, cautery, or radiation, *acquired cervical stenosis* or *cervical occlusion* may be the cause. Dysmenorrhea after uterine curettage may be due to *intrauterine synechiae* (Asherman's syndrome). Secondary dysmenorrhea due to *endometriosis* is usually late in onset (beginning when the patient is in her 30s) and worsens with age. Endometriosis is uncommon in teenagers. *Adenomyosis* may be a cause of secondary dysmenorrhea, particularly in parous women over age 40, especially if menorrhagia is present.

Nature of Symptoms

Pain that begins with menstrual flow or a few hours before flow commences and lasts for 6 hours to 2 days is most characteristic of *primary dysmenorrhea.* The pain is usually crampy but may be a dull ache. It is normally located in the midline of the lower abdomen just above the symphysis. It occasionally radiates down the anterior aspect of the thighs or to the lower back.

In teenagers, endometriosis may mimic the pain of primary dysmenorrhea in that the pain may be limited to the first day of menstruation. Likewise, endometriosis should be suspected if pelvic pain occurs at times other than menstruation, such as with defecation, during intercourse, or midcycle.

The pain of *secondary dysmenorrhea* often begins several hours or even a few days before menses and is often relieved by the menstrual flow. This pain is usually a dull, continuous, diffuse, lower abdominal pain but may be crampy. Like the pain of primary dysmenorrhea, it can radiate down the thighs and into the back.

When *pelvic inflammatory disease* causes dysmenorrhea, the pain is greatest premenstrually and is relieved with the onset of vaginal bleeding. A common cause of secondary dysmenorrhea is *endometriosis.* Symptoms in these patients become progressively more severe with each cycle; the pain usually begins (and increases in severity) 2 to 3 days premenstrually and persists for more than 2 days after the onset of flow. It is most severe on the first and second days of bleeding. The usual drop in basal body temperature, which normally occurs 24 to 36 hours after menses, is delayed until the second or third menstrual day.

Despite the differences between primary and secondary dysmenorrhea, their symptoms can overlap, vary greatly in intensity, and do not necessarily occur with every menstrual period. The physician must recognize that patients with primary dysmenorrhea may develop pelvic pathology and have additional, superimposed symptoms of secondary dysmenorrhea. These patients can have constant, crampy pain beginning 1 to 2 days before menstrual flow and continuing for 2 to 3 days after menstrual flow.

Associated Symptoms

Systemic symptoms such as nausea, vomiting, diarrhea, headache, fatigue, nervousness, and dizziness are more characteristic of *primary dysmenorrhea* than of secondary dysmenorrhea. If menorrhagia and colicky pain are associated with menstruation, *uterine fibroids* should be suspected, although fibroids seldom are responsible for menstrual pain. If a nonpregnant patient with an enlarged, soft uterus complains of menorrhagia and dysmenorrhea, *adenomyosis* should be suspected. Bleeding from glandular tissue located deep within the myometrium has been implicated as the cause of the pain.

The pain of *endometriosis* may continue into the intermenstrual period. Rectal pain on defecation during the menstrual period also suggests endometriosis as a cause of dysmenorrhea. When dysmenorrhea is associated with dyspareunia, rectal pain, tenesmus, backache, and urgent micturition, endometriosis should be suspected.

Precipitating and Aggravating Factors

Primary dysmenorrhea is aggravated by *PMS. IUDs* may cause secondary dysmenorrhea and, in some patients, aggravate preexisting primary dysmenorrhea. *Menstrual flow* that continues longer than 8 days and *emotional stress* also appear to intensify dysmenorrhea. By itself, retroversion does not cause dysmenorrhea; however, some conditions that cause retroversion also cause dysmenorrhea.

Ameliorating Factors

Dysmenorrhea is not consistently alleviated by any known physical measure. Some patients may state that lying on the floor in the knee-chest position gives some relief. Dysmenorrhea that occurs soon after the onset of menarche frequently disappears as the menstrual cycles become more regular. Pregnancy often relieves primary dysmenorrhea and secondary dysmenorrhea due to endometriosis. The pain may be alleviated for several months or, on occasion, permanently.

Oral contraceptives often alleviate the pain of primary dysmenorrhea and endometriosis. Spontaneous alleviation of dysmenorrhea may occur with advancing age, but this is not usually the case.

Physical Findings

In patients who have primary dysmenorrhea, no physical abnormalities are usually found. In patients with secondary dysmenorrhea, physical findings depend on the specific cause.

The practitioner must perform a careful physical examination to check for pelvic infection, endometriosis, pelvic mass, uterine enlargement, and other pelvic disease. When evidence of endometriosis is being sought, the pelvic examination should ideally be performed in the late luteal phase, immediately before menstruation, when the endometrial implants (often in the uterosacral ligaments) are largest and therefore most palpable. Using a laxative to promote bowel evacuation facilitates pelvic examination for endometrial implants. **Special attention should focus on genital development, vaginal discharge, stigmata of pelvic infection, appearance of the cervix, and the size, shape, consistency, and position of the uterus.**

Diagnostic Studies

A Papanicolaou test as well as chlamydial and gonococcal cultures should be obtained for all patients with secondary dysmenorrhea. A fern test and basal body temperature may help diagnose endometriosis. Abdominal and transvaginal ultrasound, uterine curettage, laparoscopy, and hysteroscopy are often useful diagnostic tools.

Less Common Diagnostic Considerations

Less common causes of dysmenorrhea include *congenital malformations, uterine hypoplasia,* and true *cervical stenosis* or *obstruction* that results from cauterization, conization, or radiation therapy. Endometrial *carcinoma* and *tuberculosis* are rare causes of secondary dysmenorrhea. A *foreign body* (e.g., an IUD or any object inserted into the vagina) can cause dysmenorrhea.

Selected References

Avant RE: Dysmenorrhea. Prim Care 15:549–559, 1988.

Banerjee R, Laufer MR: Reproductive disorders associated with pelvic pain. Semin Pediatr Surg 7:52–61, 1998.

Coupey SM, Ahlstrom P: Common menstrual disorders. Pediatr Clin North Am 36:551–571, 1989.

Dawood MY: Dysmenorrhea. Clin Obstet Gynecol 33:168–178, 1990.

Friederich MA: Dysmenorrhea. Women Health 8(2–3):91–106, 1983.

Differential Diagnosis of Menstrual Pain

CAUSE	NATURE OF PATIENT	NATURE OF SYMPTOMS	ASSOCIATED SYMPTOMS	PRECIPITATING AND AGGRAVATING FACTORS	AMELIORATING FACTORS	PHYSICAL FINDINGS	DIAGNOSTIC STUDIES
Premenstrual syndrome		Begins 2–12 days before menses and subsides at onset or during first days of period Diffuse, dull, pelvic ache May coexist with dysmenorrhea	Irritability Nervousness Headaches Swelling of breasts and extremities Bloating and weight gain Breast tenderness	Emotional stress Dysmenorrhea	Menses	Breasts tender to palpation	
Primary dysmenorrhea	30%–50% of young women 95% of adolescents	Most common menstrual disorder, especially in adolescents Begins within 3–12 months of menarche with ovulatory cycles Becomes more severe with age *Pain:* Just precedes or begins with menstrual flow Lasts for 6 hours to 2 days Is crampy or a dull ache Is usually in midline of lower abdomen May radiate down thighs and to lower back	Nausea and vomiting Diarrhea Headache Fatigue Nervousness Dizziness	PMS IUD Emotional stress	Pain may lessen as menstrual cycles become regular Pregnancy Oral contraceptives Nonsteroidal antiinflammatory drugs	None	

Secondary dysmenorrhea	Over age 20 Often a history of recurrent pelvic inflammatory disease	Secondary to organic disease Begins years after menarche; may occur with anovulatory cycles *Pain:* Begins several hours before menses Is a dull, continuous, diffuse, lower abdominal pain May be crampy Can radiate down thighs and into back		Cervical stenosis secondary to cervical conization or radiation IUD	Menses	Depends on cause of secondary dysmenorrhea	Papanicolaou test Gonorrhea and chlamydia culture Laparoscopy Ultrasound for myomas and ovarian cysts
Endometriosis	Usually over age 30 Uncommon in teenagers	Symptoms worsen with each cycle *Pain:* Begins 2–3 days before menses and persists for 2 days after May continue into intermenstrual period	Rectal pain with defecation Dyspareunia Tenesmus Backache Urgent micturition		Pregnancy Oral contraceptives	Pelvic examination best done in late luteal phase Nodularity felt in uterosacral ligaments or other sites of endometrial implants	Fern test Basal body temperature Laparoscopy Ultrasonography
Fibroids		Uncommon cause of dysmenorrhea	Menorrhagia			Uterine mass	Ultrasonography
Pelvic inflammatory disease		Pain is greatest premenstrually	Menorrhagia	Onset at menses		Cervical discharge Chandelier sign	Gonorrhea culture Leukocytosis Chlamydial culture

Heinrichs WL, Adamson GD: A practical approach to the patient with dysmenorrhea. J Reprod Med 25:236–242, 1980.

Johnson SR: Clinician's approach to the diagnosis and management of premenstrual syndrome. Clin Obstet Gynecol 35:637–657, 1992.

Renaer M, Guzinski GM: Pain in gynecologic practice. Pain 5:305–331, 1978.

Smith RP: Cyclic pelvic pain and dysmenorrhea. Obstet Gynecol Clin North Am 20:753–764, 1993.

Steiner M: Premenstrual syndromes. Annu Rev Med 48:447–455, 1997.

CHAPTER 22

Nausea and/or Vomiting Without Abdominal Pain

Nausea is a vague, unpleasant sensation; it may herald the onset of vomiting or occur without vomiting. *Vomiting* is the forceful expulsion of gastric contents through the mouth and must be differentiated from *regurgitation.* The latter is an effortless backflow of small amounts of ingested food or liquid during or between meals or feedings. Dribbling of milk from a child's mouth is an example of regurgitation. When a patient complains of vomiting, it is helpful for the physician to distinguish acute from chronic and cyclic vomiting.

The most common cause of acute nausea and vomiting in adults and children is *gastroenteritis.* Other common causes include *gastritis, excessive alcohol ingestion,* certain *drugs, motion sickness,* and, in children, *otitis media.* Common causes of chronic nausea and vomiting include *gastritis, drugs* (especially codeine, digitalis glycosides, quinidine, salicylates, theophylline, chemotherapeutic agents, and antibiotics), *uremia,* and *hepatic failure.* Recurrent nausea that occurs without vomiting is often a reaction to *environmental* or *emotional stresses.* This form of nausea is temporally related to the stressful period and usually disappears when the stress is removed.

Nature of Patient

In neonates, vomiting with the first feeding suggests *esophageal atresia* or some other congenital gastrointestinal (GI) anomaly (e.g., malrotation, Hirschsprung's disease). The most common causes of vomiting in the first year are *feeding problems, GI infection, urinary tract infection* (UTI), and *septicemia.* When projectile vomiting occurs in infants less than age 3 months (usually ages 2 to 3 weeks), *pyloric stenosis* must be considered. Although uncommon, recurrent vomiting of bile-stained material in neonates may indicate *intestinal obstruction* due to atresia, stenosis, or volvulus of the small bowel.

The most common causes of vomiting in children are *viral* and *bacterial infections, high fevers* of any cause, and *otitis media.* Otitis media has its highest incidence in young children and may present with unexplained vomiting and fever. **Cyclic vomiting, with or without typical migraine symptoms, may be caused by abdominal migraine, which is more common in children.**

In adults, the common causes of acute nausea or vomiting are *gastritis* (alcohol or drug induced), *viral gastroenteritis, psychogenic conditions,* and occasionally *labyrinthine disorders.* Nausea and vomiting can also be the presenting symptoms in patients with *hepatitis, myocardial infarction,* and *diabetic ketoacidosis.* Chronic vomiting in adults usually results from *gastritis, mechanical obstruction, gut motility disorders* (including *diabetic gastroparesis), achalasia, drugs, labyrinthine disorders,* and *uremia.*

Both *food contamination* and *chemical poisoning* must be considered as causes of vomiting, particularly if several people are affected at the same time; in cases of food poisoning, usually more than one person is experiencing symptoms. Nausea and vomiting of *pregnancy* must be considered in women of reproductive age; some pregnant women experience morning sickness in the first trimester of pregnancy, often before they are aware of their condition.

Self-induced vomiting should be suspected in neurotic patients. If these patients are questioned carefully, they may admit to a feeling of nausea, which they attempt to relieve by gagging themselves to produce vomiting. If an elderly patient presents with persistent vomiting, gastric or intestinal obstruction secondary to *neoplasm* should be suspected.

Nature of Symptoms

When vomiting is painless or has preceded abdominal pain by a considerable time, a surgical lesion is unlikely. Repeated episodes of unexplained vomiting and nausea may indicate *pancreatitis,* which is not always associated with abdominal pain. Persistent vomiting without any bile staining is an indication of *pyloric obstruction.* In children this may be caused by *pyloric stenosis* and in adults by ulcer scarring or tumor. Vomiting or regurgitation of undigested food indicates *esophageal obstruction.* Vomiting secondary to *increased intracranial pressure* (ICP) is often projectile and not preceded by nausea.

Nausea and vomiting are frequent manifestations of *digitalis toxicity.* These symptoms are not necessarily from high serum levels of the digitalis glycoside; a GI adverse effect of the drug may occur at normal serum levels. Although many patients with *gastritis* have abdominal pain, some patients experience unexplained nausea or vomiting without pain. *Substance abuse* (alcohol, caffeine, and drugs) also may be associated with unexplained nausea or vomiting.

When children vomit more than four times per hour, cyclic vomiting due to abdominal migraine is probable. It usually occurs a few times a month. Chronic vomiting, once or twice an hour, occurs around 30 times a month and is usually caused by peptic or infectious GI disorders.

The timing of vomiting may be of diagnostic importance. Patients with *uremia, pregnant women,* and *chronic alcoholics* often experience early-morning nausea and vomiting. Vomiting immediately before food is ingested may be a manifestation of *neurosis,* whereas vomiting shortly after eating may be a consequence of *gastric outlet obstruction* caused by a pyloric channel ulcer, adenocarcinoma, or other infiltrative lesions.

Postprandial vomiting may also be of *functional origin,* although organic gastric disease should be suspected. Vomiting soon after eating occurs frequently in patients with *gastritis* and in those with *digitalis toxicity.* Vomiting that begins 20 to 40 minutes after meals suggests *gastric atony* associated with diabetes, prior gastric surgery, or peritonitis. If vomiting begins 1 to 2 hours after a meal, disease of the biliary tract or pancreas may be the cause. In these latter instances, pain usually is not relieved by vomiting. Recurrent vomiting that occurs 1 to 4 hours after eating may be due to gastric or duodenal lesions causing *gastric outlet obstruction.* Vomiting that follows and relieves an episode of epigastric pain is usually caused by an *intragastric lesion* or *pyloric spasm.*

The odor of vomitus may also provide a clue to the cause. If the vomitus lacks the pungent odor of gastric acid, a *dilated esophagus* (possibly from a stricture or achalasia) may be the cause. Patients frequently vomit in the morning and vomit or regurgitate undigested food. If vomitus has a fecal odor, *intestinal obstruction* or *gastrocolic fistula* should be suspected.

Associated Symptoms

If headache (especially a unilateral one) is associated with nausea or vomiting, *migraine* should be suspected. Occasionally, recurrent or cyclic nausea and vomiting may be the only manifestation of migraine; acephalic migraine is more common in children and adolescents. If vertigo and tinnitus are associated with nausea and vomiting, *Meniere's disease* or other middle ear disturbances should be considered. If symptoms of depression are present with little or no weight loss despite a history of longstanding emesis, psychogenic vomiting is probable. As with *anorexia nervosa,* women experience psychogenic vomiting more often than men.

If chest pain or other symptoms of myocardial infarction (MI) are associated with vomiting, the vomiting is probably caused by MI. Nausea and vomiting often precede the development of chest pain. Rarely, chest pain and vomiting are caused by a strangulated diaphragmatic hernia. In these instances, electrocardiographic (ECG) abnormalities may erroneously suggest posterior infarction.

Acute nausea and vomiting associated with diarrhea and occasionally abdominal pain are most often caused by *gastroenteritis.* When vertigo accompanies vomiting, *labyrinthine disorders* should be suspected. When vomiting, without vertigo, is induced by a recumbent posture, a *posterior fossa lesion* should be suspected. Vomiting may be the initial manifestation of *diabetic ketoacidosis.* It is a particularly common presentation in juvenile diabetic patients.

Precipitating and Aggravating Factors

Nausea and vomiting are frequently precipitated by *medications* such as digitalis, theophylline, quinidine, potassium preparations, chemotherapeutic agents, antibiotics, and antihypertensives. Iron preparations, salicylates, and nonsteroidal antiinflammatory agents (NSAIDs) also cause nausea and occasionally vomiting.

Nicotine poisoning and excessive use of nicotine patches and gum may cause vomiting. *Radiation therapy* may also cause nausea and vomiting.

Anticipatory nausea and vomiting may occur before radiation therapy or chemotherapy, especially in anxious patients. *Postoperative nausea and vomiting,* no longer attributed to anesthetic agents, occurs often and is usually caused by central mechanisms and perioperative medications. If vomiting is preceded by a cough, it may be the primary manifestation of *asthma* when wheezing is trivial or not present.

Ameliorating Factors

Vomiting usually relieves the symptoms of fullness and pain caused by pyloric obstruction. Vomiting relieves nausea if it is being caused by nauseating substances in the stomach. It does not usually alleviate nausea caused by gastroenteritis, gastritis, uremia, or drugs that cause nausea through a central effect.

Physical Findings

The presence of fever in a vomiting patient suggests that *infection* is causative. In children, physical findings of *otitis media* suggest that this is the probable cause of the vomiting. A walnut-size mass may be palpable in the epigastrium of infants with *hypertrophic pyloric stenosis.* A cloudy sensorium or papilledema suggests an *intracranial lesion,* whereas nystagmus suggests a labyrinthine cause. Jaundice or hepatomegaly suggests *hepatitis* or *cirrhosis* as the cause. A distended abdomen accompanying nausea and vomiting may indicate *paralytic ileus* or *mechanical obstruction* of the intestine. Abdominal tenderness, distention, and occasionally visible peristalsis suggest *GI obstruction.* A succussion splash suggests *diabetic gastroparesis.* The location of abdominal pain may provide clues about which organ is responsible for the symptoms.

Chronic vomiting results in weight loss. If a patient's weight is maintained despite a history of chronic nausea and vomiting, the origin of symptoms is probably *psychogenic.* Decreased skin turgor suggests that the vomiting has caused significant fluid loss. Physical findings consistent with congestive heart failure (e.g., tachycardia, gallop, peripheral edema) suggest that nausea may be from *hepatic capsule distention* and *mesenteric congestion.*

Diagnostic Studies

Studies to confirm a visceral origin of nausea and vomiting include survey films of the abdomen, upper GI series, cholecystography, and endoscopy. Ultrasonography is the diagnostic procedure of choice for the diagnosis of *infantile hypertrophic pyloric stenosis.* Detailed neurologic studies, including spinal tap and computed tomography (CT) scan, should be performed only if an intracranial process is suspected. A metabolic cause may be suspected if laboratory tests indicate abnormal serum levels of substances such as urea nitrogen, creatinine, glucose, bilirubin, and calcium. An elevated serum amylase level suggests *pancreatitis.* Digitalis excess may be diagnosed on the basis of elevated serum digitalis levels. Toxicology screening may detect toxins and drugs that cause vomiting.

More sophisticated tests include radioisotope studies of liquid and solid gastric emptying, esophageal and GI manometry, and electrogastrography (Table 22–1). Psychiatric assessment, including the Minnesota Multiphasic Personality Inventory test, may also be helpful.

Less Common Diagnostic Considerations

Several authors have categorized the causes of vomiting as follows: allergies, cerebromedullary factors, toxins, visceral problems, deficiency states, and motion sickness. *GI allergies* should be considered if sudden nausea or vomiting consistently follows ingestion of specific food. The less common *cerebromedullary causes* include increased ICP, trauma, cerebral tumors, abscesses, hydrocephalus, intracranial hemorrhage, and acephalic migraine. *Hepatic coma* and *Addison's disease*

■ TABLE 22.1 Tests That May Be Necessary in Diagnosis of Unexplained Vomiting

History, including psychiatric assessment and family history
Physical examination, with particular attention paid to:
- Orthostatic hypotension
- Succussion splash, rash, Raynaud's phenomenon
- Neurologic assessment, especially cranial nerves, vestibular and pupillary function, peripheral neuropathy, extrapyramidal signs

Laboratory tests
- Routine hematologic and biochemical screening
- Amylase
- Drug screening, such as digoxin levels
- Hormonal levels: thyroxine, thyroid-stimulating hormones, plasma cortisol, orthostatic catecholamines
- Serum (and urine) protein electrophoresis
- Immunologic tests: rheumatoid factor, DNA-binding titer, autoantibody screening
- Gastric intubation for residual volume after overnight fast

Radiologic tests
- Plain abdominal radiograph
- Gastrointestinal tract contrast series
- Intravenous urogram
- Computed tomography scan of abdomen and head

Upper gastrointestinal tract endoscopy
Gastric emptying tests
- ^{99m}Tc chicken liver (absorbable solid)
- ^{131}I-fiber (nondigestible solid)
- ^{111}In-pentetic acid (aqueous phase)

Conventional esophageal and anorectal manometry
Gastrointestinal manometry and electrogastrography
- Manometry: low compliance perfusion system (peroral or intraoperative)
- Electrogastrography: internal, external, intraoperative

Formal psychiatric assessment, such as Minnesota Multiphasic Personality Inventory and inpatient evaluation
Laparotomy and full-thickness biopsy of small bowel, including electrophysiologic study of muscle

From Malagelada JR, Camilleri M: Unexplained vomiting: a diagnostic challenge. Ann Intern Med 101:211–218, 1984.

Differential Diagnosis of Nausea and/or Vomiting Without Abdominal Pain

CAUSE	NATURE OF PATIENT	NATURE OF SYMPTOMS	ASSOCIATED SYMPTOMS	PRECIPITATING AND AGGRAVATING FACTORS	PHYSICAL FINDINGS	DIAGNOSTIC STUDIES
Gastroenteritis	Most common cause at any age	Acute nausea and vomiting	Diarrhea Fever Abdominal pain		Hyperactive peristalsis	
Gastritis		Acute or chronic nausea and vomiting occur postprandially	Abdominal pain	Viral infection Alcohol or drug induced		Endoscopy
Viral or bacterial infection	Common cause of vomiting in children	Acute nausea and vomiting	Fever		High temperature	
Drugs		Acute or chronic nausea and vomiting Postprandial vomiting		Cytotoxic Codeine Digitalis glycosides Quinidine Salicylates Theophylline Antihypertensives Antibiotics Iron preparations NSAIDs Nicotine (also patches, gum)		Serum drug levels
Otitis media	Children	Acute nausea and vomiting	Fever Earache		Inflamed tympanic membrane	
Excessive alcohol ingestion	Alcoholics Social drinkers	Early-morning vomiting				Gastroscopy

Uremia		Chronic nausea and vomiting Usually in early morning				Elevated blood urea nitrogen and creatinine levels
Morning sickness	Pregnant females	Early-morning nausea and vomiting Usually in first trimester				Serum human chorionic gonadotropin
Environmental or emotional stresses		Episodic nausea usually without vomiting				
Diabetic gastroparesis	Diabetic				Succussion splash	Radiograph of abdomen
Pyloric obstruction	In infants aged <3 months may be due to pyloric stenosis In adults may be secondary to ulcer scarring or tumor	Projectile vomiting	Abdominal pain		Palpable mass Succussion splash	Ultrasonography
Esophageal obstruction and achalasia		Vomiting or regurgitation of undigested food Odorless vomitus Usually occurs in early morning or after large meals				Esophageal radiograph Endoscopy
Increased intracranial pressure		Projectile vomiting not preceded by nausea			Papilledema	Neurologic examination Spinal tap CT scan
Pancreatitis	Alcoholics	Repeated episodes of unexplained nausea and vomiting	Abdominal pain	Excessive alcohol intake		Elevated serum amylase level CT scan of pancreas

are less common causes of nausea and vomiting. *GI disorders* such as ulcers, obstructive tumors (particularly those of the stomach and proximal small bowel), adhesive bands, volvulus, and gastritis may also cause nausea and vomiting. *Blood* in the GI tract is another cause.

Patients with *pyelonephritis* and *pelvic inflammatory disease* may present with a chief complaint of vomiting, particularly if they also have reflex ileus. Patients with *anorexia nervosa,* particularly in the early stages, may self-induce vomiting. Because anorectic patients seldom complain of this symptom, however, it may be difficult for the physician to diagnose the condition before pronounced weight loss has occurred. Vomiting may also be caused by conditions that alter neural control of gut motility.

Selected References

Bockus H: Gastroenterology, 4th ed. Philadelphia, WB Saunders Co, 1985.

Bramble MG, Record CO: Drug-induced gastrointestinal disease. Drugs 15:451–463, 1978.

Bruppacher R, Gyr N, Fisch T: Abdominal pain, indigestion, anorexia, nausea and vomiting. Baillieres Clin Gastroenterol 2:275–292, 1988.

Camilleri M: Gastrointestinal problems in diabetes. Endocrinol Metab Clin North Am 25:361–378, 1996.

Fleisher DR, Matar M: The cyclic vomiting syndrome: a report of 71 cases and literature review. J Pediatr Gastroenterol Nutr 17:361–369, 1993.

Fuchs S, Jaffe D: Vomiting. Pediatr Emerg Care 6:164–167, 1990.

Hanson JS, McCallum RW: The diagnosis and management of nausea and vomiting: a review. Am J Gastroenterol 80:210–218, 1985.

Katelares PH, Jones DB: Chronic nausea and vomiting. Dig Dis 7:324–333, 1989.

Malagelada JR, Camilleri M: Unexplained vomiting: a diagnostic challenge. Ann Intern Med 101:211–218, 1984.

Pfau BT, Li BUK, et al: Differentiating cyclic from chronic vomiting patterns in children: quantitative criteria and diagnostic implications. Pediatrics 97:364–368, 1996.

Rollins MD, Shields MD, Quinn RJM, Wooldridge MAW: Value of ultrasound in differentiating causes of persistent vomiting in infants. Gut 32:612–614, 1991.

Rosenthal RH, et al: Diagnoses and management of persistent psychogenic vomiting. Psychosomatics 218:722–730, 1980.

Valman HB: The first year of life—vomiting. Br Med J 280:620–623, 1980.

CHAPTER 23

Pain in the Foot

Foot pain is usually caused by local disease or abnormality but occasionally results from referred pain. Therefore, examination of the foot should begin with the spine and proceed distally. Foot pain is most often caused by *muscular* or *ligamentous strain* associated with *trauma,* unaccustomed or strenuous *physical activity,* and *sport.* New shoes or change in heel size also may cause foot pain. Other common causes include *gout, rheumatoid arthritis, plantar warts, callosities,* and *metatarsal stress fracture (march fracture).* Isolated pain in the heel can result from *plantar fasciitis, subcalcaneal syndrome, arterial insufficiency, Achilles tendinitis* or *bursitis,* and *jogger's trauma.* In adolescents, pain in the heel may be caused by *calcaneal apophysitis.*

Nature of Patient

Foot pain in children is rare. When it does occur, it usually results from acute bone and ligament injuries or chronic bone-tendon disorders. Rarely, it is caused by tumors, infections, or arthritis.

Because foot pain usually results from *muscular* or *ligamentous strain,* it is more likely to occur in people who are physically active, particularly those who are unaccustomed to physical exercise and muscular strain in their feet, such as unconditioned athletes and weekend sportsmen. The gradual development of forefoot pain in a new military recruit suggests a *metatarsal stress fracture,* which is most common in the second metatarsal, followed by the third and fourth metatarsals. Joggers and runners may develop *Achilles tendinitis, tarsal tunnel syndrome,* or *plantar fasciitis.*

Gout is more common in men over age 40 but does occur in women, especially those who are postmenopausal. The patient may present with a history of previous attacks of painful joints or urolithiasis. Often a family history of gout may be elicited.

Pain in the heel caused by *plantar fasciitis* and its associated soft tissue irritation is most common in obese patients over age 40. When adolescents complain of pain in the heel, it most likely is caused by *calcaneal apophysitis. Achilles tendinitis,* which also causes heel pain, is usually caused by trauma (e.g., injury from jogging), although the trauma may not be recalled by the patient. Achilles tendinitis is more common in patients with Reiter's syndrome and ankylosing spondylitis who are HLA-B27 positive, even without a history of trauma. In patients with *rheumatoid arthritis,* foot pain is second in frequency only to knee pain, which is most common.

Nature of Symptoms

As with other types of pain, a careful history of the location (forefoot, midfoot, or hindfoot) and quality of the pain (how it began, what intensifies it) is most helpful in determining its cause.

Forefoot pain, generally referred to as *metatarsalgia,* has many causes. They include metatarsal stress fracture, interdigital neuroma, Freiberg's infraction, gout, sesamoiditis, synovitis or dislocation of the metatarsophalangeal (MTP) joint, plantar warts, and atrophy of the plantar fat pad. *Midfoot pain* is an infrequent complaint but usually results from tendinitis or acquired flatfoot. *Heel pain* is often used to describe *hindfoot pain.* This common complaint can be caused by plantar fasciitis, calcaneal apophysitis, heel pad fat atrophy, nerve entrapment, Achilles tendinitis, and arterial insufficiency.

Foot pain described as a dull ache is probably caused by *foot strain.* This is more likely to occur in older adults, overweight people, those wearing new shoes, and those who are on their feet for much of the day. It is critical that the physician establish the precise location of the ache because this will determine which ligaments, tendons, or fascia are involved (torn or under strain). For example, pain below the ankle on the inner aspect of the heel suggests a tear or strain of the ligamentous fibers attached to the internal malleolus. Symptoms of burning, tingling, or numbness suggest a *neuropathy.*

Plantar warts and *callosities* can cause severe pain, particularly with weight bearing. These typically are located on the plantar surface of the foot in the metatarsal region. Pain from a *calcaneal spur* or *plantar fasciitis* is usually continuous, although it may worsen with weight bearing. The spur is usually located in the center of the undersurface of the heel, about 2.25 cm from the back of the foot; the pain, however, may be more toward the back of the heel. The condition called *jogger's foot* or *tarsal tunnel syndrome* may produce complaints of a burning pain in the heel, aching in the arch, or diminished sensation in the sole behind the large toe.

The pain of *Achilles tendinitis* is usually over the Achilles tendon and may be associated with tenderness to palpation and swelling.

With *gout,* the pain is usually acute, frequently recurrent, and often agonizing, although atypical cases of gout may present with less severe symptoms. The attacks usually have a sudden onset and characteristically start during the early hours of the day while the patient is still in bed. Before gout is diagnosed, the patient may attribute the bouts of pain to minor trauma such as "stubbing the toe" or "spraining the involved joint." Once the diagnosis of gout has been established, the patient usually recognizes subsequent attacks. Although the MTP joint of the big toe is classically affected, one or more other joints, including the ankle, may also be affected.

In general, systemic causes of foot pain such as gout, rheumatoid arthritis, or diabetes occur at rest, whereas biomechanical causes of foot pain such as sprains or calcaneal spur occur with ambulation and decrease with rest.

Precipitating and Aggravating Factors

Most foot pain is precipitated by *trauma,* unaccustomed or strenuous *physical activity,* and *sport.* Change in occupation or work that involves constant jarring of the foot or walking or standing on concrete floors may lead to foot strain. Constant vibration or jarring frequently leads to heel pain that may result from calcaneal periostitis. Likewise, new shoes or change in heel size can lead to foot strain.

Gouty pain in the foot may have no particular precipitating factors, although several reports have indicated that a gouty diathesis may be caused by minor trauma to the involved joint.

Physical Findings

In addition to careful examination of the foot for local discoloration, coldness, hair loss, swelling, and areas tender to palpation, patients who complain of foot pain should have a careful examination of the lower back and legs, since foot pain may result from referred pain.

When pain is caused by *foot strain,* the forefoot may flatten on weight bearing, and calluses under the metatarsal heads may be present. With *metatarsal stress fracture,* the head of the involved metatarsal is tender to palpation. With *interdigital neuroma,* pain often radiating to the toe can be reproduced by palpating interdigitally with one hand while applying side-to-side pressure with the other hand. When the pain is from *gout,* there is usually a warm, violaceous, tender, swollen joint, typically the MTP joint of the big toe or the ankle. Tophi may be present in the foot, other joints, or the ear lobe.

When the pain is from a *calcaneal spur* or *plantar fasciitis,* there may be spot tenderness with deep palpation, particularly on the undersurface of the heel. If this is associated with radiographic evidence of calcaneal spur, the diagnosis is obvious. In cases that present no radiographic confirmation of a calcaneal spur, this pain may be caused by plantar fasciitis.

Although the diagnosis of *ankle sprain* is usually obvious by history, patients may not remember the traumatic incident. Sprained ankles most often result from an inversion injury and have tenderness and swelling over the anterior talofibular ligament. Likewise, *fractures* are usually associated with a history of significant trauma. A radiograph is usually necessary to diagnose small fractures of the ankle. In patients with a history suggesting a sprained ankle, the physician should suspect an associated fracture if the swelling appears disproportionate to the severity of the sprain.

Bunions can also cause foot pain, particularly at the MTP joint. This pain is usually worse with extension of the big toe. *Heel fasciitis,* also called *calcaneal periostitis,* may produce chronic pain in the bottom of the foot. Patients with this condition usually have pain and tenderness localized to the insertion of the long plantar tendon into the base of the calcaneus. When *peripheral ischemia* gives rise to isolated heel pain without other evidence of peripheral vascular disease, there is often cornification of the heel skin and coolness in this area.

Diagnostic Studies

Doppler studies help the physician detect arterial insufficiency. Radiographs may demonstrate calcaneal spurs and fractures, including small stress fractures, although magnetic resonance imaging (MRI) is often required to detect sress fractures. Quantitative scintigraphs help the physician identify abnormal weight distribution and its associated fasciitis. Occasionally, computed tomography (CT) scan, MRI, or arthroscopic examination is helpful. Bone scans may detect avascular necrosis, stress fracture, osteomyelitis, or rarely metastatic carcinoma.

Less Common Diagnostic Considerations

Metatarsalgia is not a cause but a symptom of pain in the forefoot (Table 23–1). *Primary metatarsalgia* is pain in the forefoot caused by a chronic disorder of weight distribution across the MTP joints. Pain in the metatarsal region can result from other local processes (e.g., plantar warts, tarsal tunnel syndrome, plantar fasciitis) or systemic disease (e.g., rheumatoid arthritis, sesamoiditis, gout). *Neuralgia* and *polyneuritis* from alcohol ingestion, lead poisoning, or diabetes may produce pain in one or both feet. In addition, affected patients frequently complain of burning sensations or paresthesias of the soles. Decreased tactile and vibratory sensations may be observed on physical examination.

If foot pain is precisely located on the plantar surface between a pair of metatarsal heads, *Morton's neuroma* should be suspected (Fig. 23–1). This relatively rare condition is more common in women than in men. The usual history is foot pain for 2 or more years that is relieved by shoe removal and unchanged by conservative measures. This pain is often described as "burning," "shooting," "needles," "daggers," or "like walking on a stone." It may radiate to the toes. Patients may complain of numbness and tingling. Physical findings include pain with compression of the toes, a palpable click after the release of pressure in the affected area, occasional swelling, and some sensory changes. The pain is precipitated by walking and is aggravated by compression of the toes and weight bearing.

Patients with *Raynaud's disease,* in addition to having tingling and numbness, may present with pain in the toes that often is associated with pain in the fingers. These pains may be precipitated by exposure to cold, emotional stress, beta blockers, and cigarette smoking. Patients with *Fabry's disease,* a recessively inherited disorder linked to the X chromosome, may present with disabling crises of burning pain in the feet and hands. Some patients with *rheumatoid arthritis* have marked prominence of the metatarsal heads with pain in this region.

Text continued on page 236.

■ **TABLE 23.1 Forefoot Pain: 23 Diagnoses in 98 Patients**

DIAGNOSIS	NUMBER
Primary metatarsalgia	
Static disorders	12
Iatrogenic (postoperative)	12
Secondary to hallux valgus	9
Hallux rigidus	3
Morton's foot (neuroma)	3
Congenital	3
Long first ray	2
Freiberg's disease	1
Total	45
Secondary metatarsalgia	11
Rheumatoid arthritis	10
Sesamoiditis	4
Posttraumatic	3
Neurogenic	2
Stress fractures	1
Gout	2
Short ipsilateral lower limb	33
Total	
Pain under forepart of foot	
Morton's neuroma	5
Plantar fasciitis	3
Causalgia	2
Tarsal tunnel syndrome	2
Tumors	2
Intermittent claudication	1
Buerger's disease	1
Plantar verrucae (warts)	4
Total	20

Modified from Scranton PE: Metatarsalgia: diagnosis and treatment. J Bone Joint Surg 62:723–732, 1980.

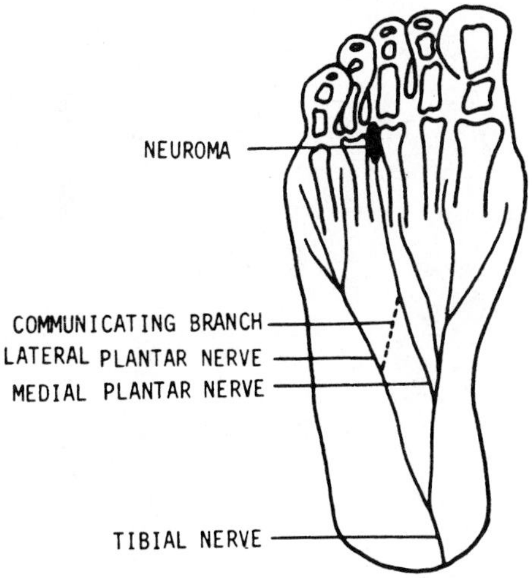

■ **Figure 23.1** Anatomy of Morton's neuroma. (From Morris MA: Morton's metatarsalgia. Clin Orthop Rel Res 127:203–207, 1977.)

Differential Diagnosis of Foot Pain

CAUSE	NATURE OF PATIENT	NATURE OF SYMPTOMS	PRECIPITATING AND AGGRAVATING FACTORS	PHYSICAL FINDINGS	DIAGNOSTIC STUDIES
Muscular and ligamentous strain	Physically active, especially those unaccustomed to exercise	Pain in region of strained muscles or ligaments	Trauma Unaccustomed or strenuous physical activity	Localized tenderness on palpation	
Foot strain	Older adults Overweight patients	Dull ache in foot, especially forefoot	New shoes Change in heel size Prolonged standing	Forefoot may splay with weight bearing	
Plantar warts and callosities		Pain in plantar surface in metatarsal region	Weight bearing	Plantar callosities	
Jogger's foot	Joggers	Burning in heel Aching in arch		Decreased sensation behind big toe	
Fractures	Patients with history of trauma Joggers		Trauma		May need radiographs or MRI to diagnose small fractures of ankle and march fractures of metatarsals

Calcaneal spur or plantar fasciitis		Pain on undersurface of heel Continuous 2.25 cm (1 inch) from back of heel	Worse with weight bearing	Worse with dorsiflexion of toes	Radiograph may show calcaneal spur
Achilles tendinitis or bursitis	Joggers	Heel pain over Achilles tendon	Trauma Running	Swelling and tenderness over Achilles tendon	
Calcaneal apophysitis	Adolescents	Pain in back of heel	Running and jumping	Pain on palpation of Achilles insertion	
Arterial insufficiency	Older adults Diabetics	Rest pain in heel or toes		Coolness Decreased pulses Cornification of heel skin	Arteriography
Gout	Males, especially over age 40 Postmenopausal females	Acute severe pain in big toe metatarsophalangeal joint, occasionally other toes or ankle	Trauma	Warm, violaceous, tender, swollen joints	Uric acid Radiographs

Foot ulcerations, which are not necessarily associated with significant pain, can occur in patients with diabetes mellitus, tabes dorsalis, leprosy, paraplegia, Raynaud's disease, and thromboangiitis obliterans (Buerger's disease). These conditions should be suspected whenever an ulcer exists without much pain. They may all cause some degree of neuropathy that interferes with pain perception.

Erythromelalgia is painful dilatation of the superficial vessels of the foot. The pain is burning in quality and may be severe. It may be seen in patients with lead poisoning, polycythemia, or syringomyelia and in some psychologically disturbed patients.

Selected References

Brown C: A review of subcalcaneal heel pain and plantar fasciitis. Aust Fam Physician 25:875–885, 1996.

Di Marcangelo MT, Yu TC: Diagnostic imaging of heel pain and plantar fasciitis. Clin Podiatr Med Surg 14:281–301, 1997.

Gibbon WW, Cassar-Pullicino VN: Heel pain. Ann Rheum Dis 53:344–348, 1994.

Karr SD: Subcalcaneal heel pain. Orthop Clin North Am 25:161–175, 1994.

Lichniak JE: The heel in systemic disease. Clin Pediatr Med Surg 7:225–241, 1990.

Pach LG, Julien PH: Differential diagnosis of lessor metatarsalgia. Clin Podiatr Med Surg 7:573–577, 1990.

Quirk R: Metatarsalgia. Aust Fam Physician 25:863–869, 1996.

Rask MR: Medial plantar neuropraxia (jogger's foot): report of three cases. Clin Orthop 134:193–195, 1978.

Stern SH: Ankle and foot pain. Prim Care 15:809–826, 1988.

Van Wyngarden TM: The painful foot. Part I. Common forefoot deformities. Am Fam Physician 55:1866–1876, 1997.

West SG, Woodburn J: Pain in the foot. Br Med J 310:860–864, 1995.

Wilkins KE: The painful foot in the child. Intr Course Lect 37:77–85, 1988.

CHAPTER 24

Pain in the Lower Extremity in Adults

To diagnose pain in the lower extremity accurately, the physician must determine whether the pain is *articular* (hip, knee, or ankle) or *nonarticular* (muscular, vascular, or neurologic). In addition, the examiner should note whether the pain is present at rest or is primarily associated with exercise. The most likely causes of pain in a child's leg are different from those in an adult. Therefore, lower extremity pain in adults and lower extremity pain and limp in children are reviewed in separate chapters.

In adults the most common causes of leg pain include *muscular* and *ligamentous strains, degenerative joint disease* (DJD, particularly of the hip and knee), *intermittent claudication* due to arterial insufficiency, *sciatica, night cramps, varicose veins, thrombophlebitis, gout,* and *trauma.* **The major clues to diagnoses are (1) the location of the pain, (2) the age of the patient, and (3) whether the pain is related to exertion.**

Nature of Patient

The most common cause of leg pain is *muscular* or *ligamentous strain,* seen frequently in weekend athletes. Questioning usually reveals a history of unusual or strenuous exercise. The usual causes of leg pain in joggers and runners are *shin splints, stress fractures,* and *compartment syndromes.* The most common is shin splints, a musculotendinous inflammation of the anterior tibia that occasionally involves the periosteum. The pain is usually on the anterior aspect of the tibia, particularly the distal third along the medial crest, but it can occur on the lateral aspect of the tibia as well. Shin splints are most common in less well-conditioned athletes and are most frequently reported early in the running season. Skiers often develop anterior knee pain due to *patellofemoral problems.*

Patellar problems are more common in young women, often beginning in adolescence. During pregnancy the common causes of painful legs include *venous insufficiency, postphlebitic syndrome, thrombophlebitis, muscle cramps,* and *trauma.*

DJD is uncommon in patients under age 40 unless it has been facilitated by unequal leg length (causing DJD of the hip) or prior trauma, such as athletic injuries of the knee. After age 40, pain in the hip or knee is typically caused by DJD. Sports injuries and overuse syndromes are also more common in adults over age 40.

In patients age 50 or older, calf pain precipitated by walking or exercise that abates with rest is most likely from *peripheral arterial insufficiency.* **Intermittent claudication pain in the hip is seen in patients with aortoiliac disease.** When exercise-induced calf pain occurs in younger adults, frequently with a history of phlebitis, *venous claudication* is probable. *Gout* is most common in older men but can occur in women, particularly those who have had an early menopause (natural or surgically induced). Patients with gout may or may not have a family history of the condition. Often a history of a prior attack can be elicited. Classic gouty pain occurs in the big toe, but it may occur in other toes or in ankles or knees; it is rare in the hip.

Nature of Symptoms

Anterior knee pain is most often caused by *patellar tendinitis, patellofemoral malalignment,* or *chondromalacia patellae.* Pain due to patellofemoral malalignment usually is aching in quality, has a gradual onset, and is located in the peripatellar region. It is often bilateral and is worse with activity such as stair climbing, hill climbing, skiing, squatting, and after prolonged sitting. Sharp pain in the knee suggests *synovial impingement* or structural difficulties such as loose bodies. Aching joint pain is usually seen in inflammatory conditions with diffuse involvement of the synovium, such as in *rheumatoid arthritis.*

Degenerative Joint Disease

When the knee or hip joints are painful and stiff in the morning, improve during the day, and worsen toward the end of the day, DJD is probable. These pains may be exacerbated by certain activities (e.g., descending stairs). Patients with osteoarthritis of the hip may present with pain in the groin or the knee. Therefore, the diagnosis of DJD of the hip must be considered in patients who present with knee or groin pain when no pathology is noted in these areas. With DJD of the hip, hip motion is usually restricted, and radiographs are abnormal. *Obturator nerve involvement* also can cause pain in the groin and medial aspect of the thigh and knee. A hernia may be suspected because of groin pain; if no hernia is found, obturator involvement should be considered.

Osteoarthritis of the hip also may present with pain in the buttock; therefore, causes of buttock pain must be considered in the differential diagnosis. Buttock pain caused by *lumbar disc disease* is worse with extension of the spine and relieved by rest in the fetal position. Buttock pain caused by osteoarthritis of the hip is not usually exacerbated by spinal extension or relieved by rest in the fetal position. Likewise, no evidence of nerve root compression is usually seen with osteoarthritis of the hip.

Sciatica

Typical sciatica causes pain in the buttock that radiates down the posterolateral aspect of the leg. It may radiate into the dorsum of the foot and tends to follow standard dermatome patterns. Sciatic pain may be sharp or burning. Frequently, it is made worse by coughing, straining at stool (if sciatica is caused by a herniated disc), or walking down steps; it may be precipitated by sudden strenuous movements. The patient may present with pain initiated by an attempt to lift a heavy object or by vigorous turning or twisting with the back flexed (e.g., pulling the rope on a lawn mower or outboard engine).

Effects of Exercise and Rest on Pain

Leg pain that develops during walking occurs in patients with arterial insufficiency, venous insufficiency, spinal stenosis, and thrombophlebitis.

Arterial insufficiency. The pain of arterial insufficiency (*intermittent claudication*) usually is described as soreness, a cramp, or a burning sensation in the calf. The discomfort also may be described as a tightness, heaviness, tiredness, or achiness rather than pain. The discomfort usually is precipitated by walking and relieved by rest. It rarely occurs while the patient is at home. It usually develops after the patient has walked a predictable (by the patient) distance and is relieved by rest in a standing position after a predictable (by the patient) time. After resting, the patient can resume walking and walk a similar distance before the pain starts again; relief is achieved again after resting.

A common mistake is the diagnosis of osteoarthritis of the hip when gluteal claudication is the problem. This error is more likely if buttock pain is not associated with pain in the calf. Some patients with vascular disease of the iliac artery complain only of the symptoms of gluteal claudication, which are usually felt when the patient walks outside.

Rest pain (often nocturnal) in the toes or heel is almost pathognomonic of arterial insufficiency. With arterial insufficiency the patient may have pallor on elevation, rubor on dependency, and loss of hair on the toes. Some men with aortoiliac disease may present with pain in the upper leg or the buttock and an inability to develop or sustain an erection. Intermittent claudication pain is usually unilateral but can be bilateral. When the pain is present bilaterally, it seldom occurs in both legs simultaneously. The onset of pain in one leg may prevent the patient from walking enough to produce symptoms in the other leg. Physical examination for evidence of arterial insufficiency must therefore be performed on both legs.

Venous insufficiency. Venous claudication is difficult to distinguish from claudication due to arterial insufficiency. In both conditions, walking causes calf pain that may be severe enough for the patient to stop walking. Patients with venous claudication usually have no physical signs of arterial insufficiency.

Spinal stenosis. Spinal stenosis is another cause of leg pain that is exacerbated by exercise. The pain is similar to that associated with arterial insufficiency; it also occurs more frequently in older men. The first clue that the pain in the leg is not caused by arterial insufficiency is the presence of normal pedal pulses. **Although both begin with exercise, the pain of spinal stenosis is less often relieved by rest than the pain of arterial insufficiency** (Table 24–1). The pain of intermittent claudication is relieved within a few minutes, whereas the pain of spinal

■ TABLE 24.1 Comparison of Symptoms and Signs in Vascular and Spinal Claudication

	VASCULAR CLAUDICATION	CAUDA EQUINA CLAUDICATION
Backache	Uncommon, occurs in aortoiliac occlusion	Common but need not be present
Leg symptoms	Quantitatively related to effort	May be brought on by effort; directly related to posture of extension of spine
Quality	Cramplike, tight feeling; intense fatigue; discomfort; pain may be absent	Numbness, cramplike, burning, paresthetic; sensation of cold or swelling; pain may be absent
Relief	Rest of affected muscle group	Rest not enough; postural alteration of spine to allow flexion is necessary in most
Onset	Simultaneous onset in all parts affected	Characteristic march up or down legs
Urinary incontinence	Does not occur	Very rare
Impotence	Common in aortoiliac disease (failure to sustain erection)	Very rare (failure to achieve erection)
Wasting of legs	Global in aortoiliac disease	Cauda equina distribution in severe cases
Trophic changes	May be present; absent in aortoiliac disease	Absent but may be present in combined disease
Sensory loss	Absent	Not uncommon; common after exercise
Ankle jerks	Often absent in patients over 60 years	Common, particularly after exercise
Straight leg raising	Full	Often full

From DeVilliers JC: Combined neurogenic and vascular claudication. SA Med J 57:650-654, 1980.

stenosis requires 10 to 30 minutes to subside. Some patients with calf pain from spinal stenosis state that they must sit or lie down with the thighs flexed to relieve the discomfort.

The pain of spinal stenosis is caused by a localized narrowing of the spinal canal due to a structural abnormality that results in *cauda equina compression.* Patients occasionally complain of backache or buttock pain as well as numbness and tingling in the feet with walking. Walking uphill is easier than walking downhill for these patients. They have no problem riding a bicycle, probably because the stooped position assumed during this activity reduces the amount of cauda equina compression. The examiner must remember that vascular claudication and spinal stenosis can coexist.

Thrombophlebitis. Unilateral pain and swelling in the calf usually are caused by thrombophlebitis. The pain is usually present at rest and seldom is worsened by exercise. In a patient with thrombophlebitis who experiences calf pain when walking, an acute exacerbation of the calf pain occurs immediately after placing the foot on the ground. Although the history and physical examination of thrombophlebitis are well known to most physicians (i.e., pain, swelling, tenderness to palpation, occasionally a history of prior trauma or previous bouts of phlebitis), this relatively common cause of leg pain often is misdiagnosed. Several studies have suggested that venography should be used to confirm the clinical diagnosis because thrombophlebitis has often been incorrectly diagnosed in the absence of venographic evidence.

Other Conditions

Other causes of painful swelling of the calf include *traumatic rupture* of the plantaris tendon or the medial head of the gastrocnemius, *muscle trauma*, and *muscle stiffness* after unaccustomed exercise. *Popliteal (Baker's) cyst*, called the "pseudothrombophlebitis syndrome," causes painful swelling of the calf, thus mimicking thrombophlebitis. Therefore, all patients with painful calf swelling should be examined for a popliteal cyst. In one large series, most patients with painful popliteal cysts also had inflammatory joint disease of the knee, usually rheumatoid arthritis (Table 24–2).

Diffuse aching in one or both calves with no relation to exercise suggests *varicose veins.* Patients with this condition frequently complain of night cramps and that their legs hurt when they go to bed at night. The pain of venous insufficiency is vague, nonspecific, and unrelated to any specific muscle groups. Superficial varicosities may suggest the diagnosis, but deep venous insufficiency may be present without noticeable superficial serpiginous varicosities.

A first attack of *gouty arthritis* of the knee (or rarely of the hip) may be difficult to diagnose unless the patient has a warm, swollen joint in the big toe (podagra) and a prior history of gout. When the first attack is a warm, swollen, painful knee, the diagnosis is less apparent and may be confused with *pyogenic arthritis.* Patients with gout do not usually have as many systemic signs and symptoms (rash, malaise, fever) as do patients with pyogenic arthritis. Gouty arthritic patients often have a hot, red, tender, swollen joint. The involved joint is sensitive to external pressure; some patients cannot even tolerate the weight of a sheet or blanket on the joint.

Associated Symptoms

Patients with *DJD* often have pain and stiffness in other joints. A limp may be present in cases of DJD of the hip. Patients with *sciatica* may have numbness, paresthesia, weakness, and sensory deficits as well as abnormal knee or ankle jerks

TABLE 24.2 Disease Entities Associated with Pseudothrombophlebitis Syndrome

Rheumatoid arthritis	Traumatic arthritis
Psoriatic arthritis	Meniscal injury
Osteoarthritis	Osteochondritis dissecans
Juvenile rheumatoid arthritis	Villonodular synovitis
Reiter's syndrome	Systemic lupus erythematosus
Gonococcal arthritis	Ankylosing spondylitis
Gouty arthritis	Mixed connective tissue disease

From Katerndahl DA: Calf pain mimicking thrombophlebitis. Postgrad Med 68(6):107-115, 1980.

(hyperactive early; diminished to absent later). Patients with *intermittent claudication* may complain of numbness in the foot, which may erroneously suggest a *peripheral neuropathy.* If they also report *impotence,* an *aortoiliac lesion* is probable.

Night cramps, edema of the legs, and stasis abnormalities suggest *chronic venous insufficiency.*

Precipitating and Aggravating Factors

Pain during activity usually is seen with structural abnormalities, whereas pain at rest or after activity suggests inflammatory processes. Bone pain occurs at rest and increases with weight bearing. The pain of *DJD* worsens with exercise and prolonged weight bearing. *Sciatic* pain is aggravated by coughing, straining at stools, sneezing, walking, stooping, lifting, and spinal extension. As mentioned earlier, both the pain of *intermittent claudication* and the pain of *spinal stenosis* are brought on by walking and exercise. Pain in the knee after sitting for a while suggests patellofemoral disorders.

Ameliorating Factors

Patients with *DJD* will report that their morning stiffness, aches, and pain often abate during the day as they move the joint. *Sciatic* pain often is alleviated by recumbency in the fetal position. The pain of *intermittent claudication* abates within a few minutes after cessation of walking; the pain of *spinal stenosis* is relieved more slowly and by spinal flexion. The pain of *varicose veins* is alleviated somewhat by elevation of the involved limb; the resting (nocturnal) pain of *arterial insufficiency* often is relieved by lowering of the involved limb. **Relief of symptoms with an adequate dose of colchicine is pathognomonic of gout.**

Physical Findings and Diagnostic Studies

A careful history and physical examination are essential in all patients who complain of pain in the extremities. The physician especially notes any history of previous joint disease, precipitating events, previous diagnoses, and medications, particularly oral contraceptives, which are associated with a higher incidence of thrombophlebitis.

Physical examination should include observation of gait, neurologic evaluation (Fig. 24–1), attempts to reproduce the pain by palpation or maneuver, determination of range of motion of all joints, measurement of both calves and both thighs, and inspection and palpation for arterial insufficiency. Examination of the knee and popliteal space should be performed in both the supine and the erect positions. Joint effusions are more readily detected in the supine position, whereas cysts are more prominent when the patient is erect.

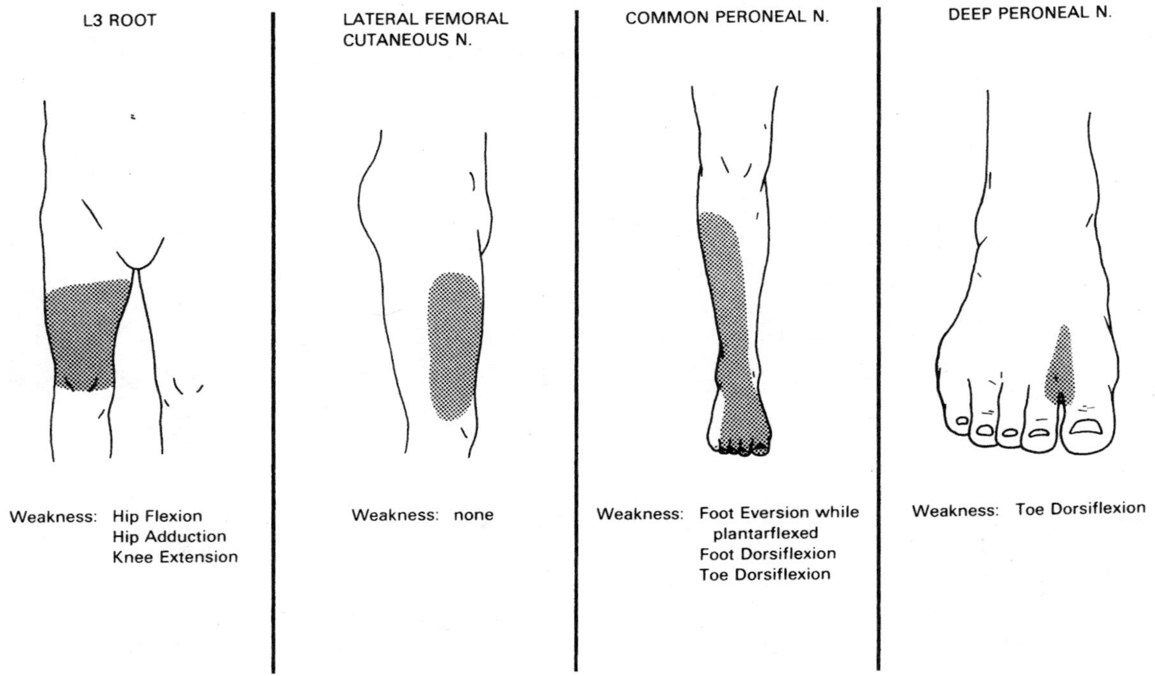

■ **Figure 24.1** Common root and peripheral nerve syndromes (lower extremity). Syndromes are usually incomplete. Dermatomes and innervations can vary in some patients. (From Birnbaum JS: The Musculoskeletal Manual, 2nd ed. Philadelphia, WB Saunders Co, 1986.)

Illustration continued on following page.

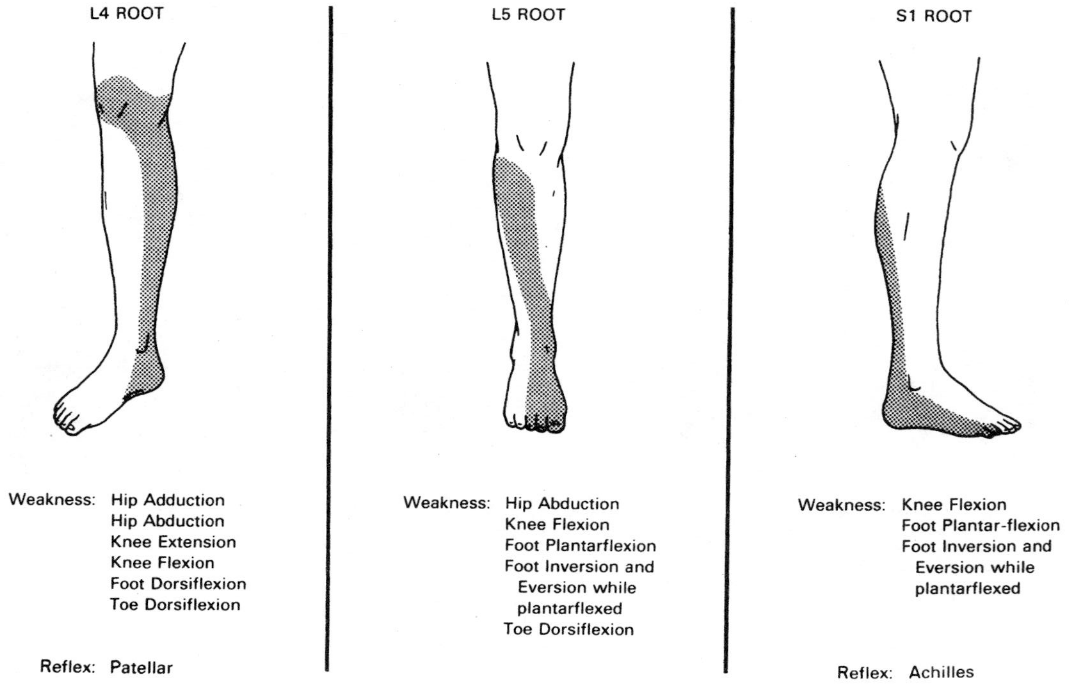

■ **Figure 24.1** *Continued*

Muscular and Ligamentous Strains and Tears

When patients complain of pain in the knee, the joint should be palpated (Figs. 24–2 and 24–3). Tenderness at the joint line suggests damage to the medial or collateral ligaments, the capsular ligament, or the meniscus. Radiographs, magnetic resonance imaging (MRI), and arthroscopic examination may be needed for an accurate diagnosis. The stability of the knee ligaments should be determined by careful physical examination (Figs. 24–4 and 24–5). Tenderness above or below the joint line suggests a muscle pull or strain (Fig. 24–6). With acute muscle tears, there usually is local tenderness, bruising, and possibly a gap in the muscle.

With *acute gouty arthritis*, the joint is usually warm, red, tender, and swollen. Although pain can be as severe as that seen in pyogenic arthritis, patients with gouty arthritis do not have comparable systemic symptoms. The serum uric acid level usually is elevated, and uric acid crystals may be seen in the joint aspirate.

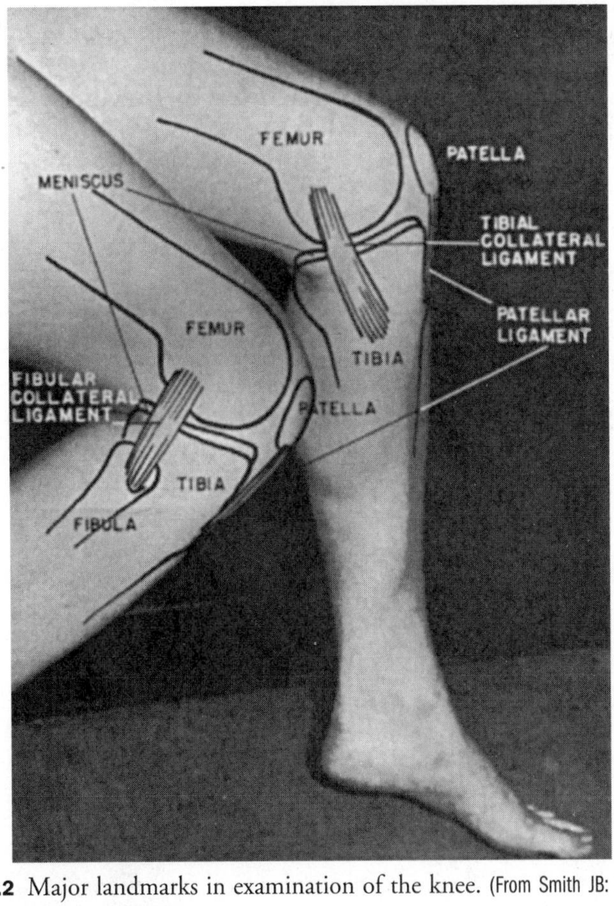

■ **Figure 24.2** Major landmarks in examination of the knee. (From Smith JB: Knee problems in children. Pediatr Clin North Am 24:4, 1977.)

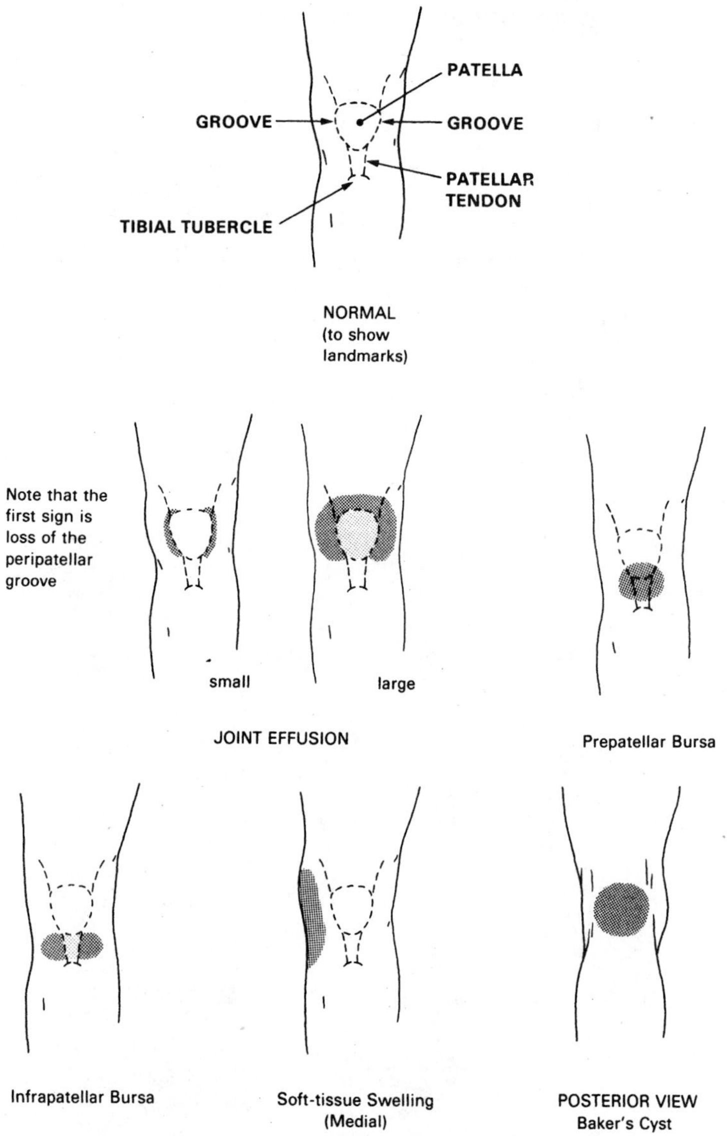

■ **Figure 24.3** Knee swelling. (From Birnbaum JS: The Musculoskeletal Manual, 2nd ed. Philadelphia, WB Saunders Co, 1986.)

Degenerative Joint Disease

Pain in the hip is frequently caused by DJD but may also result from other common conditions (Fig. 24–7). The major physical findings that suggest DJD of the knee include joint crepitus, limitation of joint movement, and elicitation of presenting symptoms at extremes of joint movement. Patients with advanced disease may have fixed flexion contractures, joint effusions, and radiographic evidence of arthritis. Patients with DJD are often in the same age group as those with vascular insufficiency, in whom the symptoms are referable to soft tissue. **The physician must remember that both conditions can coexist. If a careful examination reveals no swelling of the joint, there probably is no serious problem inside the joint.**

Sciatica

Some common physical findings in sciatica include restriction of spinal movement (hyperextension often reproduces sciatic pain), limitation of straight leg raising,

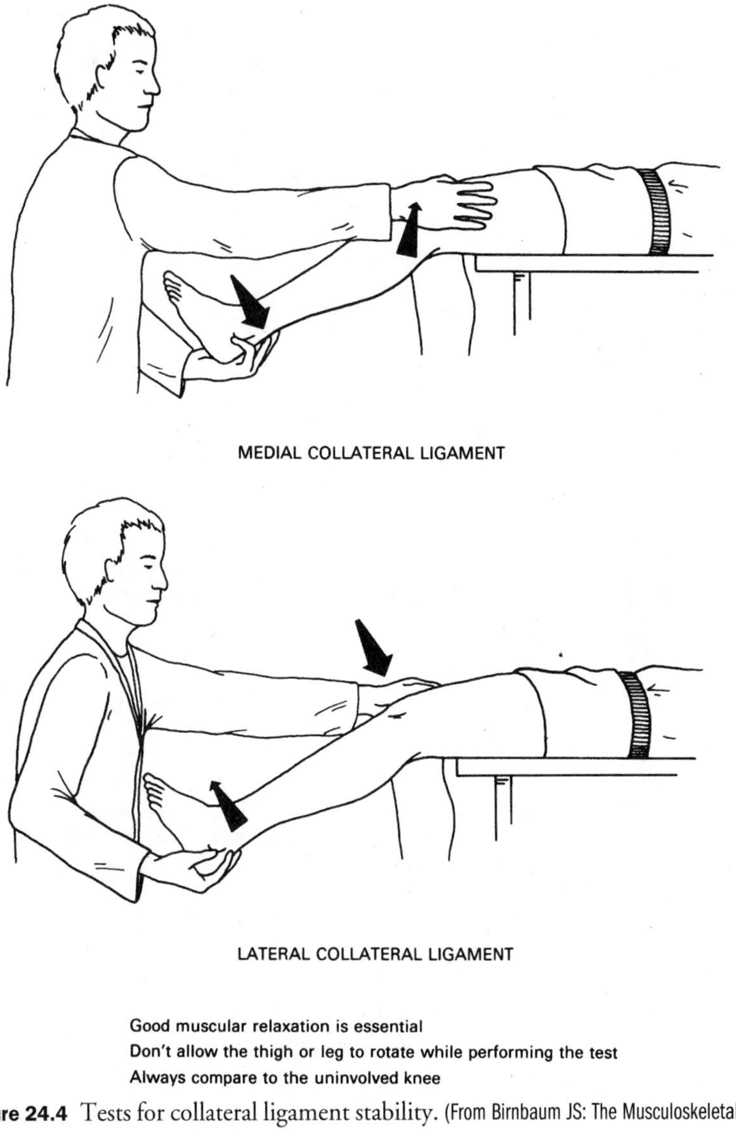

■ **Figure 24.4** Tests for collateral ligament stability. (From Birnbaum JS: The Musculoskeletal Manual, 2nd ed. Philadelphia, WB Saunders Co, 1986.)

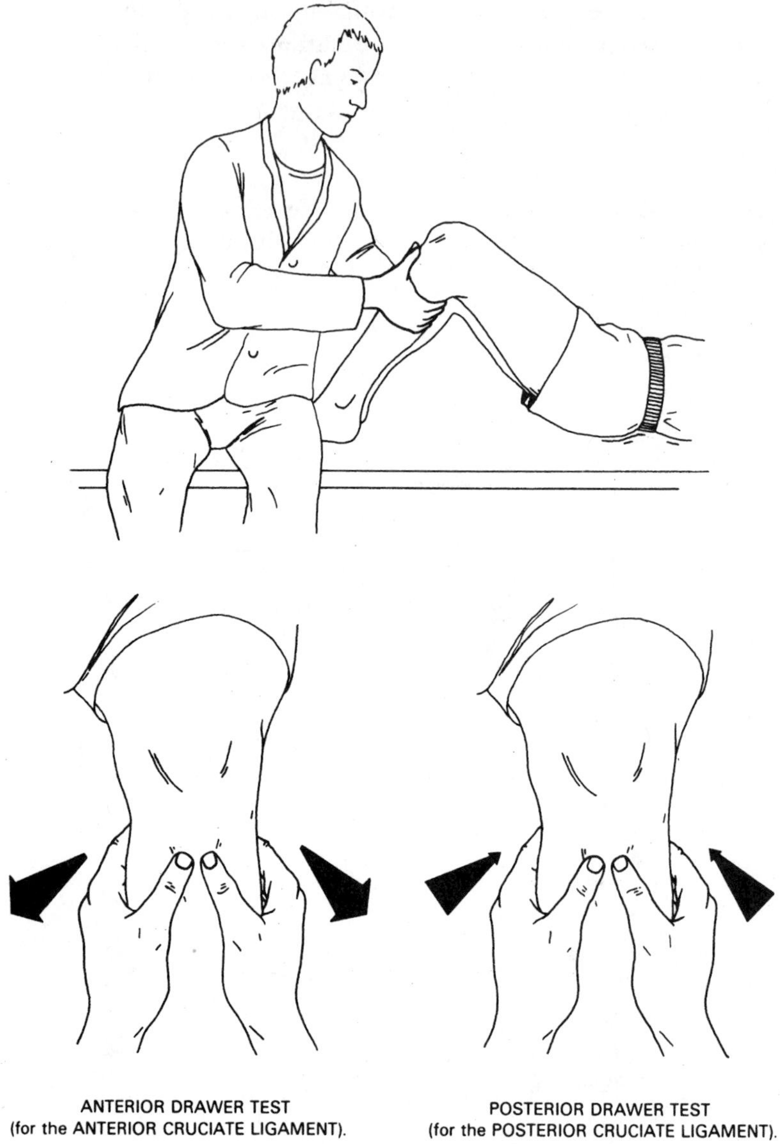

■ **Figure 24.5** Drawer tests to evaluate cruciate ligament stability. (From Birnbaum JS: The Musculoskeletal Manual, 2nd ed. Philadelphia, WB Saunders Co, 1986.)

and spasm over the sacrospinal muscles (which may be tender to palpation). Changes in reflex activity may occur, as well as sensory or motor loss over the involved segments (see Fig. 24–1). Myelograms and computed tomography (CT) scans are rarely necessary for diagnosis. They are used to determine the extent of the spinal cord compression.

Intermittent Claudication

Physical findings in intermittent claudication include pallor on elevation, rubor on dependency (most noticeable in the toes and sole), loss of hair on the toes, and diminished arterial pulsations. The presence of normal pedal pulses at rest and after walking virtually rules out arterial insufficiency.

Patients with *venous claudication* usually have varicose veins. Occasionally they can identify a tender point in the calf, but examination is nonrevealing. These

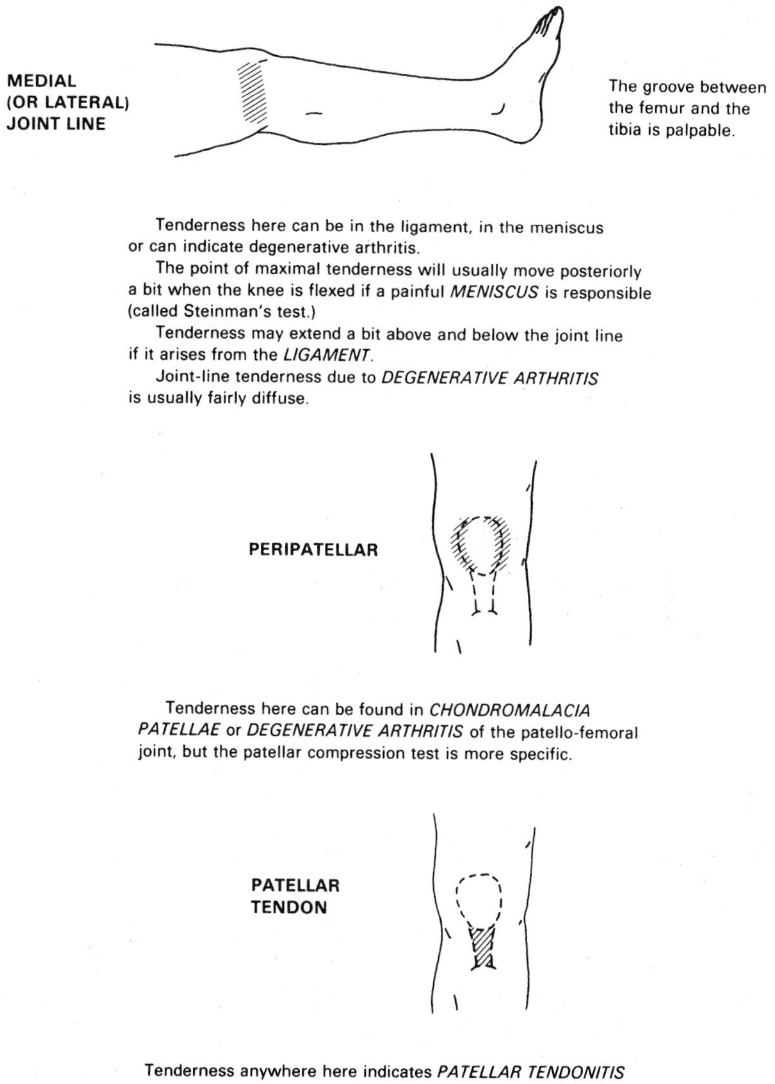

■ **Figure 24.6** Sites of tenderness around the knee. (From Birnbaum JS: The Musculoskeletal Manual, 2nd ed. Philadelphia, WB Saunders Co, 1986.)

Illustration continued on following page.

TIBIAL
TUBERCLE

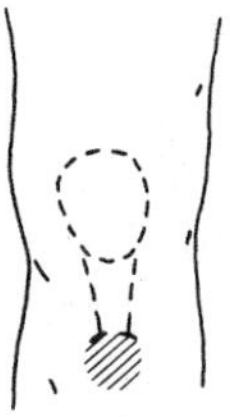

Tenderness (and sometimes swelling) here in a teenager implies *OSGOOD-SCHLATTER'S DISEASE*

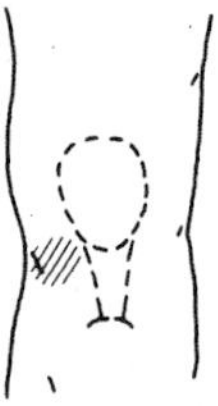

The bony prominence where the anserine tendons insert is easily palpable inferior to the joint line on the antero-medial tibia.

Tenderness here indicates *ANSERINE TENDONITIS*.

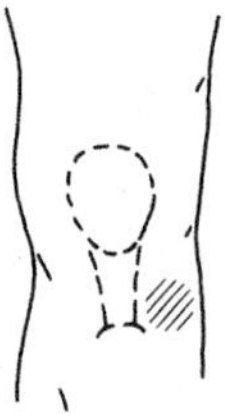

GERDY'S TUBERCLE
on the anterolateral tibia

Tenderness here indicates *ILIOTIBIAL BAND TENDONITIS*

■ **Figure 24.6** *Continued*

patients should be exercised to the point of discomfort, at which time a group of varices may be noted. Venography may be required for diagnosis.

Thrombophlebitis

The classic findings in patients with thrombophlebitis are swelling and a measurable increase in calf circumference when compared with that of the opposite side. The clinician often can palpate a tender cordlike vein between the heads of the gastrocnemius muscle. The patient may have dilatation of other veins, edema, erythema, and Homans' sign. These findings are variable and not always reliable for the diagnosis of thrombophlebitis. Inflation of a sphygmomanometer around each calf until pain is produced is a sensitive test. The single most important test is venography. **Because thrombophlebitis may coexist with a popliteal (Baker's) cyst, a venogram should be obtained for all patients with popliteal cysts.**

Other Conditions

The diagnosis of *joint sprain* is made by demonstrating instability of the joint. Tears of joint ligaments often can be demonstrated by the use of stress-view radiographs of the joint involved. With suspected *fractures,* a radiograph that includes the joints at both ends of the fractured bone always should be performed. Instability of joints suggests ligamentous tears. Angulation in valgus or varus with knee slightly flexed suggests either medial or lateral ligament instability. Abnormal forward or backward shift of the tibia on the femur is indicative of anterior

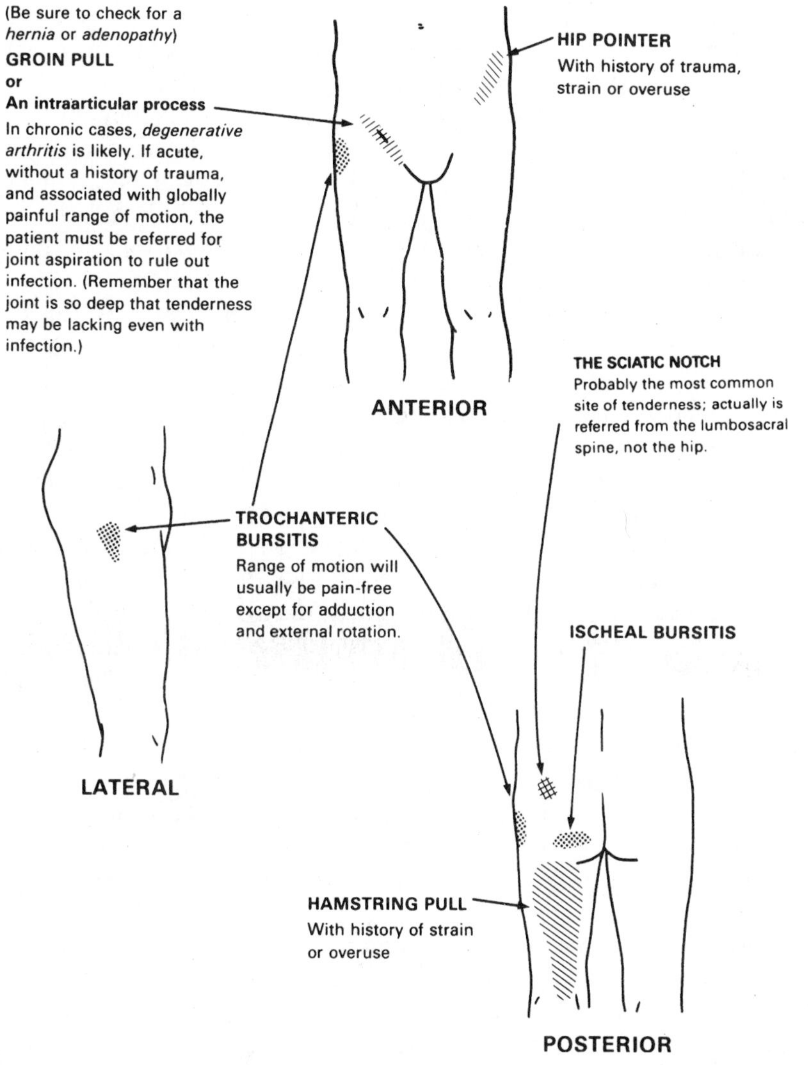

■ **Figure 24.7** Sites of tenderness around the hip. (From Birnbaum JS: The Musculoskeletal Manual, 2nd ed. Philadelphia, WB Saunders Co, 1986.)

cruciate or posterior cruciate ligament instability, respectively (see Fig. 24–5). Occasionally, abnormal rotations may be present; these suggest a complicated combination injury of the knee.

If the diagnosis is still unclear after a complete physical examination is conducted with special attention to the musculoskeletal, vascular, and nervous systems, noninvasive and invasive studies of the vascular system, electromyography, CT scanning, and myelography may be helpful.

Less Common Diagnostic Considerations

Sudden onset of pain in the leg, especially the lower leg and sometimes associated with paralysis, paresthesia, pallor, or absence of arterial pulsation, suggests acute arterial *embolism.* The likelihood of this diagnosis is increased by the presence of atrial fibrillation. Vague arthralgias and muscle aches often are seen with viral and flulike *infections,* but no joint abnormality can be detected on physical examination in these cases. Primary bone *tumors* are rare in adults; pain from metastatic bone disease, however, frequently is seen in patients with breast, lung, and prostatic tumors.

Because cellulitis of the calf can mimic thrombophlebitis, the two conditions must be differentiated. In patients with *cellulitis* the pain is described as being on the surface, no palpable cord is present, and Homans' sign is absent. Careful examination reveals that pain is induced by light palpation rather than deep palpation over the course of the vein. Likewise, the area of erythema is more clearly demarcated, occasionally with an associated open wound. An inflated sphygmomanometer requires high pressure to reproduce the pain of cellulitis, and often no difference exists between the two calves. These findings contrast with those reported in patients with thrombophlebitis.

Chondromalacia patellae, although more common in adolescents than in adults, may be seen in patients in their 40s and 50s. These patients characteristically have pain, stiffness, grating, or locking of the knee. The pain is worse when the knee is weight bearing in flexion. Crepitation and pain with manipulation of the patella over the femoral condyle are characteristic. Pain is exacerbated when the patient tenses the quadriceps with the knee in free extension while the examiner depresses the upper pole of the patella.

Meralgia paresthetica, which is slightly more common in men than in women, is caused by entrapment of the lateral femoral cutaneous nerve by the tensor fasciae latae. The patient complains of pain, burning, or tingling over the lateral aspect of the thigh that occasionally is worse at night or after exercise. It is alleviated by rest, particularly in the sitting position.

Peripheral neuropathies are more common in diabetic patients but may be seen in others. Patients complain of burning, tingling, and numbness, particularly in the feet. They may have a sensation of coldness, but no decrease in vascular pulsations is noted in those with a pure peripheral neuropathy. Diabetic patients with a peripheral neuropathy often have an associated vascular insufficiency.

Physical findings include sensory loss (often symmetric), muscle wasting, weakness, decreased tendon reflexes, and signs of arterial insufficiency.

Obturator hernias, an uncommon cause of pain, occur more frequently in elderly debilitated women than in other patients. The female/male ratio is 6:1. Patients usually present with pain along the anteromedial aspect of the thigh. This pain is increased by adduction of the thigh. Pain also may be felt in the hip or knee. The pain may be associated with intermittent bouts of nausea, vomiting, abdominal pain, and distention, all signs of small bowel obstruction. **Obturator hernia should be given particular consideration in elderly women who complain of pain in the hip or knee with no objective evidence of DJD or other common causes.**

Iliopsoas bursitis, a rare condition, should be suspected if the patient has gradual onset of groin pain that is exacerbated by flexion or internal rotation of the hip.

Half of patients with *pseudothrombophlebitis* due to a popliteal (Baker's) cyst have rheumatoid arthritis. Among patients with a confirmed popliteal cyst, only 50% had palpable masses, and 12% had masses below the popliteal space in one study. **A Baker's cyst should be suspected in all patients with thrombophlebitis and rheumatoid arthritis and in all patients with suspected thrombophlebitis but no evidence of phlebitis on venography.** An arthrogram is essential to the diagnosis of a popliteal cyst. Ultrasonography may help the physician diagnose an intact cyst, but it is not often useful in the diagnosis of a ruptured popliteal cyst.

Rheumatoid arthritis is a relatively uncommon cause of pain in the lower extremity. The joint pain usually lasts for a few weeks, with characteristic morning stiffness, joint tenderness, and pain with motion. Frequently the patient has joint effusion, soft tissue swelling, and synovial thickening. Pseudothrombophlebitis should be suspected when calf pain occurs in any patient with rheumatoid arthritis, especially if active inflammation of the knee is present.

Spinal stenosis (neurogenic claudication, cauda equina claudication) is often difficult to differentiate from intermittent claudication due to arterial insufficiency. The patient's history is particularly important because both conditions affect the same age group. Patients with calf pain due to spinal stenosis state that the pain starts insidiously, is exacerbated by walking, and is particularly related to extension of the spine. They may have associated backache or buttock pain, which is relatively uncommon in patients with intermittent claudication. A paresthetic quality to the pain suggests a neurogenic origin. Patients with spinal stenosis do not experience prompt relief of pain with cessation of exercise (as do those with arterial insufficiency); they feel greater relief when they lie or sit down with their thighs flexed. Patients do not have pain when riding a bicycle because the spine is in a flexed position. In any patient who has signs of intermittent claudication and who rides a bicycle without difficulty, spinal stenosis should be suspected.

Musculotendinous rupture of the gastrocnemius or plantaris, particularly during athletic activities such as jogging, running, and tennis, is characterized by a sudden onset of pain in the leg ("felt like I got a shot in the leg"). Frequently the physician can palpate the retracted end of the plantaris muscle.

Text continued on page 258.

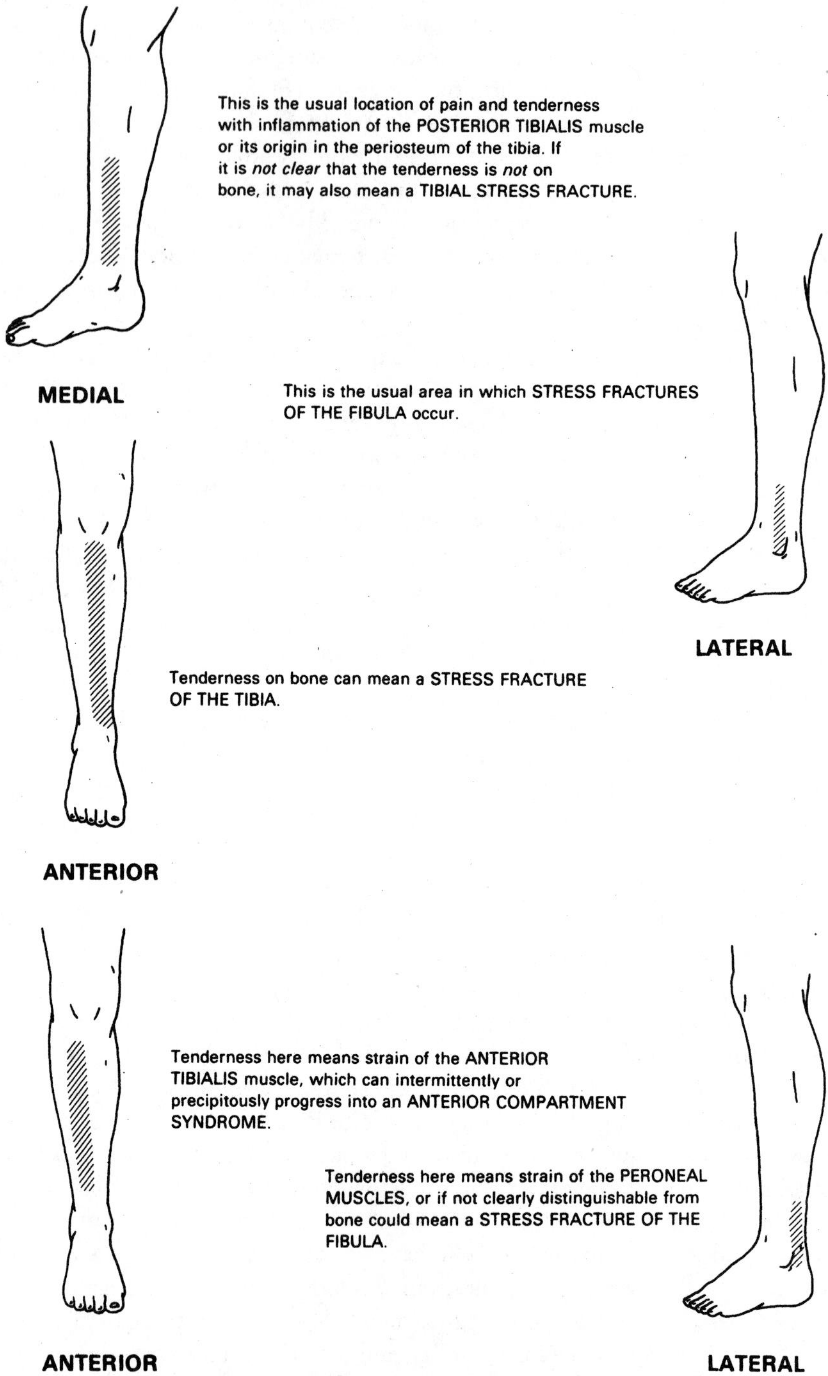

■ **Figure 24.8** Pain in the shin, often seen in runners.

Differential Diagnosis of Lower Extremity Pain in Adults

CAUSE	NATURE OF PATIENT	NATURE OF SYMPTOMS	ASSOCIATED SYMPTOMS	PRECIPITATING AND AGGRAVATING FACTORS	AMELIORATING FACTORS	PHYSICAL FINDINGS	DIAGNOSTIC STUDIES
Muscular or ligamentous strain	Weekend athletes Those with trauma			Unaccustomed or strenuous muscular activity		With ligamentous injury of joint, possible tenderness at joint line and swelling of joint Local tenderness	MRI for injury of knee, especially meniscal and ligamentous
Degenerative joint disease	Over age 40 (except those with prior trauma)	Knee or hip pain Morning stiffness Gradual onset	Pain and stiffness in other joints Occasional limp	Standing and weight bearing Descending stairs	Movement	Buttock pain not worse with hyperextension No evidence of nerve root compression Crepitation of joint Joint limitation of movement, effusion	Radiographs Arthroscopy of knee MRI

Table continued on following page.

Differential Diagnosis of Lower Extremity Pain in Adults *Continued*

CAUSE	NATURE OF PATIENT	NATURE OF SYMPTOMS	ASSOCIATED SYMPTOMS	PRECIPITATING AND AGGRAVATING FACTORS	AMELIORATING FACTORS	PHYSICAL FINDINGS	DIAGNOSTIC STUDIES
Lumbar disc disease (sciatica)	More common in men over age 40	Pain in buttock and posterolateral aspect of leg Acute onset Lancinating or like toothache Less severe previous episodes	Paresthesias Dysesthesias Weakness	Lifting Turning Twisting Spinal extension Coughing Straining	Fetal position	Spasm of hamstrings Positive straight or flexed leg signs Neurologic signs in lower leg Reversal of lordotic curve Pain of sciatic distribution with spinal hyperextension Asymmetric limitation of motion	CT scan Electromyography MRI
Anterior compartment syndrome (shin splint)	Runners	Achy Tightness Claudication type of pain	Occasional muscle weakness or sensory symptoms	Exercise	Rest	Tenderness to palpation over medial border of shin	Isotopic bone scan
Varicose veins		Diffuse aching of one or both calves Worse at night	Edema and stasis abnormalities		Elevation of limb	Varicose veins may or may not be apparent	Venography Doppler studies

Thrombophlebitis	History of phlebitis Use of oral contraceptives	Unilateral Pain at rest	Swelling	Placing foot on ground		No evidence of arterial insufficiency Swelling of calf with tenderness and warmth Palpable cord	Venography Doppler studies
Arterial insufficiency	Over age 50, earlier in diabetics	Pain in calf with walking Intermittent claudication of hip with aortoiliac disease Rest pain in calf, toes, or heel suggests severe arterial insufficiency Usually unilateral	Impotence with aortoiliac disease	Walking	Rest Dependency of involved limb	Decreased pulses Pallor on elevation, rubor on dependency Cool Loss of hair on toes	Arteriography Doppler studies MRI
Spinal stenosis	Older men	Calf pain induced by walking and leg exercise	Paresthesias Backache Buttock pain	Exercise Not precipitated by exercise with spine flexed (bicycling)	Not quickly relieved by rest Spinal flexion	Good pedal pulses Transient neurologic deficit	Electromyography CT scan MRI
Gout	More common in men	Acute onset Toe and knee pain Rare in hip		Occasionally precipitated by trauma		Joint warm, swollen, exquisitely tender	Serum uric acid test Uric acid crystals in joint aspirate

Trochanteric bursitis, a relatively uncommon cause of leg pain, usually presents with pain over the greater trochanter, in the buttock, and in the lateral thigh along the distribution of the second lumbar dermatome. On physical examination, the patient may limp and usually has marked point tenderness over the greater trochanter. The differential diagnosis consists of arthritis of the hip or lumbar spine problems. The major factors in differential diagnosis include pain with palpation over the trochanteric bursa and the absence of sensory loss, which would be seen with lumbar disc disease. The pain is not exacerbated by coughing and sneezing but by squatting, climbing stairs, and sitting with the painful leg crossed over the other one. It is alleviated by infiltration of the trochanteric bursa with local anesthetics or steroids or both.

Cyclic hip pain that coincides with menstruation suggests *endometriosis.* The pain is usually unilateral.

The Leg and Sports Medicine

The most common causes of chronic leg pain in runners include *shin splints, stress fractures,* and *compartment syndromes* (Fig. 24–8). Shin splints represent muscle tenderness, inflammation, and probably subclinical periosteal reaction. With stress fractures there is usually point tenderness over the involved bone, and the diagnosis may be confirmed radiographically. Stress fractures are more common in experienced long-distance runners, particularly in those who attempt to run more than 20 to 30 miles per week. These fractures may occur in the tibia, fibula, or the metatarsus.

Compartment syndromes occur when the fascial compartment is too small to accommodate the approximately 20% increase in muscle size that occurs with strenuous exercise. This results in a limited venous outflow and tends to produce an ischemic pain of the involved tissue. Patients with compartment syndromes usually present with a gradual onset (over 1 or more years) of pain that is progressive, dull, aching, and particularly worse after long runs. Paresthesias also may be present. The anterior compartment of the leg usually is affected; the next most likely affected is the posterior compartment, followed by the posterior superficial compartment. Physical findings include tenderness in the muscle mass itself but not as much in the bone and tendons. Elevated compartment pressures are diagnostic.

Selected References

Alvarez JA, Hardy RH: Lumbar spine stenosis: a common cause of back and leg pain. Am Fam Physician 57:1825–1834, 1998.

Barry NN, McGuire JL: Acute injuries and specific problems in adult athletes. Rheum Dis Clin North Am 22:531–549, 1996.

Birnbaum JS: The musculoskeletal manual, 2nd ed. Philadelphia, WB Saunders Co, 1986.

Detmer DE: Chronic leg pain. Am J Sports Med 8(2):141–144, 1980.

Goodreau JJ, et al: Rational approach to the differentiation of vascular and neurogenic claudication. Surgery 84(6):749–757, 1978.

Katerndahl DA: Calf pain mimicking thrombophlebitis. Postgrad Med 68(6):107–115, 1980.
Lee RV, McComb LE, Mezzadri FC: Pregnant patients, painful legs: the obstetrician's dilemma. Obstet Gynecol Surv 45:290–298, 1990.
McCune WJ, Matteson EL, MacGuire A: Evaluation of knee pain. Prim Care 15:795–808, 1988.
Noble J, Abernathy PK: The painful knee. Br J Hosp Med 22(2):169–176, 1979.
Polisson RP: Sports medicine for the internist. Med Clin North Am 70:469–489, 1986.
Post WR, Fulkerson JP: Anterior knee pain—a symptom not a diagnosis. Bull Rheum Dis 42:5–7, 1993.
Provan JL, Moreau P, MacNab I: Pitfalls in the diagnosis of leg pain. Can Med Assoc J 121:167–171, 1979.
Roberts WN, Williams RR: Hip pain. Prim Care 15:783–793, 1988.
Ruffin MT, Kiningham RB: Anterior knee pain: the challenge of patellofemoral syndrome. Am Fam Physician 47:185–194, 1993.
Styf J: Diagnosis of exercise induced pain in the anterior aspect of the lower leg. Am J Sports Med 16:165–169, 1988.
Thorne RP, Curd JG: Radiating leg pain in the older patient. Hosp Pract 26:61–64, 69–72, 1991.

CHAPTER 25

Pain in the Lower Extremity and Limp in Children

The physician should approach leg pain or limp in children as in adults, that is, determine whether it originates in joints or in soft tissue. The most common causes of leg pain originating in the soft tissue are unusual or strenuous *exercise* and *trauma.* Other common causes of leg pain include *growing pains, Legg-Calvé-Perthes disease, Osgood-Schlatter disease, chondromalacia patellae,* and *ossification of Achilles insertion.* Limp can be due to pain, weakness, or structural abnormality.

Nature of Patient

If a limp occurs when a young child begins to walk, *congenital dislocation* of one or both hips should be considered. *Toddler's fracture,* an undisplaced fracture of the distal tibia, may occur when weight bearing first occurs (9 months to 3 years). It may present as a limp or inability to bear weight on the affected leg. *Legg-Calvé-Perthes disease* (epiphysitis of the hip) usually occurs between ages 5 and 7 years. In adolescents, *slipped femoral epiphyses* and *patellar problems* are more common. In children between ages 12 and 14, pain in the heel is most often caused by a painful *bursitis* or *irregular ossification* of *calcaneal apophysis.*

Nature of Symptoms

Growing pains is a general diagnosis that is being made less frequently as physicians become more expert in making specific diagnoses. Growing pains do exist, however, and they are now thought to be a form of *myalgia.* The aching pain is intermittent and usually located in the leg muscles, particularly in the front of the thigh, the calf, and the back of the knee. The pain is deep and localized to areas outside joints. It is usually bilateral and typically occurs late in the day, although it may awaken the child from a sound sleep. Growing pains may be exacerbated by excessive running during the day, but exercise is not usually a factor. **The findings that the pain is nonarticular, bilateral, and usually unrelated to activity are essential to the accurate diagnosis of growing pains.** Children with growing pains show no abnormal physical findings.

Most serious diseases that cause leg pain in children (except slipped capital femoral epiphyses) are usually unilateral. Pain in the hip may result from *Legg-Calvé-Perthes disease,* a disturbance of the epiphyseal ossification of the femoral head in children ages 4 to 12 (peak age, 5 to 7 years). It often is associated with a limp. Occasionally, the pain is referred to the medial aspect of the knee.

The most common causes of knee pain in children are *acute trauma, Osgood-Schlatter-disease,* and *chondromalacia patellae.* Osgood-Schlatter disease is an abnormality of the epiphyseal ossification of the tibial tubercle. It is most common in children ages 10 to 15. This condition involves painful swelling of the tibial tubercle at the insertion of the patellar tendon. The pain is worse with contraction of the quadriceps against resistance. It is exacerbated by activity and relieved by rest.

Chondromalacia patellae is just one of several causes of anterior knee pain. (Some believe the term should be discarded, but its use is still commonplace.) It results from chronic *patellofemoral dysfunction* and is an extremely common syndrome in active children and adolescents. It may be a precursor of adult patellofemoral arthritis. In this condition, the patellar cartilage degenerates, not because of primary cartilaginous disease, but because of abnormal mechanical forces acting on it.

These abnormal forces may result from direct or indirect trauma. Direct injury may occur when a force is applied to the anterior aspect of the patella; this usually results from a fall on the flexed knee. Indirect trauma is more common. This is usually the result of strenuous or repetitive quadriceps activity to which the patient is unaccustomed (e.g., hiking, jogging, calisthenics, skiing). **The most characteristic symptom of indirect trauma is pain in the lower pole of the patella and adjacent patellar tendon that is precipitated by strenuous activity, especially running, jumping, or squatting.** After resting with the knee flexed, patients with indirect trauma experience a marked increase in pain when they initially extend the knee and begin to move around, but they usually find some relief after standing still or walking a short distance. Patients often describe a grating sensation that may be detected on physical examination when the knee is flexed and extended. The grating is noted particularly when the knee is extended against resistance. Radiographs are usually normal but may show fragmentation of the lower pole of the patella.

Chondromalacia patellae must be differentiated from *patellar osteochondritis, jumper's knee,* and *partial rupture of patellar tendon.* Children with chondromalacia patellae usually have localized tenderness at the lower pole of the patella and the adjacent patellar tendon (see Fig. 24–2). Occasionally the physician may note separation of the patellar tendon from the lower pole and a palpable defect at that point.

Other conditions that give rise to knee pain include *patellar subluxation, patellar dislocation,* and *meniscal injuries. Rheumatoid arthritis* and *popliteal cysts,* although uncommon, can occur in children.

Limping is a common complaint among children. It is never normal, although its causes are many, ranging from poorly fitting shoes to a sprained

ankle to the earliest manifestation of a malignant tumor. To determine the exact cause of limping, the physician must approach the problem methodically and thoroughly, obtaining a detailed history and performing a careful examination of the child's gait.

Associated Symptoms

Although limping is often caused by trauma and the most common cause of leg pain is traumatic injury to the joints or soft tissue, these facts may be misleading in some cases. **In general, when pain or limp is caused by mild trauma, the symptoms should disappear within 2 to 3 weeks.** If the symptoms do not disappear, despite a report of trauma, the physician must obtain a thorough history and perform a complete physical examination to rule out more serious entities. The physician must determine whether the limp is (1) intermittent or constant, (2) present at the end of the day or in the morning, (3) made worse by climbing stairs, and (4) present only after vigorous exercise (which may be the first clue to an impending stress fracture).

The location of leg pain often provides clues to its cause, particularly in cases of referred pain. Lower back pathology most commonly refers pain to the buttocks and lateral thigh, whereas hip pathology often refers pain to the groin, medial thigh, or knee. For example, Legg-Calvé-Perthes disease is a common cause of knee pain and limp in children.

Physical Findings

Range of motion of each joint from the hip down should be noted and compared with that of the opposite side, with careful attention given to the patellae. Leg lengths should be measured; a discrepancy of 1.25 cm (½ inch) or more can cause a *pelvic tilt* and subsequent limp.

When the patient complains of lower leg pain, particularly with a limp, the gait should be examined first. Gait consists of two phases: stance and swing. In the stance phase the foot is in contact with the floor, and one limb bears all the body weight. In the swing phase the foot is not touching the floor. This phase begins when the toe comes off the floor and ends with heel strike. A child with a stiff hip would have a short swing phase because of limited hip joint movement. During each phase, the physician should observe one or two of the involved anatomic components: first the feet, then the knees, pelvis, and trunk. The sound of the walk may suggest a steppage gait, with slapping of the foot from footdrop. The shoes should be inspected for abnormal wear. Excessive wear of the toes of the shoes suggests *toe walking,* and excessive wear of the medial aspects of the shoes indicates severe *flat feet.*

With joint effusion the physician must suspect an infectious process, especially if systemic signs exist. Infections may be caused by gonococci, staphylococci, *Haemophilus* spp., or in endemic areas, Lyme disease.

■ Differential Diagnosis of Lower Extremity Pain and Limp in Children

CAUSE	NATURE OF PATIENT	NATURE OF SYMPTOMS	ASSOCIATED SYMPTOMS	PRECIPITATING AND AGGRAVATING FACTORS	AMELIORATING FACTORS	PHYSICAL FINDINGS	DIAGNOSTIC STUDIES
Epiphysitis of hip (Legg-Calvé-Perthes disease)	Ages 4–12 (5–7 peak incidence) Usually male Rare in blacks	Unilateral hip pain often referred to medial aspect of knee	Limp			Limitation of hip motion	Radiograph of hip Bone scintigraphy
Epiphysitis of knee (Osgood-Schlatter disease)	Ages 10–15	Painful swelling of tibial tubercle		Quadriceps contraction against resistance	Rest		Radiograph of knee
Chondromalacia patellae	Children and adolescents	Pain in lower pole of patella and adjacent patellar tendon		Running Jumping Squatting	Quiet standing or walking	Grating of knee with flexion and extension	Radiograph of knee
Trauma	History of sports participation	Joint or soft tissue			2–3 weeks of rest	Local tenderness	Sonography for synovitis of hip
Growing pains		Intermittent myalgia, especially of thigh, calf, and back of knee Nonarticular and bilateral Not related to activity				No abnormal findings	
Slipped capital femoral epiphysis	Usually males, ages 12–15 More common in blacks	Hip pain Only knee pain in 25%	Limp Trendelenburg gait			Bilateral in 25%	Radiograph of hip Bone scintigraphy

Diagnostic Studies

A complete blood count and erythrocyte sedimentation rate (ESR) should be ordered. An ESR greater than 50 mm per hour in a child with a limp suggests a serious disease. In selected cases a Lyme titer, rheumatoid factor, HLA-B27, or culture of joint effusion may be diagnostic. Plain radiographs (ordered first), bone scan, ultrasound, computed tomography (CT), or magnetic resonance imaging (MRI) may also be diagnostic.

Less Common Diagnostic Considerations

Rheumatoid arthritis, popliteal cyst, quadriceps malalignment, supracondylar cortical avulsion, and traumatic epiphyseal injury may cause leg pain or limp, or both. *Herpes zoster*, although uncommon in children, frequently involves the lower extremity and may cause pain, burning, or itching before the typical herpetic lesion appears. Usually children with herpes zoster of the leg have only a rash and experience no pain. Rarely, spinal problems, appendicitis, and hernias may cause a limp.

Selected References

Dabney KW, Lipton G: Evaluation of limp in children. Curr Opin Pediatr 7:88–94, 1995.

Goldberg B: Chronic anterior knee pain in the adolescent. Pediatr Ann 20:186–193, 1991.

Hollingworth P: Differential diagnoses and management of hip pain in childhood. Br J Rheumatol 34:78–82, 1995.

Myers MT, Thompson GH: Imaging the child with a limp. Pediatr Clin North Am 44:637–658, 1997.

Peterson H: Growing pains. Pediatr Clin North Am 33:1367–1372, 1986.

Smith JB: Knee problems in children. Pediatr Clin North Am 24(4):841–855, 1977.

Sty JR, Wells RG, Smith WB: The child with acute leg pain. Semin Nucl Med 18:137–158, 1988.

CHAPTER 26

Pain in the Upper Extremity

Shoulder

After backache, upper extremity pain is the next most common type of musculoskeletal pain. It usually occurs in the joints (shoulder, elbow, and wrist), with the shoulder being the most common site. Arm pain is frequently caused by occupational *repetitive strain injury.* Shoulder pain can be referred from the neck, chest, or diaphragmatic region; it usually is caused by a local process. The "shoulder joint" includes three large bones (clavicle, scapula, humerus) and four joints (sternoclavicular, acromioclavicular, glenohumeral, thoracoscapular) (Figs. 26–1 to 26–3).

Terms used to describe painful disorders of the shoulder refer to variations of the same basic process and include *supraspinatus tendinitis, rotator cuff tendinitis, subacromial bursitis, bicipital tendinitis, painful arc syndrome, impingement syndrome, calcific tendinitis, calcific bursitis,* and *calcific bicipital tendinitis.*

Pain may originate in the bursa as well as in the shoulder joint. Many authors suggest that the only significant bursa in the shoulder is the subacromial bursa and that the subdeltoid, subcoracoid, and supraspinatus bursae are extensions of the subacromial bursa.

The initial process with shoulder pain is usually a *supraspinatus tendinitis* with extension to other muscles of the rotator cuff. With severe or continuing damage, the inflammatory process spreads first to the subacromial bursa and then to the joint capsule and intraarticular and extraarticular structures. **The greater the area of pain in the arm and shoulder and the greater the spontaneity of pain (i.e., onset without aggravating events), the greater is the likelihood of an extensive lesion.**

Pain in the shoulder (as well as in the elbow and wrist) can be caused by *tendinitis, bursitis, trauma, arthritis,* or *referred pain.* Cartilage and bone are not very sensitive to pain. The following are listed in order of decreasing degrees of pain sensitivity: tendons, bursae, ligaments, synovial tissue, capsular reinforcements, and muscles.

Nature of Patient

Acute subacromial bursitis, which is painful enough to cause marked limitation of movement, is more common in younger patients. *Calcific tendinitis* is also more common in younger people and seldom is associated with tears; it is more often

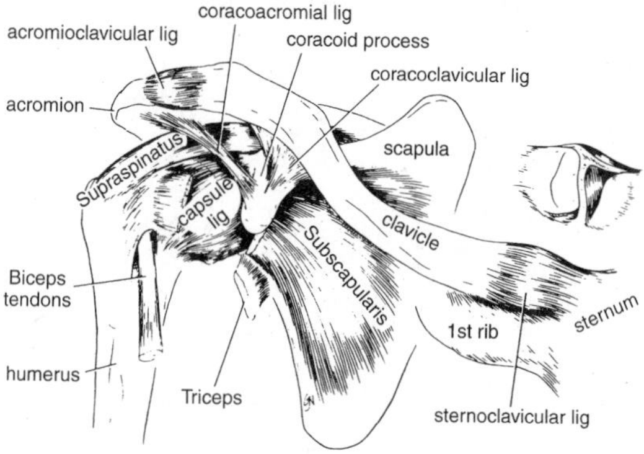

■ **Figure 26.1** Glenohumeral, acromioclavicular, and sternoclavicular joints. The thoracoscapular joint is between the anterior scapular surface and the chest wall. (From Bland JH, et al: The painful shoulder. Semin Arthritis Rheum 7:21-47, 1977.)

seen as a sequela to acute bursitis. A *supraspinatus tear,* which permits some movement, is more common in people over ages 40 to 50 years. *Dislocation of the shoulder* is also more common in people over age 50. First-time dislocations after ages 40 to 50 have a much higher incidence of a rotator cuff tear, which is rare before age 40.

Nature of Symptoms

In general, most shoulder problems cause pain in the fifth cervical (C5) dermatome, particularly around the deltoid insertion. The exception is the acromioclavicular joint, which causes pain in the C4 dermatome, especially on the superior

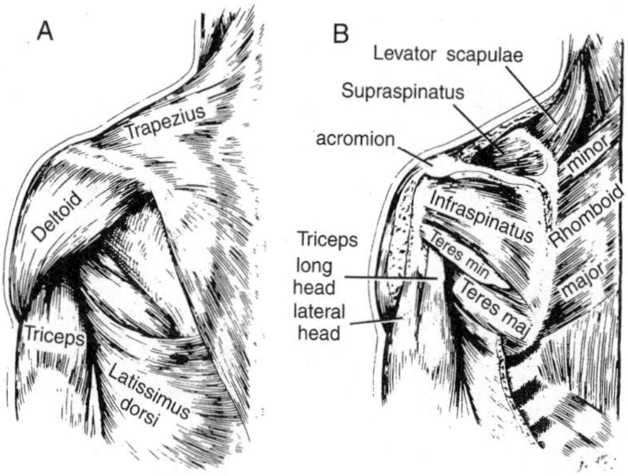

■ **Figure 26.2** Posterior view of the shoulder. *A,* Surface muscles, all groups. *B,* Rotator cuff; subcapularis not shown (medial rotator). Note that the rhomboids and levator scapulae displace the scapula medially toward the midline, whereas the scapulohumeral group rotates the humerus laterally. (From Bland JH, et al: The painful shoulder. Semin Arthritis Rheum 7:21-47, 1977.)

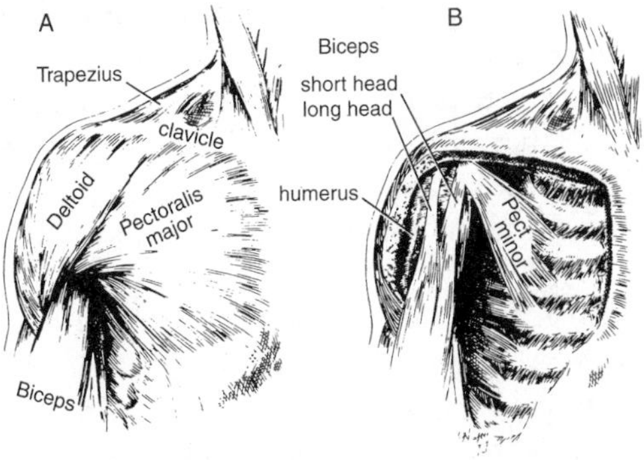

■ **Figure 26.3** Anterior view of the shoulder. *A,* Surface muscles. *B,* Deep layer of muscles. (From Bland JH, et al: The painful shoulder. Semin Arthritis Rheum 7:21–47, 1977.)

aspect of the shoulder or the joint itself. *Intracapsular lesions* of the glenohumeral joint, such as from arthritis or capsulitis, typically restrict active and passive range of motion. The more common *extracapsular lesions,* such as rotator cuff injuries or tendinitis, cause pain on active or resisted motion, whereas passive motion is usually maintained. When *impingement* causes inflammation of the superior part of the cuff, pain develops with resisted abduction and external rotation.

Shoulder pain, referred from the cervical spine, is not affected by shoulder movement but may be influenced by neck movement. The pain may also be felt in the neck and may radiate down the arm to below the elbow.

Involvement of supraspinatus tendon. Shoulder pain is most often located in the lower part of the deltoid region; this is the referral area for pain originating in the supraspinatus tendon. When a dull ache in the region of the deltoid insertion is exacerbated with abduction to 60 degrees or more (painful arc), internal rotation, reaching overhead, or putting on a coat, the physician should suspect *supraspinatus tendinitis.* Characteristically, patients report that the pain is worse at night or when they lie on the affected shoulder.

Involvement of teres minor, infraspinatus, and subscapularis muscles. If the shoulder is diffusely tender and if moving the humerus posteriorly causes pain, teres minor or infraspinatus muscle involvement should be suspected. If there is pain with resisted medial rotation, the subscapularis muscle may be involved. In patients with teres minor, infraspinatus, and subscapularis involvement with diffuse shoulder tenderness, pain usually does not radiate into the arm or neck and usually is absent or minimal when the arm is dependent.

Tears and ruptures of rotator cuff. If the patient has a sudden onset of shoulder pain in the deltoid area that intensifies within 6 to 12 hours after the initial trauma, a rotator cuff tear should be suspected. The patient may have extreme tenderness over the greater tuberosity as well as pain and restricted motion in one plane of movement at the glenohumeral joint. Patients with these findings and recurrent severe pain that awakens them at night may have a rotator cuff tear, even if the arthrogram is normal. In cases of complete rotator cuff rupture, the patient has severe pain and is totally unable to abduct the arm.

Calcific tendinitis. After a rotator cuff tear, patients may develop calcification and calcific tendinitis of the rotator cuff. Calcification has been reported in the rotator cuff in 8% of the asymptomatic population over age 30. Despite this, studies have shown that 35% of all patients with calcific tendinitis have had symptoms at some time. If 8% of the population have calcific tendinitis and 35% of these people develop symptoms, about 3% of patients over age 30 will eventually present with pain referable to a calcific tendinitis. Some studies have related the extent of the symptoms to the size of the calcific area. If the diameter of the calcific mass reaches 1 to 1.5 cm (about ½ inch), patients invariably develop symptoms. Patients have an abrupt onset of severe, aching pain and find all shoulder movement painful.

Bicipital and tricipital tendinitis. When the patient has generalized tenderness anteriorly in the region of the long head of the biceps (the region of the anterior subacromial bursa), particularly if the pain seems to be worse at night, bicipital tendinitis should be suspected. This pain resembles that of adhesive capsulitis, except that patients with bicipital tendinitis have relative freedom of abduction and forward flexion. Resisted forearm supination causing anterior shoulder pain is a hallmark of bicipital tendinitis. If there is pain in the triceps region with resisted extension of the elbow, tricipital tendinitis is probable.

Bursitis. When the patient has point tenderness over the subacromial bursa (often associated with swelling and warmth), subacromial bursitis is probable. Pain in the acromioclavicular joint suggests that this joint is the source of pain. Patients with subacromial bursitis experience particular pain when performing activities such as lifting objects and combing hair. Virtually all cases of subacromial bursitis are preceded by tendinitis or tenosynovitis in the rotator cuff, biceps, or biceps tendon sheath. When acute onset of excruciating pain occurs in the subdeltoid region of such severity that shoulder movement is totally limited, *calcific bursitis* is probable. Friction of an inflamed bursal surface may be detected with passive motion if the patient is unable to abduct or rotate the upper arm. This acute inflammatory process is probably secondary to calcific deposits in the coracoacromial arch, which ultimately ruptures into the bursal sac and leads to an acute bursitis.

Frozen shoulder. A frozen shoulder should be suspected when the patient has gradual onset of pain with limitation of motion at both the glenohumeral and the scapulothoracic joints and has limitation of abduction, external rotation, and forward flexion. Although a frozen shoulder is most often caused by inflammation of the capsule or rotator cuff, it has many other possible causes. The hallmark of frozen shoulder is a spontaneous onset of pain that worsens gradually and insidiously. The pain may radiate into the neck and arm, but pain below the elbow is unusual.

Subluxation or dislocation. When pain in the shoulder follows severe trauma (as opposed to the minor trauma of everyday activity and routine athletic endeavors), it may be caused by subluxation or dislocation of the shoulder joint. Patients may state that their shoulder "doesn't feel right," that "something popped," or that "something feels out of place." If this occurs in a child, particularly with other evidence of external trauma, child abuse should be considered.

Impingement syndrome. An impingement syndrome secondary to sports trauma usually occurs in the vulnerable, avascular region of the supraspinatus and biceps tendon. It usually starts as an irritation in the avascular region of the supraspinatus tendon and progresses to an inflammatory response (tendinitis) that involves the biceps tendon and subacromial bursa and then the acromioclavicular joint. This inflammation may finally result in rotator cuff tears and calcification. The most reliable sign of an impingement syndrome is that the pain is reproduced when the arm is flexed forward forcibly against resistance with the elbow extended (Fig. 26–4). Magnetic resonance imaging (MRI) suggests that subacromial bursitis, supraspinatus tendinitis, and impingement syndrome are variants of a single entity.

Site of pain. The location of pain is also useful in differential diagnosis (Fig. 26–5). Pain in the acromioclavicular joint suggests that the source of pain is that joint. Pain that occurs in any other part of the arm, shoulder, or neck or in the C5 dermatome may be caused by many other shoulder lesions. With supraspinatus tendinitis the initial symptom frequently is pain in the deltoid insertion area that is precipitated by abduction. As the inflammation spreads to the subacromial bursa, the pain may extend to the distal arm and occasionally into the forearm. Pain that involves the forearm as far as the wrist suggests that the inflammatory process has spread to the capsule and has been present for 3 to 6 months. If the entire arm is painful and motion is extremely limited, the inflammation has spread to involve the capsule and synovia (frozen shoulder).

Fibrositis syndrome. A form of nonarticular rheumatism, fibrositis syndrome is a common cause of pain in multiple locations, including the upper extremity (Fig. 26–6). Although some physicians doubt the existence of this syndrome, others have demonstrated exaggerated, reproducible tenderness at specific anatomic locations in patients with this condition. Even though these sites are normally tender on palpation, these patients often complain of spontaneous pain over the upper border of the trapezius, the lateral epicondyle of the humerus (the site of tennis elbow pain), and the origin of the supraspinatus muscle near the medial border of the scapula. These patients often complain of insomnia as well. Both the pain and the insomnia of fibrositis may respond to tricyclic antidepressants.

Pain from vigorous physical activity. Although they recognize the traumatic aspects of severe falls and motor vehicle accidents and the recurrent trauma of competitive sports (e.g., swimming, tennis), examiners may overlook that shoulder trauma can result from ordinary, vigorous physical activity (e.g., polishing a

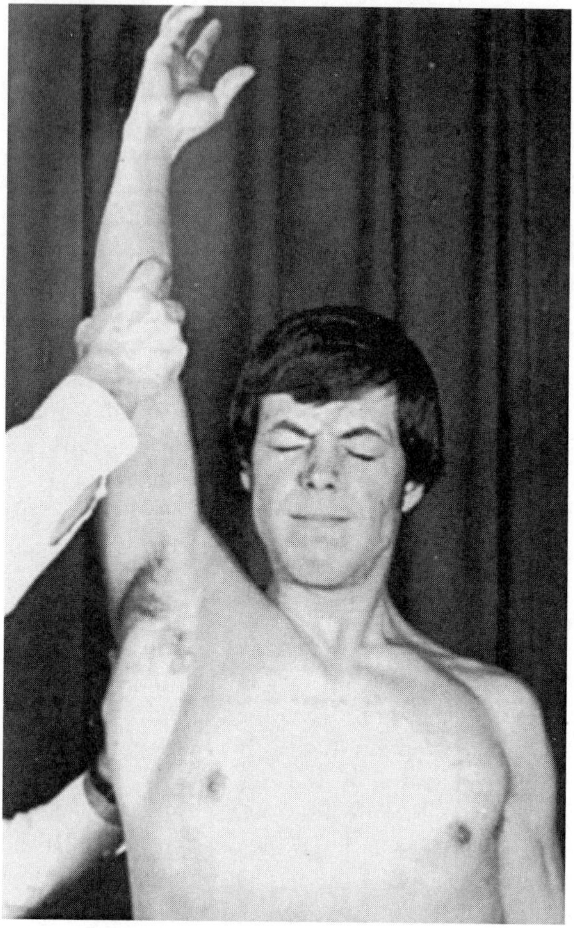

■ **Figure 26.4** Positive impingement sign. The examiner forcibly forward flexes the humerus, jamming the greater tuberosity against the anterior inferior acromial surface. The patient's facial expression on reproduction of the pain confirms the presence of impingement. This may be relieved by the injection of lidocaine directly into the subacromial bursa. (From Hawkins RJ, Kennedy JC: Impingement syndrome in athletes. Am J Sports Med 8:151–158, 1980.)

car for a few hours). Such physical exertion may cause rotator cuff injuries or subacromial bursitis and severe pain. At rest, pain may be poorly localized; the physician can better determine the source of pain by having the patient repeat the type of activity that apparently induced the pain.

Arthritis. Arthritis of the shoulder is uncommon but is usually superimposed on a previous injury. With arthritis of the acromioclavicular joint, the pain worsens with adduction of the arm across the chest or with circumduction. As with other forms of degenerative arthritis, this pain is often worse in the morning and improves as the day progresses.

Nonarticular pain. This arm pain is most often caused by *overuse syndromes (repetitive strain injury).* Other common causes are *thoracic outlet, cervical disc,* and *carpal tunnel syndromes* (Table 26–1).

Associated Symptoms

Weakness and atrophy of muscles are uncommon with *supraspinatus tendinitis.* With *rotator cuff tears,* supraspinatus and infraspinatus atrophy may occur in

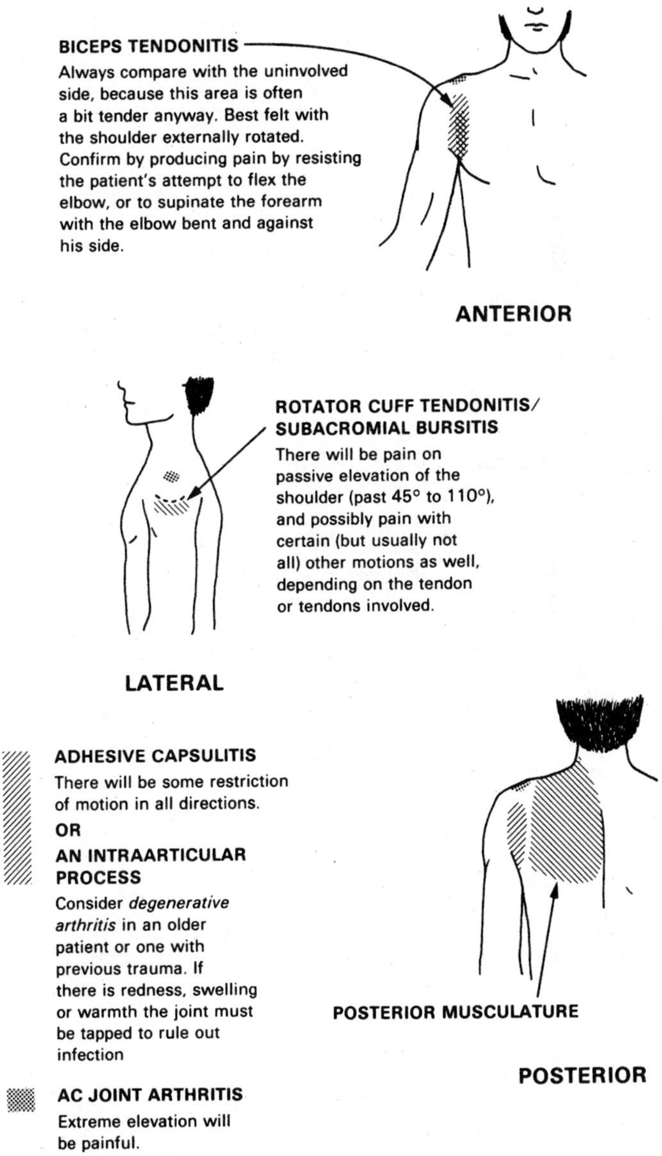

■ **Figure 26.5** Sites of shoulder tenderness. (From Birnbaum JS: The Musculoskeletal Manual, 2nd ed. Philadelphia, WB Saunders, 1986.)

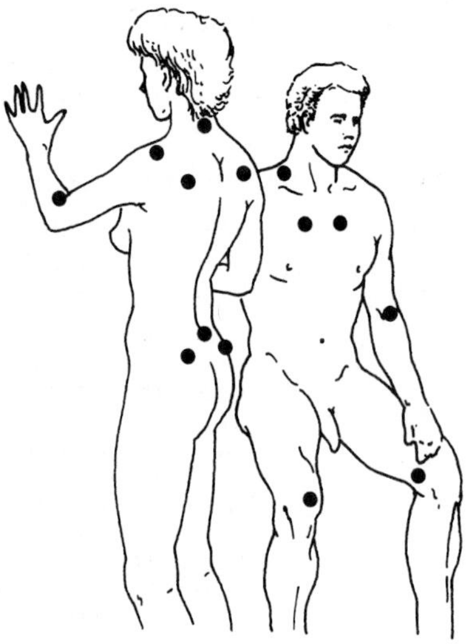

■ **Figure 26.6** Location of 14 typical sites of deep tenderness in fibrositis. (From Smythe HA, Moldofshy H: Two contributions to understanding of the "fibrositis" syndrome. Bull Rheum Dis 28(1):928, 1977-1978.)

about 3 weeks. With prolonged *frozen shoulder,* several shoulder muscles may atrophy. Patients with *acute bursitis* resist any passive or active shoulder motion.

Arthritis should be suspected if other joints are involved. If paresthesia or hyperesthesia in the region of C8 or T1 (first thoracic) is noted, especially with atrophy of the hypothenar eminence, *thoracic outlet syndrome* should be suspected. Patients with this condition also may demonstrate Raynaud's phenomenon.

Precipitating and Aggravating Factors

Prolonged and sustained immobilization with the arm at the side may lead to a *frozen shoulder.* This immobilization may have been recommended by the physician, or the patient may have avoided movement for some other reason for a prolonged period. The *impingement syndrome* often is precipitated by repetitive use of the arm above the horizontal position (as in throwing a baseball or in football, swimming, or tennis). Isolated arthritis of the sternoclavicular joint may be caused by trauma or weight lifting. *Septic arthritis of the sternoclavicular joint* has been reported in heroin users and in patients with gonococcal arthritis.

Ameliorating Factors

Full trunk and hip flexion that allows the arm to hang limp or supporting the forearm in flexion may help alleviate the pain of *rotator cuff tears.* This finding may also help the physician establish the diagnosis.

Physical Findings

A careful physical examination with implementation of specific maneuvers is essential to effective diagnosis and management of pain in the upper extremity. In most cases the diagnosis can be made without radiography or arthrography.

TABLE 26.1 Differential Diagnosis of Thoracic Outlet, Cervical Disc, and Carpal Tunnel Syndromes

	THORACIC OUTLET	CERVICAL DISC	CARPAL TUNNEL
Symptoms			
Pain	Neck, shoulder, and arm (intermittent)	Neck, shoulder, and arm (constant)	Wrist, volar forearm, fingers 1, 2, and 3 (intermittent)
Numbness	Ulnar nerve or whole hand or arm asleep	Radial nerve (dorsal web between fingers 1 and 2)	Median nerve, fingers 2, 3, and 4
Awkwardness	All fingers or 4 and 5	Thumb	Fingers 1, 2, and 3
Aggravation	Arm elevation	Neck turn or arm stretch	Sustained grasp, pinch
Color	Normal, pallid, cyanotic, or splotchy	Normal or splotchy	Normal, red, or splotchy
Edema	May be present	Absent	May be present
Signs			
Pain on percussion	Brachial plexus	Neck at disc level	Tinel sign (volar wrist)
Pain on compression	Brachial plexus	Neck and brachial plexus	Phalen sign (wrist flexion)
Symptoms reproduced	Arm elevation and brachial plexus compression	Head turn and tilt, cranial compression	Wrist and finger flexion
Nerve conduction	Positive or negative (unreliable if negative)		Positive or negative (unreliable if negative)
Radiographs	Normal, long C7 process, anomalies (venoarteriogram)	Degenerative arthritis, disc space narrowed to 85% of normal on myelogram	Normal, arthritis, or old trauma

Modified from Stabile MJ, Warfield CA: Differential diagnosis of arm pain. Hosp Pract 25:55–58, 61, 64, 1990.

Patients with *supraspinatus tendinitis* have pain on resisted abduction, limitation of joint motion (with or without disruption of the scapulohumeral rhythm), and a normal passive range of motion. Pain is absent or minimal when the arm is dependent. Pain is usually located in the deltoid region, where the supraspinatus tendon inserts.

Patients with *rotator cuff tears* usually have a full range of passive movement and experience pain at extremes of motion. They have pain and restricted movement at the glenohumeral joint and experience pain and weakness with resisted movement. These patients also may demonstrate the "drop arm" sign: weak ability to maintain abduction after passive abduction support is removed. Radiographs may show that the humeral head is high in the glenoid when the arm is in full adduction. Patients with *calcific rotator cuff tendinitis* experience pain with all movements of the shoulder. They usually have associated muscle spasm throughout the shoulder.

Patients with *bicipital tendinitis* experience exacerbation of pain on resisted forearm supination, which causes anterior shoulder pain. Likewise, pain occurs with resisted flexion of the shoulder at about 80 degrees.

Elbow

Overuse syndromes may involve the elbow. These muscle strains may be vocational or recreational due to weight lifting, throwing, or racquet sports. *Tennis elbow* is a *lateral epicondylitis* of the humerus that may appear in tennis players of any age or level of expertise, especially those over age 40. It also may occur in people who do not play tennis. Lateral epicondylitis is caused by overexertion of the finger and wrist extensors, which originate in the region of the lateral epicondyle. Pain and acute tenderness arise at the origin of the forearm extensor muscles, which attach just distal to the lateral epicondyle of the humerus. The pain may radiate down the back of the forearm. Patients with epicondylitis also experience pain when performing an activity such as opening a door or lifting a cup or glass.

Lateral epicondylitis has been referred to as "backhand tennis elbow" and medial epicondylitis as "forehand tennis elbow." Medial epicondylitis also occurs in golfers and baseball pitchers (Fig. 26–7).

If pain and swelling are noted in the posterior aspect of the elbow, *olecranon bursitis* should be suspected. This may occur after a forced, vigorous extension of the elbow joint or from repeated microtrauma. Acute olecranon bursitis can be differentiated from acute arthritis of the elbow in that passive extension is unimpaired in bursitis. Patients with septic olecranon bursitis are usually febrile and have a skin lesion overlying the bursa, with bursal tenderness. If a child develops pain in the elbow after being swung around by the hand or after having the elbow pulled suddenly while the arm is pronated and extended, *radial head dislocation* is probable. *Rheumatoid arthritis* occasionally involves the elbow (Fig. 26–8).

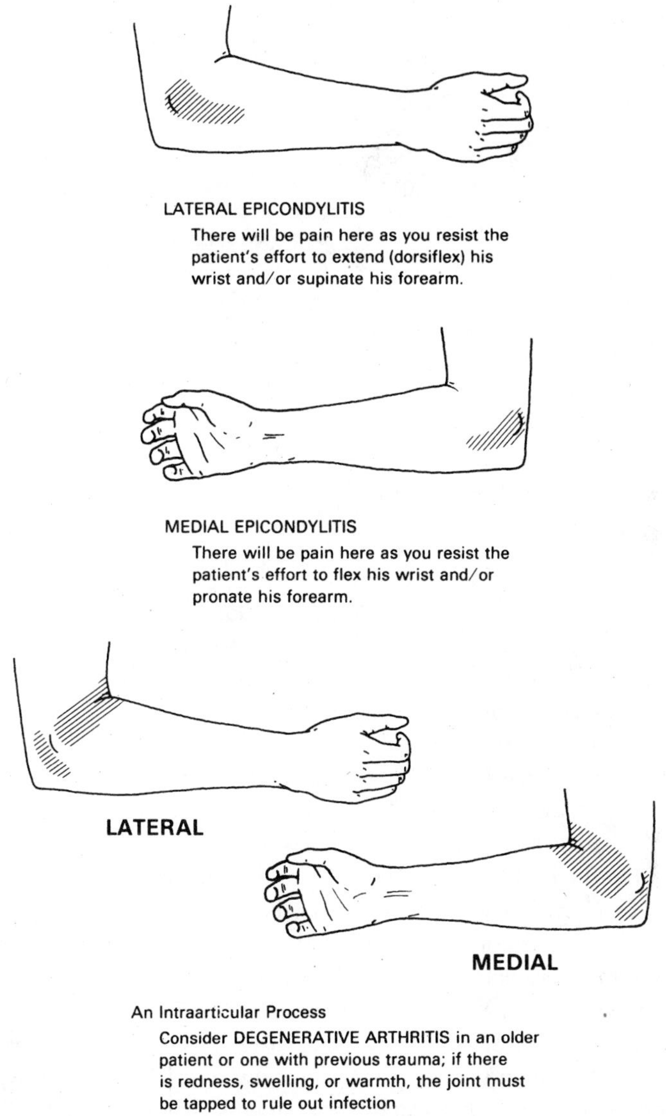

■ **Figure 26.7** Sites of elbow tenderness. (From Birnbaum JS: The Musculoskeletal Manual, 2nd ed. Philadelphia, WB Saunders Co, 1986.)

Hand and Wrist

Pain at the base of the thumb aggravated by movement of the wrist or thumb and reproducible by flexion of the thumb is called *de Quervain's disease* (Fig. 26–9). This is a *tenosynovitis* of the thumb abductors and extensors. Pain in the palm at the base of the third and fourth digits, often associated with a catching or fixation of fingers in flexion, is known as *Dupuytren's contracture.* Examination reveals a

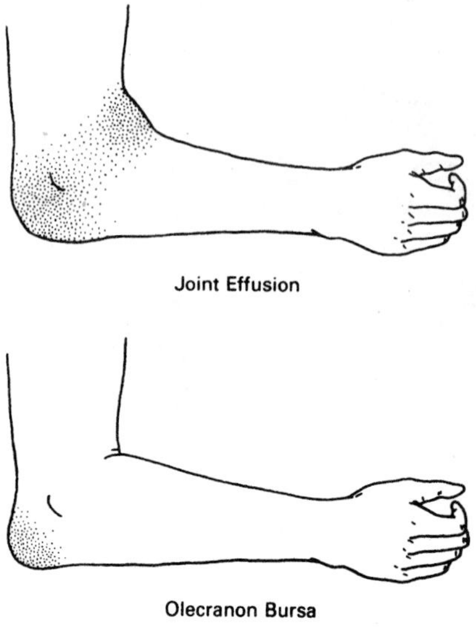

■ **Figure 26.8** Elbow swelling. (From Birnbaum JS: The Musculoskeletal Manual, 2nd ed. Philadelphia, WB Saunders Co, 1986.)

painless thickening of the palmar fascia or tendon sheath. If the pain is in the anatomic snuff box, it can be assumed to be due to *navicular bone fracture* unless another cause is determined. Pain or numbness of the fingers is seen in *Raynaud's disease* and associated conditions including *Buerger's disease, systemic lupus erythematosus* (SLE), and *scleroderma.*

Peripheral nerve entrapment syndromes, such as carpal tunnel syndrome (median nerve), may cause pain, numbness, or both in the wrist, hand, or forearm. *Carpal tunnel syndrome* is the most common cause of nocturnal hand pain and often occurs in the later stage of pregnancy and rheumatoid arthritis.

Thoracic outlet syndrome (previously referred to as scalenus anticus syndrome, neurovascular compression syndrome, and hyperabduction syndrome) is most common in middle-aged women and usually occurs on the left side. This syndrome presents with intermittent pain, numbness, or weakness in the hand (occasionally the forearm) after the arm or arms have been in a hyperabducted state for a time. Patients often experience this discomfort after working an extended period with the arms over the head or after sleeping with the arms folded behind the neck. Physical examination is normal except when specific maneuvers are employed. For example, forcing the shoulders back and down while the patient is in forced inspiration may obliterate the radial pulse on the affected side. Likewise, the radial pulse may be obliterated by Adson's maneuver.

Degenerative arthritis usually involves the distal interphalangeal joints, whereas *rheumatoid arthritis* most often involves the proximal interphalangeal and metacarpophalangeal joints. Rheumatoid arthritis also can involve the elbow and the wrist; it seldom involves the shoulder. Patients with active rheumatoid arthritis usually have joint stiffness as well as warmth, swelling, and tenderness. The pain is usually polyarticular and migratory rather than monoarticular.

Pain in the wrist is most often caused by *trauma.* Wrist sprains, and less commonly fractures, are occurring more frequently with the increased popularity of in-line skating and home trampolines. Falls on the outstretched arm with the wrist extended often result in a *scaphoid bone fracture.* Classically there is pain in the anatomic snuffbox, but early radiographs may be negative and special scaphoid views or a bone scan may be required. **Because symptoms may be mild and radiographs negative, this diagnosis must be kept in mind since an overlooked scaphoid fracture is a common cause of litigation.**

Diagnostic Studies

Precise clinical examination is more useful than radiography in the evaluation of soft tissue injuries. Arthroscopy and MRI are useful in the diagnosis of shoulder

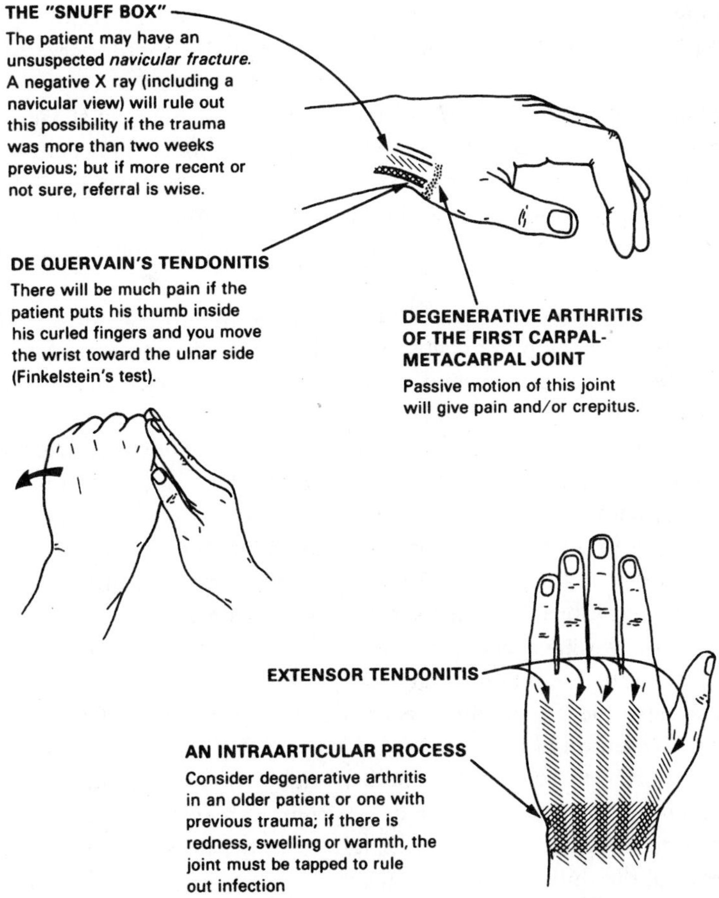

■ **Figure 26.9** Sites of wrist tenderness. (From Birnbaum JS: The Musculoskeletal Manual, 2nd ed. Philadelphia, WB Saunders Co, 1986.)

disorders. Arthrography and computed tomography (CT) scans are occasionally helpful. Radiographs and occasionally bone scans should be obtained if fracture is suspected. Electromyography and nerve conduction studies are helpful tools in the diagnosis of neural entrapment syndromes.

Less Common Diagnostic Considerations

Less common sources of pain in the upper extremity include some types of local discomfort and referred pain. Apical lung tumors (Pancoast's tumor), cervical disc disease, and cervical spondylosis all can produce shoulder pain. *Cervical spondylosis* can result from intervertebral disc protrusion or primary spondylosis. If radiculitis is present, the pain will be sharp and well localized. The patient may have paresthesias and numbness in the sensory distribution of the compromised nerve root. Fasciculations also may be present, and the pain may be exacerbated by movement of the cervical spine. Despite shoulder pain, a full range of motion may be possible. Cervical spondylosis often can be identified by tenderness over the motor point (where the motor nerve enters the muscle).

Sternoclavicular joint arthritis is rare but occurs in a small number of patients with rheumatic diseases as well as in weight lifters. This pain is usually an anterior chest discomfort that may radiate to the shoulder or arm. When there are significant soft tissue swelling and warmth in a wide area around the joint, the possibility of a septic arthritis, particularly gonococcal, must be considered.

Shoulder pain can be referred from *neck lesions* and *visceral lesions,* including mediastinal disease, subphrenic abscess, and gallbladder disease. *Neural entrapment syndromes* (e.g., median and ulnar nerve compression) cause pain in the distribution of these nerves. Median nerve compression syndrome is caused by compression of the median nerve as it passes beneath the flexor retinaculum, and its symptoms are those of carpal tunnel syndrome. This condition is most common in middle-aged and elderly women. Patients usually complain of pain and paresthesias in the thumb and in the index and middle fingers. They also may report that they feel clumsy when performing fine movements such as sewing and picking up small objects. Patients may have a sensory loss of median nerve distribution and weakness of the thenar muscles. Both the pain and the paresthesia may be worse at night and on awakening.

Cervical spine and *cervical cord lesions* often produce referred pain in the upper extremity. Herniation of the disc at C5–C6 or C6–C7 causes pain from the back of the neck, across the back of the shoulder, and down the arm and forearm to the wrist. Patients may have a history of recurrent stiff neck. Their pain is often aggravated by movement, particularly flexion, of the neck. They also may have paresthesias of the thumb and index finger.

Cervical spine spondylosis can cause pain and stiffness in the neck and a radicular distribution of pain in one or both arms. Compression of the cervical cord can

Text continued on page 283.

Differential Diagnosis of Upper Extremity Pain

CAUSE	NATURE OF PATIENT	NATURE OF SYMPTOMS	ASSOCIATED SYMPTOMS	PRECIPITATING AND AGGRAVATING FACTORS	AMELIORATING FACTORS	PHYSICAL FINDINGS
Shoulder						
Supraspinatus tendinitis	Over age 40	Pain in lower part of deltoid region, which is referral area for pain from supraspinatus tendon		Reaching overhead and lying on affected shoulder		Pain worse with resisted abduction and with abduction to 60 degrees and internal rotation
Subacromial bursitis	Under age 40	Severe pain with marked limitation of motion Pain may radiate to distal arm and even forearm		Lifting objects or combing hair		Point tenderness over subacromial bursa, which may be warm and swollen
Bicipital tendinitis		Generalized tenderness anteriorly in region of long head of biceps (anterior subacromial bursa)				Resisted forearm supination causes anterior shoulder pain Free abduction and forward flexion
Calcific tendinitis	Younger adults	Usually a sequela to acute bursitis				
Rotator cuff tear	Adults	Sudden onset Pain in deltoid area that intensifies 6–12 hours after initial trauma	Recurrent pain		Arm hanging limp	Restricted motion in one plane at glenohumeral joint Weakness and atrophy of supraspinatus and infraspinatus Pain over greater tuberosity

Table continued on following page.

Differential Diagnosis of Upper Extremity Pain *Continued*

CAUSE	NATURE OF PATIENT	NATURE OF SYMPTOMS	ASSOCIATED SYMPTOMS	PRECIPITATING AND AGGRAVATING FACTORS	AMELIORATING FACTORS	PHYSICAL FINDINGS
Shoulder *Continued*						
Teres minor or infraspinatus tendinitis		Diffuse shoulder pain	No pain radiation into arm or neck		Arm dependent	Pain on moving humerus posteriorly
Subscapularis tendinitis		Diffuse shoulder pain	No pain radiation into arm or neck		Arm dependent	Pain with resisted medial rotation
Frozen shoulder		Gradual onset of pain with limitation of motion at glenohumeral and scapulothoracic joints Limitation of abduction, extension, rotation, and forward flexion Pain may radiate into neck and down arm to elbow	Some atrophy of shoulder muscles	Prolonged immobilization		Marked restriction of motion of shoulder in all directions
Impingement syndrome	Athletes (e.g., baseball, swimming, tennis)	Tendinitis of biceps and/or supraspinatus tendon progressing to subacromial bursitis and inflammation of acromioclavicular joint				Pain on forward flexion of arm with elbow extended

Fibrositis syndrome	Ages 20–60	Pain at midpoint of upper border of trapezius, origin of supraspinatus near medial border of scapula, 2–3 cm distal to lateral epicondyle of humerus	Sleep disturbance Diffuse musculoskeletal pain		Tricyclic antidepressants	Multiple tender points
Lesion of cervical spine and cord	Referred pain to upper extremity: back of neck, back of shoulder, down arm, forearm					Pain and hypesthesia along dermatome distribution
Elbow						
Lateral epicondylitis	Often in tennis players, especially those over age 40	Pain over lateral epicondyle that may radiate down back of forearm		Resisted extension of wrist and supination of forearm		Tender to palpation over lateral epicondyle
Bursitis		Pain in back of elbow				Swelling, warmth, and tenderness over back of elbow
Radial head dislocation	Child			Swing child around by arms		Radial head palpable in displaced position

Table continued on following page.

Differential Diagnosis of Upper Extremity Pain *Continued*

CAUSE	NATURE OF PATIENT	NATURE OF SYMPTOMS	ASSOCIATED SYMPTOMS	PRECIPITATING AND AGGRAVATING FACTORS	AMELIORATING FACTORS	PHYSICAL FINDINGS
Hand and Wrist						
Tenosynovitis of abductors and extensors of wrist (de Quervain's disease)		Pain at base of thumb		Flexing thumb		
Tenosynovitis of flexors of fingers (Dupuytren's contracture)		Pain in palm at base of third and fourth digits				Catching or fixation of third or fourth digits in flexion Painless thickening of palmar fascia or tendon sheath
Thoracic outlet syndrome	More common in middle-aged women	Hand pain, weakness, or numbness (usually left) after arms are hyperabducted or on awakening	Numbness of ulnar distribution or whole hand	Prolonged hyperabduction		Decreased radial pulse with Adson's and other maneuvers
Gout and pseudogout	Adults	Wrist often involved in pseudogout				
Carpal tunnel syndrome	More common in women	Pain in wrist radiating to hand and forearm				Tinel and Phalen tests may be positive Thenar wasting

cause weakness, wasting, and fibrillations in the upper limbs; paresthesias in the arms or legs; and, occasionally, evidence of pyramidal involvement (e.g., weakness, spasticity, increased deep tendon reflexes, and a positive Babinski sign). The combination of atrophic weakness in the arms and spastic weakness in the legs may suggest *amyotrophic lateral sclerosis.* Spondylosis can be distinguished from amyotrophic lateral sclerosis by a history of paresthesias and the presence of sensory impairment in the former condition.

Meningeal tumors, Pott's disease, and primary or secondary *vertebral body tumors* may produce upper extremity pain as a result of root compression. Rarely, benign and malignant tumors cause pain in the elbow, forearm, and wrist. When this occurs in a young athlete, sports injury is often diagnosed erroneously. In elderly patients, *herpes zoster* may cause pain in the arm. Many of these patients have a history of an eruption and residual pigmented scars.

Angina pectoris is a common cause of pain in the arm and shoulder. This pain is most frequently located in the left upper arm and is usually associated with precordial pain. A history of pain in the arm with exertion is the major diagnostic clue for angina pectoris.

Arteritis of the great vessels, Norwegian pulseless disease, is a rare condition that can produce intermittent claudication of one or both arms. It is most common in young women and should be considered in those patients who have diminished blood pressure in one or both arms, especially if they also experience transient episodes of blindness or other cerebral incidents.

Painful swelling of the wrist not due to trauma may be caused by acute *gout* or acute *pseudogout.* Both are more common in adult or elderly individuals.

Selected References

Birnbaum JS: The Musculoskeletal Manual, 2nd ed. Philadelphia, WB Saunders Co, 1986.

Bland JH, Merrit JA, Boushey DD: The painful shoulder. Semin Arthritis Rheum 7:21–47, 1977.

Doherty M, Jones A: Fibromyalgia syndrome. Br Med J 310:386–389, 1995.

Fongemie AE, Buss DD, Rolnick SJ: Management of shoulder impingement syndrome and rotator cuff tears. Am Fam Physician 57:667–674, 1998.

Guidotti TL: Occupational repetitive strain injury. Am Fam Physician 45:585–592, 1992.

Heron CW: Imaging the painful shoulder. Clin Radiol 41:376–379, 1990.

Jenkins DG: Clinical features of arm and neck pain. Psychotherapy 65:102–105, 1979.

Lascelles RG, Mohr PD, Neary D, Bloor K: The thoracic outlet syndrome. Brain 100:601–612, 1977.

Matsen FA, Kirby RM: Office evaluation and management of shoulder pain. Orthop Clin North Am 13:453–475, 1982.

Polisson RP: Sports medicine for the internist. Med Clin North Am 70:469–489, 1986.

Richardson AB, Jobe FW, Collins HR: The shoulder in competitive swimming. Am J Sports Med 8:159–163, 1980.

Salzman KL, Lillegard WA, Butcher JD: Upper extremity bursitis. Am Fam Physician 56:1797–1806, 1997.

Schmerling RH: Finger pain. Prim Care 15:751–766, 1988.

Semble EL, Wise CM: Fibrositis. Am Fam Physician 38:129–139, 1988.

Spiegel TM, Crues JV: The painful shoulder: diagnosis and treatment. Prim Care 15:709–724, 1988.
Stabile MJ, Warfield CA: Differential diagnosis of arm pain. Hosp Pract 25:55–58, 61, 64, 1990.
Turner-Stokes L: Clinical differential diagnosis of shoulder pain. Br J Hosp Med 56:73–77, 1996.
Wade JP, Bell JG: Wrist pain. Prim Care 15:737–749, 1988.
Watrous BF, Ho G: Elbow pain. Prim Care 15:725–735, 1988.

CHAPTER 27

Palpitations

Palpitations are defined here as skipped heartbeat, irregular heartbeat, rapid or slow heartbeat, or increased awareness of the heartbeat. A patient's awareness of the heartbeat occurs most frequently at rest (e.g., while watching television or while lying in bed). In bed the mattress serves as a resonator; this facilitates an awareness of the heartbeat, which may be fast, slow, irregular, or normal.

The most common causes of palpitations are *anxiety, stimulants* (e.g., caffeine, alcohol), *drugs* (e.g., amphetamines, cocaine, digitalis glycosides, psychotropic agents, thyroid hormone), and *cardiac disease* (e.g., valvular disease, ischemia, myocardiopathy, mitral valve prolapse). Other common causes include *conduction abnormalities* (e.g., Wolff-Parkinson-White syndrome, sick sinus syndrome), *panic disorder, hypoglycemia, reactive hypoglycemia, hyperthyroidism, hypoxia,* and *hyperventilation.*

If the palpitations occur infrequently or only once, are not associated with other symptoms (e.g., chest pain, syncope, dizzy spells), and develop in an otherwise healthy patient, concern or extensive workup is probably unnecessary. **If palpitations are frequent, disturbing to the patient, or associated with syncope, dizzy spells, chest pain, activity, or evidence of heart disease, further investigation is required and should include electrocardiography performed with the patient at rest, exercise electrocardiography, and often 24-hour Holter monitoring or event monitoring.**

Nature of Patient

In children and adolescents, the complaint of palpitations is most often a sign of *anxiety.* If a rapid arrhythmia is suspected or if the problem is recurrent, the physician should perform electrocardiographic studies and Holter monitoring to determine whether *Wolff-Parkinson-White syndrome* is present. The most common arrhythmias in children are supraventricular tachycardias. Children, adolescents, and young adults should be specifically questioned about the use of *stimulants* such as tobacco, snuff, caffeine, alcohol, and illegal drugs.

In adults who have no clinical evidence of heart disease or other systemic disease, the complaint of palpitations is often only an awareness of their normal heartbeat or an occasional atrial or ventricular contraction. The patient should be questioned carefully about excessive use of tobacco and about stimulants such as caffeine, alcohol, and other agents, including recreational drugs, amphetamines, psychotropic agents, over-the-counter weight-reducing agents, and thyroid replacement therapy. **Increasing age often brings a decreasing tolerance to**

agents such as caffeine, alcohol, and drugs. Although previously tolerated without symptoms, these agents may induce palpitations as the patient gets older. Occasionally, palpitations (often paroxysmal atrial fibrillation) are noted by a patient during the day after unusual but not necessarily excessive alcohol ingestion, a phenomenon known as "holiday heart syndrome." The most common causes of palpitations in elderly patients include supraventricular and ventricular premature beats, sick sinus syndrome, and atrial fibrillation.

Patients with known cardiac disease who complain of palpitations are more likely to have serious arrhythmias, such as *atrial fibrillation, ventricular tachycardia,* and *sick sinus syndrome.* If a patient with a wide-complex tachycardia has a history of heart failure, myocardial infarction, or recent-onset angina, the tachycardia is more likely to be ventricular in origin rather than supraventricular with aberration. Those who have poor left ventricular function are particularly prone to ventricular arrhythmias and sudden death. *Mitral valve prolapse* occurs most frequently in young women. One study revealed that the average age of patients with mitral valve prolapse is 38 and that 70% of patients are women.

Palpitations occur more frequently and are of greater clinical significance in patients with the "click-murmur syndrome" than in those with only an echocardiographic diagnosis of mitral value prolapse. Well-conditioned athletes often have a *resting bradycardia* (sometimes marked). This may be associated with premature ventricular contractions, first-degree atrioventricular (AV) block, and second-degree AV block; these arrhythmias disappear with exercise.

Nature of Symptoms

All patients should be questioned about the characteristics (fast, slow, irregular, etc.) of the palpitations, mode of onset, mode of termination, precipitating factors, frequency, and results of any prior therapy. Patients may complain of a forceful, fast, slow, or irregular heartbeat. It is often useful to have the patient tap out what the rhythm feels like. If the patient cannot do this, the physician can tap out a selection of rhythms—slow and regular, slow and irregular, fast and regular, fast and irregular, and the beat of a premature contraction followed by a compensatory pause—to assist patients in describing what they mean by "palpitations."

The sudden onset of a regular tachycardia with a rate greater than 160 beats per minute suggests a supraventricular tachycardia. A rate of 150 beats per minute suggests atrial flutter with a 2:1 conduction ratio. A rapid irregularly irregular tachycardia with a pulse deficit suggests atrial fibrillation. The precise nature of the arrhythmia must be documented by electrocardiography or Holter monitoring.

Various types of arrhythmias are typically found at different times in the same patient. Arrhythmias that recur in late afternoon and early evening suggest that they are precipitated by *reactive hypoglycemia.* For any patient with unexplained recurrent arrhythmias that occur several hours after eating, the physician should perform a 5-hour glucose tolerance test to rule out reactive hypoglycemia. These arrhythmias are usually supraventricular in origin. Arrhythmias in insulin-dependent diabetic patients that occur near the time of peak insulin activity are also frequently induced by hypoglycemia. Patients with diabetes often have accelerated coronary artery disease, which is another possible cause of arrhythmias.

Associated Symptoms

Fatigue, confusion, and syncope may be noted in patients with *sick sinus syndrome,* which occurs frequently in elderly patients. Sweating, tremors, and other symptoms of *hypoglycemia* suggest that this is contributing to the arrhythmia. When palpitations are associated with anxiety, dyspnea, dizziness, and tingling in the hands or face, *hyperventilation* may be the cause.

Sticking chest pains that do not usually coincide with the arrhythmia should suggest *mitral valve prolapse,* a condition in which arrhythmias are common. Chest pain, congestive heart failure, syncope, and dizziness all suggest a clinically significant arrhythmia such as *paroxysmal atrial tachycardia, complete heart block,* or *ventricular tachycardia. Generalized anxiety disorder* or *panic attack* should be suspected if the patient with palpitations also complains of symptoms such as shortness of breath, nervousness, gastrointestinal upset, muscle aches, tension, or insomnia.

Precipitating and Aggravating Factors

Although exercise may induce arrhythmias in a normal heart, arrhythmias that increase with exercise are probably caused by *cardiac disease,* especially coronary artery disease, mitral valve prolapse, and cardiomyopathy (both hypertrophic and dilated forms). When premature ventricular contractions decrease with exercise (and its associated increase in sinus rate), they are probably benign.

Digitalis-induced arrhythmias can be in the form of premature beats, tachyarrhythmias or bradyarrhythmias, supraventricular arrhythmias, supraventricular tachycardia with block, or ventricular tachycardia. Digitalis arrhythmias can be precipitated by increased digitalis dosage, hypokalemia, hypomagnesemia, or decreased renal function. *Antiarrhythmic drugs,* particularly the class I agents (e.g., quinidine, procainamide, lidocaine, disopyramide, phenytoin), can both precipitate and suppress arrhythmias. Their prolongation of the Q–T interval makes the patient more vulnerable to the torsades de pointes type of ventricular tachycardia, which the patient may perceive as palpitations or dizzy spells. Ventricular arrhythmia can be caused by cocaine, phenothiazines, diphenhydramine, propranolol, propoxyphene, tricyclic antidepressants, amiodarone, and class I agents.

Most of the beta blockers, lithium, many of the antihypertensive agents (e.g., reserpine, methyldopa, clonidine), and the calcium channel blockers cause bradycardia. Hydralazine and minoxidil can cause sinus tachycardia. Sometimes discontinuation of drugs (e.g., clonidine, phenytoin, beta blockers, antiarrhythmics) is associated with the development of palpitations.

Ameliorating Factors

If the palpitations abate with cessation of stimulants or other drugs, the arrhythmias most likely were caused by the discontinued agent or agents. Some patients find that performing Valsalva's maneuver, pressing on their carotid sinus, or gagging themselves to induce vomiting terminates the arrhythmias. In these patients the arrhythmias are probably supraventricular in origin.

Physical Findings

Auscultation of a midsystolic click or late systolic murmur is found in patients with *mitral valve prolapse.* Premature atrial or ventricular contractions occur most often in patients with mitral valve prolapse; supraventricular tachycardia or ventricular tachycardia occurs in about 12% of these patients. Signs of dilated cardiomyopathy or congestive heart failure suggest the palpitations may be ventricular tachycardia or atrial fibrillation. A holosystolic murmur heard at the left sternal border that increases with Valsalva's maneuver suggests hypertrophic obstructive cardiomyopathy, which is often associated with ventricular tachycardia and atrial fibrillation.

Many clinical signs and maneuvers (well documented in cardiology texts) may help the physician determine the nature of arrhythmias. **Precise diagnosis requires electrocardiographic documentation.** In anxious patients who complain of palpitations, the arrhythmias may be precipitated by *hyperventilation.* If this is suspected, the physician can instruct the patient to hyperventilate forcibly for 3 or 4 minutes to determine whether this activity induces an arrhythmia that should be recorded.

Diagnostic Studies

If arrhythmias cannot be documented clinically or electrocardiographically, and if they are frequent or associated with dizziness, syncope, or other cardiac symptomatology, Holter monitoring or event recording must be performed. Several studies of 24-hour Holter monitoring have shown that a significant number of patients note palpitations when no abnormality is detected on their Holter tape and, conversely, that many patients demonstrate arrhythmias on their Holter tape but are unaware of palpitations at that time.

Other studies that may help the physician determine the cause of palpitations include thyroid function tests, the 5-hour glucose tolerance test, drug screens, determination of serum digitalis and arterial blood gas levels, echocardiography, invasive cardiac electrophysiologic tests, and rarely coronary arteriography.

Text continued on page 292.

Differential Diagnosis of Palpitations

CAUSE	NATURE OF PATIENT	NATURE OF SYMPTOMS	ASSOCIATED SYMPTOMS	PRECIPITATING AND AGGRAVATING FACTORS	PHYSICAL FINDINGS*	DIAGNOSTIC STUDIES†
Anxiety	Most common cause of palpitations in children and adolescents		Sweaty palms	Hyperventilation	Have patient hyperventilate for 3–4 min to see whether arrhythmias can be induced	
Ingestion of stimulants or drugs (caffeine, alcohol, amphetamines, cocaine)	Patients have decreased tolerance to these agents with increased age		Nervousness Tremor	Caffeine Alcohol Drugs (e.g., amphetamines, psychotropic agents, thyroid hormone)	Premature ventricular contractions Tachycardia	Toxicology screening tests
Digitalis glycosides			Nausea Anorexia	Increased digitalis dose Hypokalemia Hypomagnesemia Decreased renal function	Premature ventricular contractions Tachyarrhythmias Bradyarrhythmias Second- or third-degree heart block	Serum digitalis levels Electrocardiography Holter monitoring Serum potassium Serum magnesium Creatinine
Beta blockers Antihypertensives Calcium channel blockers	Patients with angina or hypertension				Bradycardia	
Hydralazine Minoxidil					Sinus tachycardia	

Table continued on following page.

Differential Diagnosis of Palpitations *Continued*

CAUSE	NATURE OF PATIENT	NATURE OF SYMPTOMS	ASSOCIATED SYMPTOMS	PRECIPITATING AND AGGRAVATING FACTORS	PHYSICAL FINDINGS*	DIAGNOSTIC STUDIES†
Hypoglycemia	Insulin-dependent diabetics	Arrhythmias occur near time of peak insulin activity	Sweating Headache Tremor Weakness	Increased insulin Decreased carbohydrate	Premature ventricular contractions Tachycardia	Blood sugar
Hyperthyroidism	More common in older men	Atrial premature contractions May be silent	Nervousness Tremors Weight loss	Heart disease	Atrial fibrillation Premature contractions Tachycardias	Thyroid function tests
Exercise	Normal More frequent in patients with coronary heart disease, hypertension, mitral valve prolapse, and cardiomyopathy			Exercise		
Reactive hypoglycemia		Recurrent arrhythmias in late afternoon and early evening Arrhythmias occur several hours after ingestion of carbohydrates	Sweating Tremors Headache	Anxiety		5-hour glucose tolerance test

Cardiac disease						
Mitral valve prolapse	Most common in young women (average age, 38 years)		Sticking chest pain	Exercise	Midsystolic click Late systolic murmur Premature ventricular contractions or premature atrial contractions Tachycardia	Echocardiography
Wolff-Parkinson-White syndrome	Often detected in children and adolescents	Recurrent palpitations Frequent paroxysmal tachycardia		Exercise Digitalis	Paroxysmal tachycardia	Electrocardiography Holter monitoring
Sick sinus syndrome	Older patients	Bradyarrhythmia Tachyarrhythmia	Chest pain Syncope Congestive heart failure Dizziness	Exercise Digoxin Beta blockers Calcium channel blockers	Bradyarrhythmia Tachyarrhythmia	Electrocardiography Holter monitoring Electrophysiologic studies
Coronary artery disease	Older patients	Palpitations	Angina pectoris Congestive heart failure		Premature ventricular contractions Paroxysmal atrial fibrillation	Exercise electrocardiography Holter monitoring

*Arrhythmias are often absent.

†All arrhythmias should be documented by electrocardiography or Holter monitoring.

Less Common Diagnostic Considerations

Less common causes of palpitations include *infiltrative myocardial diseases,* such as amyloidosis, sarcoidosis, and tumors. *Hypothyroidism* can cause sinus bradycardia; *hyperthyroidism* can cause sinus tachycardia, paroxysmal atrial tachycardia, and paroxysmal atrial fibrillation.

Selected References

Brugada P, Gursoy S, Brugado J, Andries E: Investigation of palpitations. Lancet 341:1254–1258, 1993.

Fogel RI, Evans JJ, Prystowsky EN: Utility and cost of event recorders in the diagnosis of palpitations, presyncope and syncope. Am J Cardiol 79:207–208, 1997.

Kopp DE, Wilber DJ: Palpitations and arrhythmias: separating the benign from the dangerous. Postgrad Med 91:241–251, 1992.

Kung G, et al: What does the symptom "palpitation" mean? Correlation between symptoms and the presence of cardiac arrhythmias in the ambulatory EKG. Z Kardiol 66:138–141, 1977.

Ladenson PW: Recognition and management of cardiovascular disease related to thyroid dysfunction. Am J Med 88:638–641, 1990.

Linzer M, Yang EH, Estes M, et al: Diagnosing syncope. Part 1. Value of history, physical examination and electrocardiography. Ann Intern Med 126:989–995, 1997.

Marcus FI, Ruskin JN, Surawicz B: Cardiovascular disease in the elderly. Arrhythmias J Am Coll Cardiol 10(2 suppl A):66A–72A, 1987.

Miller MB: Arrhythmias associated with drug toxicity. Emerg Med Clin North Am 16:405–417, 1998.

Oakley CM: Mitral valve palpitations. Aust N Z J Med 22:562–565, 1992.

Rodriguez RD, Schlocken DD: Update on sick sinus syndrome: a cardiac disorder of aging. Geriatrics 45:26–30, 33–36, 1990.

Toff WD, Joy M, Comm AJ: Exercise-induced arrhythmias. Eur Heart J 9(suppl G):119–126, 1988.

Zeldis SM, et al: Correlation with cardiac arrhythmias on 24-hour electrocardiographic monitoring. Chest 78:456–461, 1980.

Zimetbaum P, Josephson ME: Evaluation of patients with palpitations. N Engl J Med 338:1369–1373, 1998.

CHAPTER 28

Shortness of Breath

Dyspnea, or breathlessness, has been defined as patient awareness of respiratory discomfort, unpleasant sensation of labored breathing, or shortness of breath. Dyspnea can be caused by increased rigidity of lung tissue, increased airway resistance, enhanced ventilation during exercise, or any combination of these factors.

Some investigators have suggested that determining the cause of dyspnea is often facilitated by first classifying it into different types, such as wheezing dyspnea, dyspnea on exertion, paroxysmal nocturnal dyspnea, hyperventilation, and dyspnea of cerebral origin. Perhaps a simpler classification is acute, chronic, or recurrent. The common causes of dyspnea include *chronic obstructive pulmonary disease* (COPD), *asthma, congestive heart failure* (CHF), *anxiety, obesity,* and *poor physical condition.*

Nature of Patient

Acute dyspnea in children is most frequently caused by *asthma, bronchiolitis, croup,* and *epiglottitis.* Rarely, it may result from *foreign body aspiration.* An acute onset of dyspnea in a woman who is pregnant or who is taking oral contraceptives suggests *pulmonary embolism.* Pulmonary embolism should also be suspected if dyspnea occurs in patients who are in the postoperative period, in people who have had prolonged recumbency, and in patients who have a history of phlebitis or cardiac arrhythmias (dysrhythmias).

The most common cause of chronic and recurrent shortness of breath in children is asthma. In elderly patients, chronic dyspnea is frequently caused by COPD or heart failure, which are rare conditions in patients under age 30. As these elderly patients develop dyspnea, they decrease their physical activity; the resultant deconditioning confounds the clinical picture.

Chronic dyspnea is more common in people who are heavy smokers because smoking is one of the most important factors in the development of *emphysema, chronic bronchitis,* and *COPD. Obese* and *physically inactive* patients frequently complain of recurrent dyspnea on minimal exertion because of their poor cardiopulmonary reserve.

Nature of Symptoms

The duration of dyspnea, precipitating factors such as exercise or exposure to allergens, nighttime and/or daytime occurrence, number of pillows used when sleeping, concomitant coughing, chest pain, and palpitations are factors that assist the physician in making an accurate diagnosis.

Acute Dyspnea

In patients with acute dyspnea the physician should consider the possibility of *pulmonary embolus, asthma, upper airway obstruction, foreign body aspiration, panic disorder, hyperventilation, pneumonia, pneumothorax, pulmonary edema,* and occasionally *respiratory failure.* Asthma is usually episodic and often precipitated by allergens, exercise, or infections. It is characterized by bilateral wheezing and a decreased respiratory flow rate.

Upper airway obstruction can be caused by *aspiration, vocal cord paralysis, tumors,* and *epiglottic* and *laryngeal edema.* In cases of *foreign body aspiration* (more common in children) the onset of respiratory difficulty is acute. When acute respiratory difficulty occurs during eating, especially in the intoxicated or semiconscious patient, foreign body aspiration is probable. When complete respiratory obstruction occurs, severe respiratory distress, cyanosis, gasping, and loss of consciousness occur quickly. Incomplete respiratory obstruction causes tachypnea, inspiratory stridor, and localized wheezing.

Patients with acute dyspnea due to *hyperventilation* are usually anxious. They often complain of numbness and tingling in the perioral region and the extremities. These patients also often complain of lightheadedness, sighing respiration, and an inability to "get enough air in."

A gradual onset of shortness of breath occurs in patients with *CHF, anemia, lung tumors,* and *parenchymatous lung disease.*

Chronic Dyspnea

Chronic dyspnea in adults is most often caused by *COPD, chronic CHF,* and *obesity.* It also may be seen with *severe anemia* and *infiltrative pulmonary carcinomatosis.*

When dyspnea occurs in one lateral position but not in the other (trepopnea), unilateral lung disease, pleural effusion, or obstruction of the proximal tracheobronchial tree should be suspected. Dyspnea in the upright position relieved by recumbency (platypnea) may be seen in patients with intracardiac shunts, vascular lung shunts, and parenchymal lung shunts.

Associated Symptoms

When dyspnea occurs in young children, especially when associated with coughing and expectoration, *cystic fibrosis* and *bronchiectasis* should be considered.

Acute Dyspnea

When chest pain accompanies acute dyspnea, *spontaneous pneumothorax, pulmonary embolism, chest trauma,* and *myocardial infarction* should be suspected.

Pulmonary embolism is a common cause of acute dyspnea in adults. Patients usually appear severely ill and may complain of chest pain, faintness, and occasionally loss of consciousness. Peripheral cyanosis, low blood pressure, and rales may be present.

When acute dyspnea is caused by severe *anemia* of acute onset, there are usually symptoms of dizziness, weakness, and sweating and possibly signs of hemorrhage (e.g., hypotension, tachycardia, rapid shallow respirations). When acute dyspnea is a manifestation of *anxiety neurosis* or *panic disorder,* the patient usually also complains of dizziness, lightheadedness, palpitations, and paresthesias. The patients do not appear dyspneic and often complain of "not being able to take in enough air." Patients who complain of dyspnea at rest have either a severe physiologic impairment or anxiety hyperventilation.

Chronic Dyspnea

The most common causes of chronic dyspnea on exertion are *cardiac* and *pulmonary.* **Although paroxysmal nocturnal dyspnea is most frequently caused by cardiac pathology, some asthmatic patients develop symptoms primarily when recumbent, usually at night.** Associated findings are often helpful in differentiating pulmonary from cardiac causes of dyspnea. When dyspnea is primarily caused by lung disease, the dyspnea is intensified by effort, there is a daily productive cough, the respirations are shallow and rapid, and postural changes have little or no effect. When dyspnea is of cardiac cause, it is intensified by recumbency, and the respirations are shallow but not necessarily rapid.

Other clues also help differentiate pulmonary from cardiac causes of dyspnea on exertion. When the cause is pulmonary, the rate of recovery to normal respiration is fast, and dyspnea abates a few minutes after cessation of exercise. Patients with dyspnea due to cardiac causes, however, remain dyspneic much longer after cessation of exercise. Likewise, in these patients the heart rate also takes longer to return to preexercise levels. Patients with pulmonary dyspnea do not usually have dyspnea at rest. Patients with severe cardiac dyspnea demonstrate a volume of respiration that is greater than normal at all levels of exercise; they also experience dyspnea sooner after the onset of exertion.

Precipitating and Aggravating Factors

Smoking is the most frequent precipitating and aggravating factor of chronic pulmonary dyspnea. When *exercise* precipitates wheezing or dyspnea, *bronchial asthma* or *CHF* may be the diagnosis. *Exposure to cold* often precipitates wheezing and shortness of breath in asthmatic patients. Bronchial asthma is also probable when *air-borne allergens, noxious fumes,* or *respiratory infections* precipitate dyspnea, cough, or wheezing.

Drugs (e.g., beta blockers) may precipitate wheezing or dyspnea in asthmatic patients. Beta blockers and calcium channel blockers may exacerbate dyspnea in cardiac patients. Less common precipitating and aggravating factors include *trauma, shock, hemorrhage,* and *gaseous anesthesia.*

Ameliorating Factors Other Than Medical Therapy

Some patients with severe COPD obtain relief by leaning forward while seated or by lying supine with their heads down. These positions increase the efficiency of diaphragmatic movement and facilitate the use of the accessory muscles of respiration. Performance of the Heimlich maneuver (abdominal thrust) may dislodge a foreign body from the upper airway.

Physical Findings

Patients with *upper airway obstruction* have coarse sonorous rhonchi and impaired inspiration. Stridor as well as suprasternal retraction may be noted with inspiration. Sibilant, whistling expiratory sounds are usually heard in asthmatic patients. Their expiration appears to be prolonged, whereas inspiration seems to be prolonged in patients with upper airway obstruction. The trachea may be shifted to the opposite side in patients with *pneumothorax* or *large pleural effusion.*

Wheezing dyspnea at rest associated with rhonchi and a productive cough suggests *asthmatic bronchitis.* In contrast, patients with a history of progressive dyspnea that precedes the development of cough or sputum production often have *emphysema.* The physical findings are a hyperinflated lung, decreased breath sounds, decreased diaphragmatic movement, increased anteroposterior chest diameter, and hyperresonance to percussion. Classically, emphysematous patients have been described as "pink puffers"; patients with chronic bronchitis are called "blue bloaters."

Bilateral wheezing usually is heard when acute dyspnea is caused by *asthma.* Bilateral wheezing also may occur with *pulmonary edema.* Wheezing frequently may be heard before the auscultation of rales at the bases and other more classic signs of CHF. Bilateral wheezing also may be heard in patients with *pulmonary emboli,* but more frequently the wheezing is limited to the side of the pulmonary embolus. Unilateral wheezing may also indicate a *bronchial obstruction* by a foreign body, polyp, or mucous plug. Other causes of dyspneic wheezing include *upper airway obstruction,* localized *bronchial obstruction,* and *hypersensitivity pneumonitis.*

Diagnostic Studies

When the cause of dyspnea is not apparent, initial studies should include an electrocardiogram, chest radiograph, hemoglobin, thyroid function tests, creatinine, and spirometry with the use of a bronchodilator. Pulmonary function tests (PFTs) are most helpful and frequently can be performed in an outpatient setting. **PFTs should be an integral part of the clinical evaluation of all patients with**

dyspnea. Patients with *simple acute bronchitis* may have a persistent productive cough but demonstrate no signs of airway narrowing on spirometry. In patients with *chronic bronchitis* and a persistent cough, spirometry may indicate widespread narrowing of the airways, but dyspnea may not be present. *COPD* may be diagnosed with simple spirometry. Occasionally, patients with COPD demonstrate airway narrowing on spirometry without any other symptoms except cough.

PFTs do not provide a specific diagnosis; rather, they demonstrate a pattern of the physiologic abnormality. Typical, but not exclusive, patterns of physiologic abnormalities are seen in most patients with chronic pulmonary diseases, in most people with diseases of pulmonary circulation, and in patients with mild cardiac or valvular disease. PFTs may help the physician differentiate dyspnea due to hyperventilation or psychological factors from pulmonary dysfunction.

PFTs demonstrate increased obstruction to inspiration with extrathoracic (upper airway) obstructive lesions and increased obstruction to expiration with intrathoracic obstructive lesions. Expiratory airway obstruction is indicated by decreased airflow rates, decreased forced expiratory volume in 1 second (FEV_1), decreased peak flow rate (PFR), decreased maximum midexpiratory flow rate (FEF_{25-75}), decreased maximum voluntary ventilation (MVV), increased tidal volume (TV), and increased residual volume (RV). These findings are often observed in patients with *asthma, bronchitis, emphysema,* and *bronchial adenoma.*

The abnormal findings of bronchospasm can usually be transiently reversed with the inhalation of a bronchodilator drug. Lung volume restriction is indicated by a decreased total lung capacity (TLC), increased respiratory minute volume, and decreased compliance. Decreased compliance is found in patients with *fibrosis, sarcoidosis, pneumoconiosis, pulmonary edema, pneumonia, pleural effusion, kyphoscoliosis, obesity,* and *ascites.* Pulmonary vascular disease is evidenced by increased ventilation (V_E) and increased dead space (V_D). Ventilation and perfusion scanning and digital subtraction angiography are useful in the diagnosis of pulmonary embolism. An electrocardiogram may show P pulmonale and right ventricular strain.

Chest radiographs may show pulmonary parenchymal disease, pleural effusions, tumors, or signs of CHF. Doppler measurement of aortic blood flow during exercise may be helpful in distinguishing CHF from COPD as the cause of dyspnea. It is significantly reduced in patients with CHF compared with COPD patients.

Less Common Diagnostic Considerations

Dyspnea is occasionally the presenting symptom in patients with *hyperthyroidism. Pregnant* patients may complain of dyspnea. Patients with *idiopathic pulmonary hemosiderosis* may present with dyspnea on exertion, chronic cough, hemoptysis, and recurrent epistaxis. People who work in grain elevators or with hay also may have severe wheezing and dyspnea. Progressive dyspnea and a nonproductive cough may be the presenting symptoms of patients with *interstitial pulmonary*

Text continued on page 302.

Differential Diagnosis of Shortness of Breath

CAUSE	NATURE OF PATIENT	NATURE OF SYMPTOMS	ASSOCIATED SYMPTOMS	PRECIPITATING AND AGGRAVATING FACTORS	AMELIORATING FACTORS	PHYSICAL FINDINGS	DIAGNOSTIC STUDIES
Acute or recurrent dyspnea							
Asthma	Most common cause of recurrent dyspnea in children	Acute dyspnea Episodic May rarely be dyspneic only at night	Cough (indicates asthmatic bronchitis)	Allergens Exercise Noxious fumes Respiratory tract infections Recumbency Exposure to cold or beta blockers		Bilateral wheezing Sibilant, whistling sounds Prolonged expiration	Pulmonary function tests (PFTS)*: Decreased PFR Decreased MVV Increased TV Pre/postbronchodilator evidence of reversible airway obstruction (>10%)
Pulmonary emboli	Women using birth control pills Patients in postoperative period Long-term recumbent patients Patients with phlebitis Patients in postpartum period	Acute onset of dyspnea	Chest pain Faintness Loss of consciousness	Oral contraceptives Prolonged recumbency		Tachypnea Peripheral cyanosis Low blood pressure Rales Wheezing (usually only on side of emboli) Pleural friction later with pulmonary infarction	Ventilation and perfusion studies Digital subtraction angiography Electrocardiogram: acute right ventricular strain Radiograph: pulmonary infarction or effusion
Hyperventilation and anxiety	Usually anxious	Acute dyspnea "Sighing" respirations	Lightheadedness Palpitations Paresthesias (especially in perioral region and extremities)	Stress Panic		Signs of anxiety but not signs of dyspnea	PFTs: usually normal

Poor physical conditioning	Obese Physically inactive	Dyspnea on minimal exertion				Obesity After exercise pulse slows very gradually	PFTs: Decreased TLC Increased respiratory minute volume Decreased compliance
Foreign body aspiration	Most common in children May occur in intoxicated or semiconscious people during eating	Acute dyspnea			Removal of foreign body Heimlich maneuver	Tachypnea Inspiratory stridor Localized wheezing Suprasternal retraction with respiration May be unilateral wheezing	Chest radiograph: atelectasis or foreign body
Pulmonary edema		Acute onset Episodic	Dyspnea on exertion Orthopnea Paroxysmal nocturnal dyspnea			Gallop rhythm Rales at bases	Decreased ejection fraction Chest radiograph: cardiomegaly with upper lobe redistribution or Kerley's B lines
Pneumothorax	Often a prior history of similar episode May be familial	Acute onset		Cystic fibrosis COPD		Decreased or absent breath sounds Tracheal shift	Chest radiograph: pneumothorax

Table continued on following page.

Differential Diagnosis of Shortness of Breath *Continued*

CAUSE	NATURE OF PATIENT	NATURE OF SYMPTOMS	ASSOCIATED SYMPTOMS	PRECIPITATING AND AGGRAVATING FACTORS	AMELIORATING FACTORS	PHYSICAL FINDINGS	DIAGNOSTIC STUDIES
Chronic dyspnea Chronic obstructive pulmonary disease (COPD)	Older adults Rarely patients under age 30 Most often smokers	Chronic dyspnea Dyspnea with exertion	Fast recovery to normal respiration after stopping exercise	Smoking Exertion Postural changes have little or no effect	Leaning forward while seated	Rapid and shallow respirations	PFTs Spirometry
Emphysema		Progressive dyspnea precedes onset of cough Usually no dyspnea at rest		Smoking		"Pink puffers" Hyperventilated lungs Decreased breath sounds and diaphragmatic movement Increased anteroposterior chest diameter Hyperresonance	PFTs: Decreased PFR Increased TV Decreased MVV Increased RV

Chronic bronchitis		Dyspnea not necessarily presenting symptom Cough precedes dyspnea	Persistent, minimally productive cough			"Blue bloaters" Rhonchi	Same as with emphysema Spirometry: widespread airway narrowing
Congestive heart failure (CHF)	Older patients	Chronic dyspnea with gradual onset Paroxysmal nocturnal dyspnea Dyspnea remains long after stopping exercise	Edema	Exercise Beta blockers Calcium channel blockers Recumbency Trauma Shock Hemorrhage Anesthesia	Nocturnal dyspnea may be relieved by sitting	Shallow respirations (not necessarily rapid) Edema Hepatomegaly Jugular venous distention Third heart sound Basilar rales	Spirometry Respiratory volume greater than normal at all exercise levels Radiograph: pulmonary congestion and cardiomegaly

fibrosis, which may result from drugs (e.g., phenytoin), sarcoidosis, and other granulomatous diseases.

Patients with recurrent *pulmonary emboli* may present with recurrent episodes of dyspnea. Patients with *interstitial pulmonary diseases* (e.g., pulmonary fibrosis, pneumoconiosis), as well as those with *constrictive cardiomyopathy* and *constrictive pericarditis,* may present with dyspnea on exertion, chronic cough, and paroxysmal nocturnal dyspnea.

Selected References

Angelillo VA: Evaluation of dyspnea: is it really present and, if so, why? Postgrad Med 73(2):336–345, 1983.

Gillespie DJ, Staats BA: Unexplained dyspnea. Mayo Clin Proc 69:657–663, 1994.

Golish JH, Ahmad M, Yarnal JR: Chronic upper airway obstruction: methods of detection and recognition. Cleve Clin Q 47:9–15, 1980.

Gulsvik A: Prevalence of and manifestations of obstructive lung disease in the city of Oslo. Scand J Respir Dis 60:286–296, 1979.

Mahler DA: Dyspnea: diagnosis and management. Clin Chest Med 8:215–230, 1987.

Morgan WC, Hodge HL: Diagnostic evaluation of dyspnea. Am Fam Physician 57:711–716, 1998.

Neff TA: The diagnosis and management of chronic obstructive lung disease. Cleve Clin Q 47:17–24, 1980.

Salzman GA: Evaluation of dyspnea. Hosp Pract, March 1997, pp 195–206.

Schmitt BP, Kushner MS, Weiner SL: The diagnostic usefulness of the history of the patient with dyspnea. J Gen Intern Med 1:386–393, 1986.

Silvestri GA, Mahler DA: Evaluation of dyspnea in the elderly patient. Clin Chest Med 14:393–404, 1993.

Spiro G: Exercise testing in the assessment of respiratory disease. Can Med Assoc J 122:890–896, 1980.

CHAPTER 29

Skin Problems

Skin problems are one of the most common reasons for which patients seek medical attention. The 10 most common skin problems leading patients to consult dermatologists are *acne, fungal infections, seborrheic dermatitis, atopic* or *eczematous dermatitis, warts,* benign and malignant *skin tumors, psoriasis, hair disorders, vitiligo,* and *herpes simplex.*

Occupational dermatoses (Table 29–1) most often appear as an eczematous *contact dermatitis,* although they occasionally present as skin cancers, vitiligo, or infectious lesions. Irritant contact dermatoses are often caused by frequent handwashing, cleansers, solvents, cutting oils used by machinists, and disinfectants. Allergic contact dermatitis is usually caused by frequent exposure to nickel chromates and epoxy resins. Other common lesions include infestations such as *scabies* and *pediculosis, contact dermatitis* (Table 29–2), *pityriasis rosea, herpes zoster,* and *seborrheic keratoses.*

These are not necessarily the most common skin problems; some of the most prevalent are handled by physicians other than dermatologists. About one third of all patients with a primary dermatologic complaint consult a general physician.

This chapter presents the most common dermatologic problems in tabular form. Because dermatologic diagnosis is based on the type of lesion, its configuration, and the distribution of the lesions, the summary table is organized accordingly. Because most of the pediatric exanthems such as measles (rubeola), German measles (rubella), and chickenpox (varicella) are easily diagnosed, they are not discussed in this chapter, and the reader therefore should consult pediatric textbooks for their description.

Skin tumors are most common later in life. The most common malignant lesions are *basal cell epithelioma* and *squamous epithelioma.* **If any uncertainty exists about whether a skin lesion is malignant, it should be biopsied.**

For the differential diagnosis of benign and malignant skin tumors, the reader is referred to several excellent texts and articles (see Selected References, p. 348).

TABLE 29.1 Potential Allergens in Contact Dermatitis from Occupational Exposure

AGENT	WHERE TYPICALLY FOUND	BODY SITE AFFECTED
Nickel	Tools, utensils, musical instruments, machinery parts, batteries, steel-toed work boots, jewelry, clothing snaps	Face, hands, eyelids, waist, umbilicus, tops of toes
Chromates	Engraving devices, lithography and photography processing materials, ceramics, glues and adhesives, shoe polishes, cement, leather, match heads, auto primer paints, catgut, electroplating solutions	Hands, wrists, forearms, feet
Epoxy resin	Adhesive and glues for industrial and household use, laminates, electrical encapsulators, eyeglass frames, paints and inks, product finishers, surface coatings, handbags	Hands, face (especially eyelids), forearms
Formaldehyde	Photography processing materials; paints; paper products; pathology fixatives; fertilizers; plastic; resins; insulation; wood composites; permanent-press fabrics; cosmetics; shampoos; medications; leather-tanning agents; smoke from cigarettes, cigars, charcoal, wood	Axillae, waist, hands, face, scalp
Mercaptobenzothiazole	Rubber products, especially shoes (soles and arch supports) and—less frequently—gloves, cutting oils, antifreeze, anticorrosive agents, cements and adhesives, detergents, fungicides, photographic film emulsion	Feet, hands
Thiuram	Rubber products, especially gloves and—less frequently—shoes, fungicides, germicides, insecticides, soaps and shampoos, disulfiram	Hands, face, scalp, feet
Paraphenylenediamine	Hair dyes, printer's ink, leather, fur dyes (cross-reacts with para-aminobenzoic acid, procaine, benzocaine, thiazides, sulfonamides)	Scalp, face, hands

Ethylenediamine	Aminophylline, hydroxyzine hydrochloride, hydroxyzine pamoate, tripelennamine, rubber products, antifreeze, dyes, fungicides, triamcinolone acetonide/nystatin and other prescription creams	Hands, face, generalized allergic reaction
Acrylates	Construction adhesives, printing materials, textiles, medical products (dental adhesives, artificial joints, heart valves, contact lenses), utensils (plexiglass, veneer), glues (superadhesive types), artificial nails, nail polish	Hands, face
Propylene glycol	Cosmetics, pharmaceuticals (topical corticosteroids, otic preparations, sterile lubricant jelly, electrocardiogram pastes, injectables), antifreeze, food coloring, flavoring agents	Face, ears, hands, genitalia, generalized allergic reaction
Polyethylene glycol	Topical medications, suppositories, shampoos, hair dressings, toothpaste, contraceptive jellies, insect repellents, glues, lubricants for rubber molds, textile fibers, metal-forming operations	Scalp, face, genitalia, anus, hands
Neomycin	Topical antibiotics (cross-reacts with kanamycin, gentamicin, spectinomycin, tobramycin, bacitracin)	Face, ears, leg ulcers, generalized allergic reaction
Benzocaine	Topical anesthetics (including creams and lozenges) for burns, hemorrhoids, poison ivy, toothaches (cross-reacts with procaine, tetracaine, procainamide, hydrochlorothiazide, sunscreens containing para-aminobenzoic acid, paraphenylenediamine, sulfonamides, sulfonylurea, para-aminosalicylic acid)	Face, genitalia, anus, generalized allergic reaction

From Prawer SE: Occupational dermatoses in primary care: a guide to recognition. Consultant 38:423–444, 1998.

TABLE 29.2 Common Areas of Involvement and Causes of Allergic Contact Dermatitis

AREA	CAUSES
Ear lobes	Earrings (nickel)
Postauricular area	Hair dye (paraphenylenediamine)
	Shampoos (formalin)
	Hearing aids or glasses (nickel or plastic)
Ear canal	Medications
Face	Hair dye (paraphenylenediamine)
	Poison ivy
	Cosmetics
	Sprays or any airborne contactant
Eyelids	Sprays or any airborne contactant
	Cosmetics
	Eyelash curlers (rubber accelerators or nickel)
	Any contactant on the hands (topical medications, formalin in nail polish)
Perioral area	Lipstick
	Toothpaste
Neck	Jewelry (nickel)
	Perfumes
	Sprays or any airborne contactants
Axilla	Deodorants
	Clothing (formalin)
Chest	Brassieres (rubber accelerators)
	Metal objects carried in pockets (nickel)
Back	Metal fasteners (nickel)
Waist	Belt buckles or snaps (nickel)
	Waist bands or girdles (rubber accelerators)
Extremities	Poison ivy
	Airborne contactants
Wrists	Jewelry (nickel)
Hands	Rings (nickel)
	Gloves (rubber accelerators)
Feet	Components of shoes (rubber accelerators, dichromates in leather)
Scrotum	Any contactant on the hands or agent applied in the groin (topical medication)

From Huff JC, Weston WL: Eczematous dermatitis. Maj Probl Clin Pediatr 19:86–122, 1978.

Differential Diagnosis of Skin Problems

NATURE OF LESION	DISTRIBUTION OF LESION	ASSOCIATED FINDINGS	NATURE OF PATIENT	LESIONS WITH SIMILAR APPEARANCE	DIAGNOSIS
Papules and pustules	Face, back, and chest	Comedones	Start at puberty and last several years		Acne (Fig. 29-1)
Papules, vesicles, and pustules	Face, head, and neck Occasionally diaper area in infants	Oozing, honeycomb-colored crusting	Mostly children	Molluscum contagiosum (Fig. 29-4) Folliculitis (Fig. 29-5)	Impetigo (Figs. 29-2 and 29-3)
Scaling and lichenification	Face, extensor surfaces, and exposed areas in children Flexural folds (antecubital, popliteal), wrists, neck, upper arms, and thighs in adults Symmetric	Often family history of hay fever or asthma Itching, erythema, often lichenification In blacks, rash tends to be more papular 10% of general population have atopic dermatitis Erythematous or with plaques Rash in adults is usually localized, dry, excoriated, or lichenified	Often begin in infancy at age 5 months Often clear spontaneously at age 5 years Rare in elderly people	Seborrheic dermatitis (different location and yellow scales) Psoriasis (typical locations and silvery scales) Contact dermatitis is usually asymmetric	Atopic dermatitis or eczema (Figs. 29-6 to 29-9)
Scaling plaques	Mostly extensor surface of extremities, back, buttocks, and hands, but can occur anywhere	Coin-shaped lesions Itching Oozing	Children and adults	Ringworm (positive KOH) Contact dermatitis (exposed areas) Psoriasis (elbows and knees)	Nummular eczema or nummular dermatitis (Fig. 29-10)

Table continued on following page.

Differential Diagnosis of Skin Problems *Continued*

NATURE OF LESION	DISTRIBUTION OF LESION	ASSOCIATED FINDINGS	NATURE OF PATIENT	LESIONS WITH SIMILAR APPEARANCE	DIAGNOSIS
Scaling plaques or patches	Trunk and proximal extremities	Herald patch (2 × 6 cm), usually on trunk, precedes generalized lesion More common in winter Salmon colored May itch Oval patches (1 × 2 cm) with long axis along skin lines giving Christmas tree pattern Collarette scaling	Children Young adults	Fungus Psoriasis Secondary syphilis Drug eruptions	Pityriasis rosea (Figs. 29–11 to 29–13)
Plaques	Usually on covered parts of body and face Often multiple	Irregular greasy surface Superficial, on top of skin ("stuck to skin") Yellow, tan, dark brown, or rarely black Sharply defined edges	Adults (mostly elderly)	Actinic keratoses occur in sun-exposed areas and are smaller	Seborrheic keratoses (Figs. 29–14 and 29–15)
Erythematous plaques	Extensor surfaces, esp. knees and elbows Scalp Coccygeal region Nails Rare on face	Silvery, loosely adherent scales Occasional itching Arthritis, esp. in distal interphalangeal joints Sharp margins Scalp lesions usually stop at hairline	Adults Rare in young children	Seborrheic dermatitis can involve scalp but extends beyond hairline Nummular eczema	Psoriasis (Figs. 29–16 to 29–20)

Scaling patches	Scalp Eyebrows Nasolabial fold Midchest Umbilicus	Yellow, greasy scaling Greasy scaling with poor margin Some erythema	More common in adults "Cradle cap" in infants	Dandruff with little erythema and no other areas involved Psoriasis involves extensor surfaces Psoriasis of scalp usually stops at hairline with well-defined plaques	Seborrheic dermatitis (Figs. 29–21 to 29–24)
Papules inflamed with excoriation and crusting Linear burrows not always seen	Finger webs Wrists Antecubital Elbows Areolar Umbilicus Lower abdomen Genitalia Gluteal cleft	Itching (worse at night) Excoriation Weeping Others in household may have same problem	Adults and children	Pediculosis pubis Nits attached to hair Lice often seen on skin	Scabies (Figs. 29–25 to 29–27)
Papules inflamed	Usually on trunk Grouped	Itching; flea bites often grouped	Sand flies and fleas in adults on lower legs Flea bites in children can be anywhere	Scabies Drug eruptions Lymphoma	Insect bites (Figs. 29–28 to 29–30)
Depigmentation	Orifices Eyes Extensor surfaces Areas of trauma	Positive Wood's light (bright white) Increased familial incidence	Familial Thyroid disease Addison's disease	Postinflammatory hypopigmentation Tinea versicolor alba Exposure to phenolic compounds	Vitiligo (Figs. 29–31 to 29–33)
Depigmentation and pink-red-brown macules	Mainly trunk Upper arms	Positive Wood's light (pale yellow) Pink-red-brown macules Scaling Positive KOH Mild itching	Young adults	Postinflammatory hypopigmentation (e.g., seborrheic dermatitis, pityriasis rosea, esp. in blacks) Other fungi	Tinea versicolor (Figs. 29–34 to 29–37)

Table continued on following page.

Differential Diagnosis of Skin Problems *Continued*

NATURE OF LESION	DISTRIBUTION OF LESION	ASSOCIATED FINDINGS	NATURE OF PATIENT	LESIONS WITH SIMILAR APPEARANCE	DIAGNOSIS
Vesicles	Anywhere (often asymmetric exposed areas) Hands Axilla	Itching, oozing May occur hours to a few days after exposure	Adults and children	Allergy to systemic medications Atopic dermatitis	Contact dermatitis (see Table 29–2) Detergents Chemicals (Fig. 29–38) Deodorant
On erythematous areas	Exposed areas (especially extremities)	Lesions often in streaks Itching	Adults and children		Plants (ivy, oak, sumac) (Fig. 29–39)
	Near hands, zippers, jewelry (e.g., wrist, ear lobe)	Itching			Nickel (Figs. 29–40 and 29–41)
	Where medication is applied (e.g., eye, hair, face, neck)			Eczema	Medications, hair preparations, cosmetics
	Hands, other exposed areas Genital region Buttocks				Industrial agents (see Table 29–1)
With erythematous base	Genital area	Pain, not itch Positive Tzanck's test	Adults Neonates		Herpes progenitalis (simplex II) (Fig. 29–42)
	Cold sore (rarely in genital area)	Pain Systemic symptoms Positive Tzanck's test		Acute contact dermatitis Erythema multiforme	Herpes simplex I (Fig. 29–43)
With dermatomal distribution	Leg most common site in children	Tingling Occasional itch Pain (usually not in children) Often sciatic distribution	Adults and children	Contact dermatitis (usually itches) Cellulitis	Herpes zoster (Fig. 29–44)

Patchy alopecia	Scalp	Hairs broken and short Positive KOH Does not fluoresce Culture in dermatology test medium (DTM) *Microsporum audouini* and *canis* give apple-green Wood's light	Preadolescents	Alopecia areata	Fungal infections mostly *Trichophyton tonsurans* (Figs. 29–45 to 29–47)
Patchy alopecia (possibly scarring)	Scalp	Pustular lesion Boggy scalp Culture in DTM	Most common in children	Fungal infection	Bacterial infection
	Scalp	Pinhead-sized nits on hair shaft May be superimposed bacterial infection Itching	More common in children but can occur in adults	Seborrheic dermatitis Bacterial infection	Pediculosis capitis (Fig. 29–48)
Erythematous Some scaling Occasional maceration and oozing	Groin	Border not sharp; pustules at edge Positive KOH	Children Diabetics	May all look similar (KOH required for differentiation) (Fig. 29–49)	Candidiasis (Figs. 29–50 and 29–51)
	Under breasts	Moist			Diaper rash (Fig. 29–52)
	Groin	Border sharp and accentuated Itch No pustular edge Positive KOH	Often complicates simple herpes rash More common in males Not seen in children		Tinea cruris (Fig. 29–53)
		Moist	Obese adults		Seborrheic intertrigo
		Border sharp Positive Wood's light (coral red) Reddish brown macules	Adults		Erythrasma (*Corynebacterium*) (Fig. 29–54)

Table continued on following page.

Differential Diagnosis of Skin Problems *Continued*

NATURE OF LESION	DISTRIBUTION OF LESION	ASSOCIATED FINDINGS	NATURE OF PATIENT	LESIONS WITH SIMILAR APPEARANCE	DIAGNOSIS
Scaling, vesicles	Feet (soles)	Scaling Itch (worse in summer) Positive KOH	Adults and children	May coexist*	Tinea pedis (dyshidrotic form) (Fig. 29–55)
Vesicles	Feet (soles, sides, dorsum)	Negative KOH Often associated with similar process in hands	Adults	May coexist*	Dyshidrotic eczema (Fig. 29–56)
Maceration	Feet (between toes, mainly 4th and 3rd spaces)	Itch (worse in summer) Positive KOH	Adults and children	May coexist*	Tinea pedis (intertriginous form) (Fig. 29–57)
Scaling	Face or feet (soles)	Erythema and fissuring Negative KOH, spares toe webs	Children		Juvenile plantar dermatitis
Erythema scaling	Feet (dorsum and toes; toe webs and soles not involved)	Negative KOH	Adults and children	Tinea pedis	Shoe dermatitis due to chrome used in leather tanning (Fig. 29–58)

Tumor	Most common on face and other sun-exposed areas	Smooth surface Atrophic center Pearly edge Roundish shape Tannish brown Telangiectasia on border	Elderly people Those often exposed to sun	Squamous cell cancer Melanoma Sebaceous nevi	Basal cell carcinoma
	Most common on sun-exposed areas (especially hands, face, and ears)	Smooth or irregular surface Firm Irregular edge May be scaling Tannish brown	Elderly people Those often exposed to sun	Basal cell cancer Warts Actinic keratoses	Squamous cell carcinoma
	Men: mostly on trunk (47%) Women: mostly on legs (39%)	Pigmented, often with different colors in same lesion (blue, purple, white, tan) Irregular border Change in size Satellites	Adults	Mole (melanocytic nevus) Pigmented lesions Seborrheic keratosis Dermatofibroma Angiokeratoma Lentigo	Malignant melanoma

*Different forms of tinea pedis may exist with each other as well as with dyshidrotic eczema.

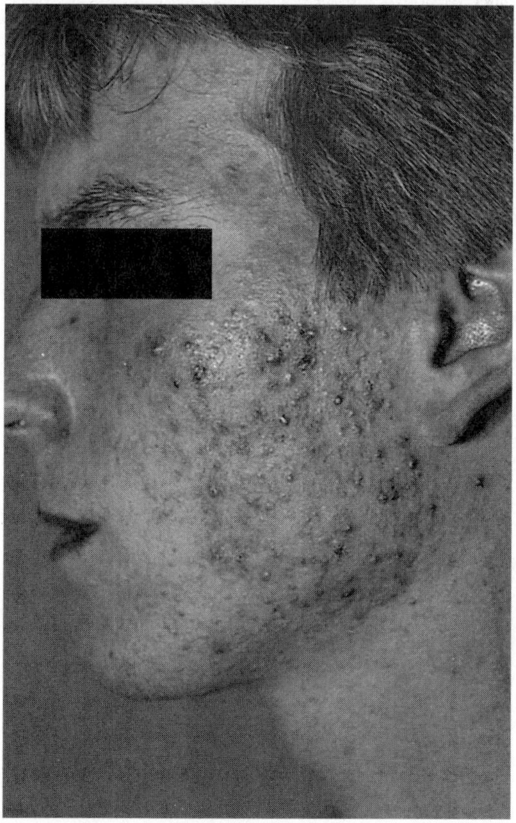

■ **Figure 29.1** Acne vulgaris of face *(above)* and back *(next page)*. (From Callen JP, et al: Color Atlas of Dermatology. Philadelphia, WB Saunders Co, 1993.)

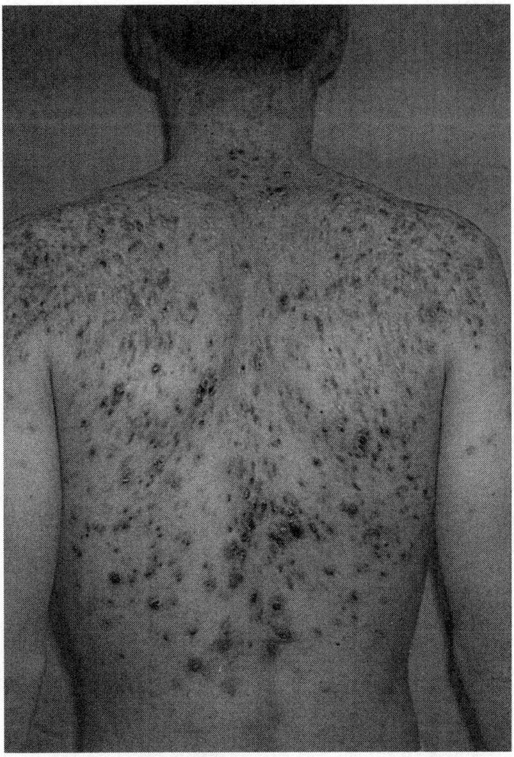

■ **Figure 29.1** *Continued*

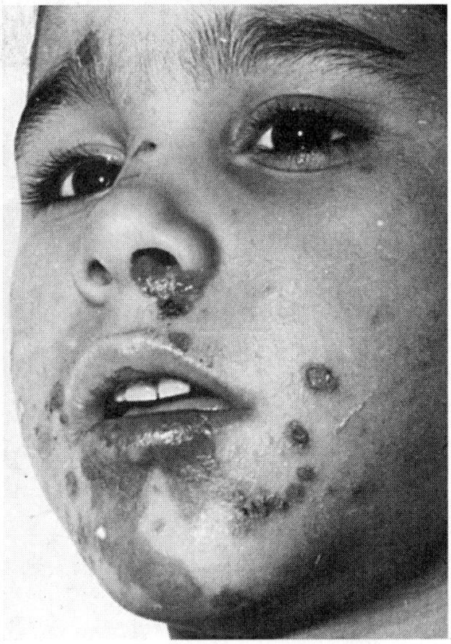

■ **Figure 29.2** Impetigo. Note serous exudation and crusting. Since impetigo is contagious, it can spread to other people and different parts of the body. It is usually caused by *Staphylococcus aureus* or less frequently by *Streptococcus pyogenes (hemolyticus).* (From Arnold HL, Odom RB, James WB: Andrews' Diseases of the Skin, 8th ed. Philadelphia, WB Saunders Co, 1990.)

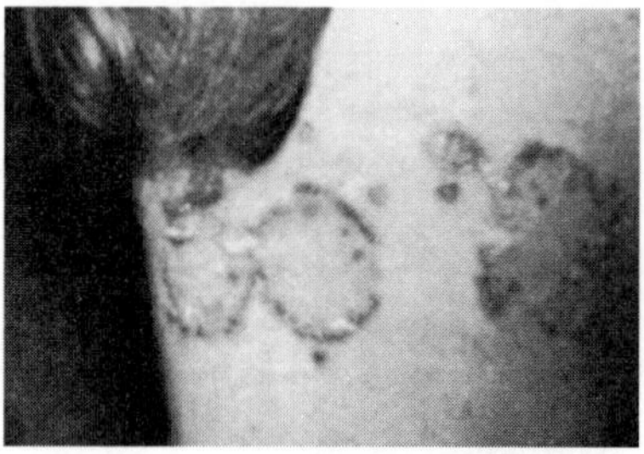

■ **Figure 29.3** Impetigo circinata. Occasionally the center of an impetiginous lesion heals, leaving a ringed, crusted edge culture from which the diagnosis can be established. (From Vickers HR: Problems of dermatological diagnoses. Br J Clin Pract 32:159-166, 1978.)

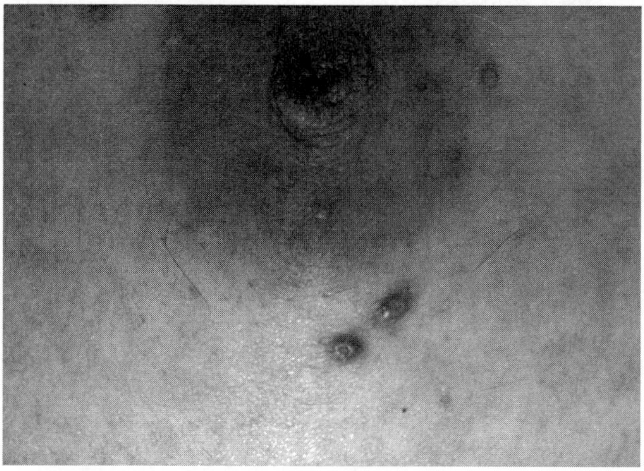

■ **Figure 29.4** Molluscum contagiosum. Papules with central umbilication. (From Callen JP, et al: Color Atlas of Dermatology. Philadelphia, WB Saunders Co, 1993.)

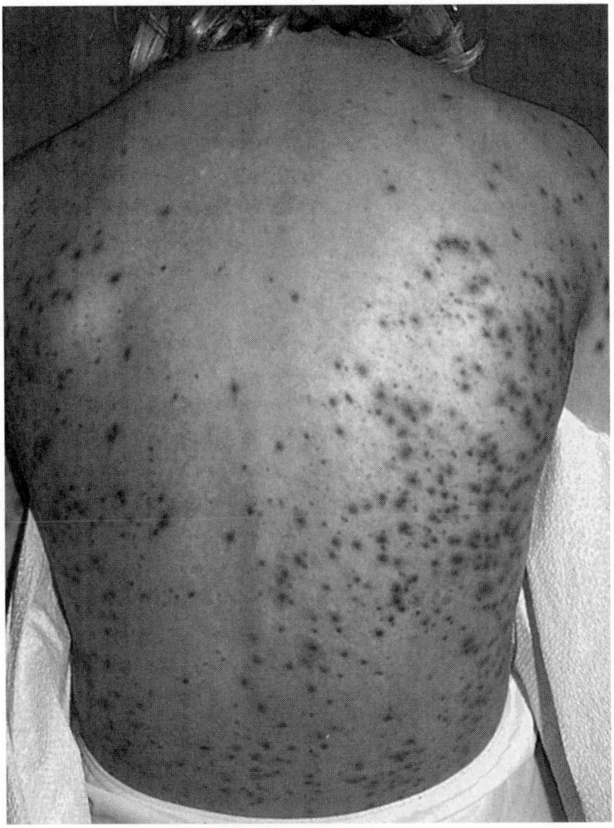

■ **Figure 29.5** Hot tub folliculitis. Papules and pustules due to *Pseudomonas* infection. (From Callen JP, et al: Color Atlas of Dermatology. Philadelphia, WB Saunders Co, 1993.)

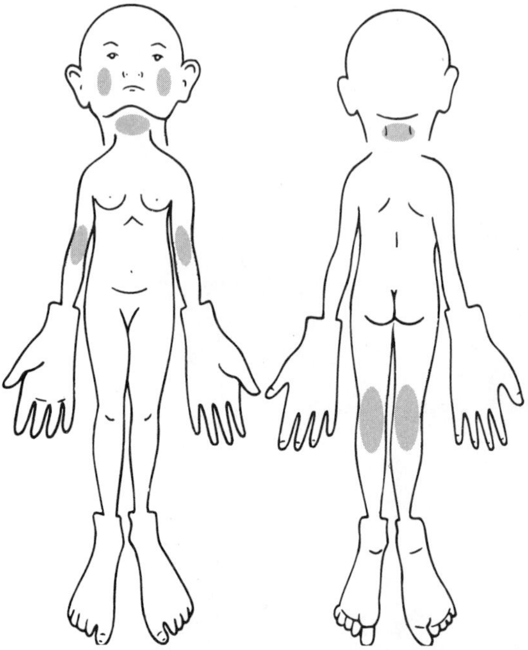

■ **Figure 29.6** Lichenified pruritic areas in flexural regions and on the face are typical locations for adult atopic dermatitis. (From Lamberg SI: Common problems of the skin. *In* Barker LR, Burton JR, Zieve PD [Eds]: Principles of Ambulatory Medicine. Baltimore, Williams & Wilkins, 1982.)

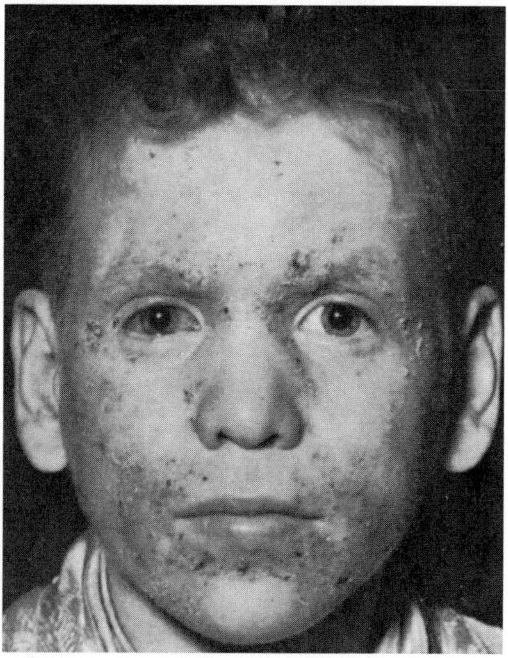

■ **Figure 29.7** Atopic dermatitis: characteristic facial appearance, chronic excoriated dermatitis, and "sad" and "strained" look. (From Huff JC, Weston WL: Eczematous dermatitis. Maj Probl Clin Pediatr 19:86-122, 1978.)

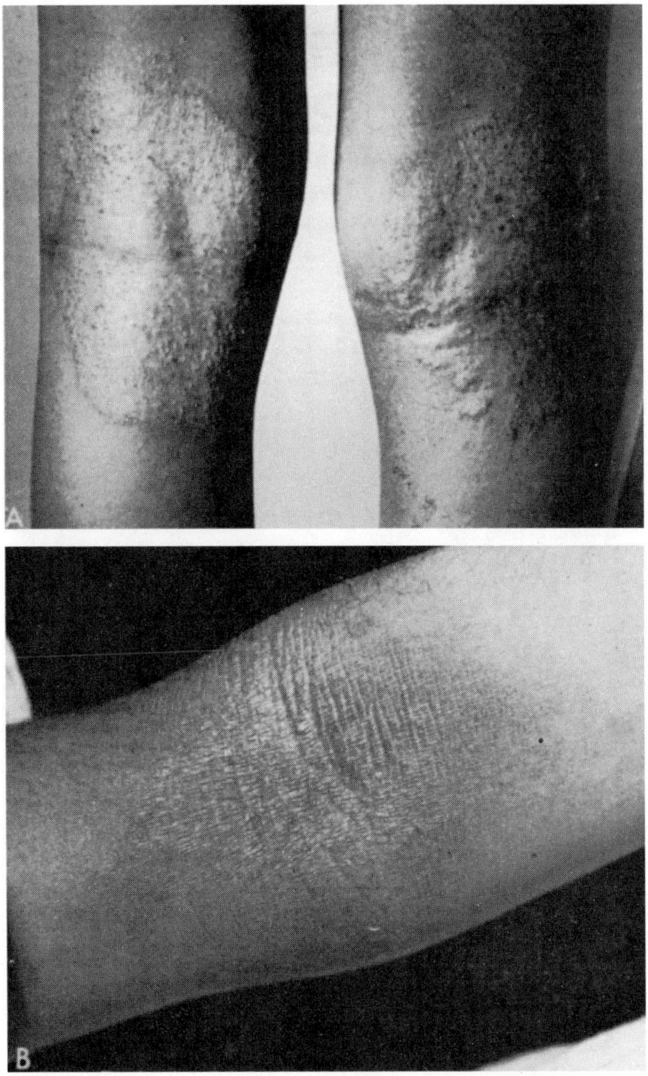

■ **Figure 29.8** Atopic dermatitis: characteristic lesions. *A,* Sharply marginated excoriated lesions of popliteal spaces. *B,* Lichenification and thickening, antecubital fossa. (From Huff JC, Weston WL: Eczematous dermatitis. Maj Probl Clin Pediatr 19:86-122, 1978.)

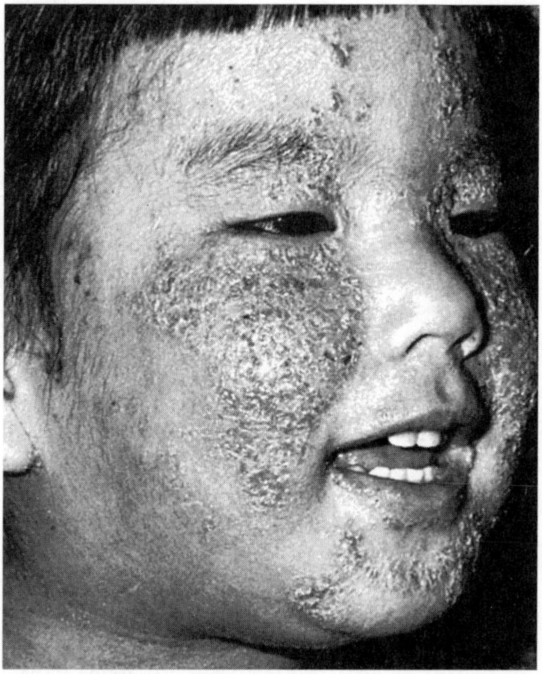

■ **Figure 29.9** Infantile atopic dermatitis of face. (From Arnold HL, Odom RB, James WB: Andrews' Diseases of the Skin, 8th ed. Philadelphia, WB Saunders, Co, 1990.)

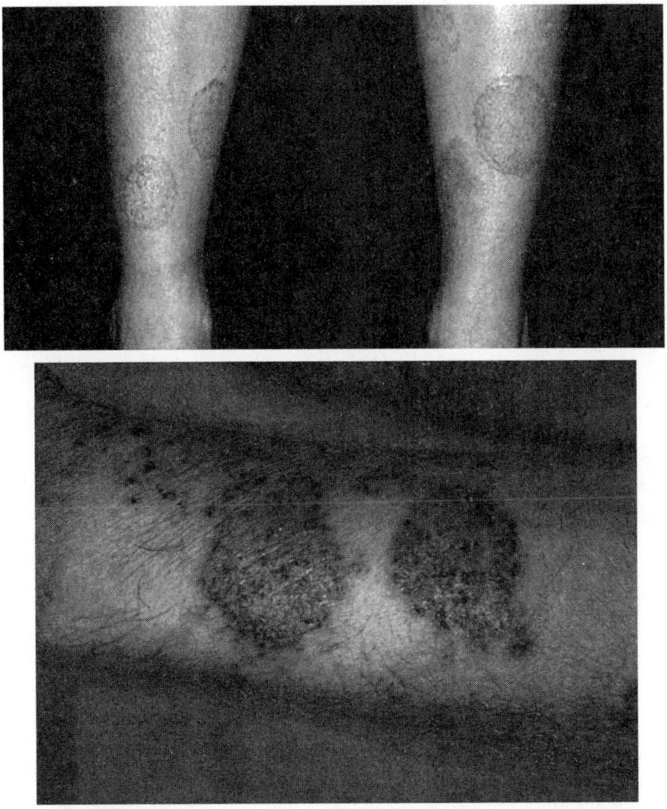

■ **Figure 29.10** Nummular eczema. (From Callen JP, et al: Color Atlas of Dermatology. Philadelphia, WB Saunders Co, 1993.)

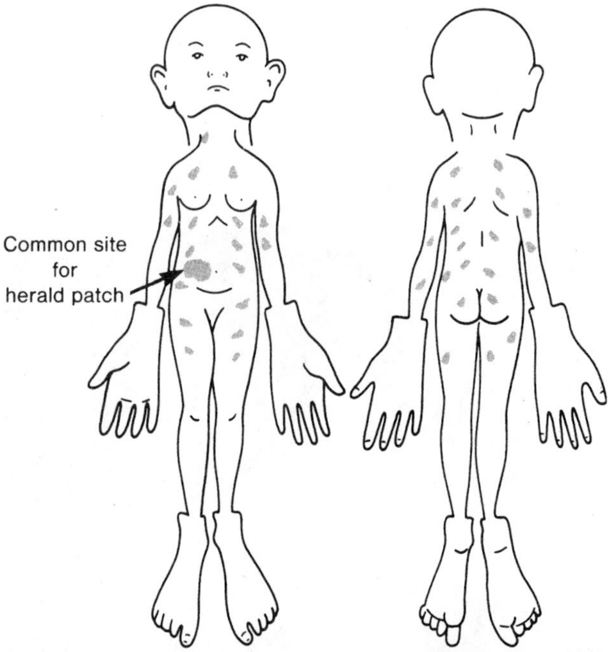

■ **Figure 29.11** Pityriasis rosea typically starts with a "herald patch" followed by oval patches in a fernlike pattern. (From Lamberg SI: Common problems of the skin. *In* Barker ZR, Burton JR, Zieve PD [Eds]: Principles of Ambulatory Medicine. Baltimore, Williams & Wilkins, 1982.)

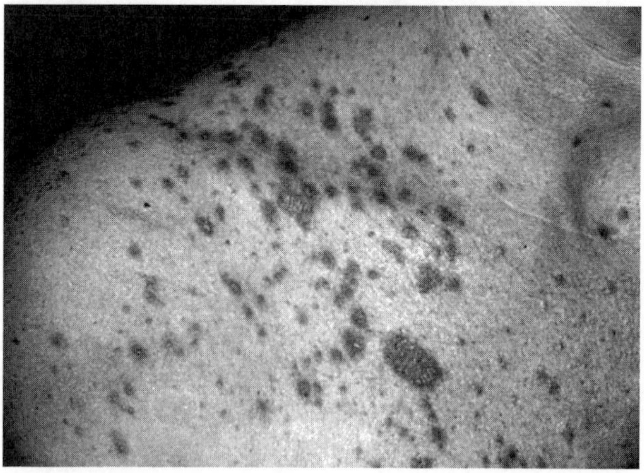

■ **Figure 29.12** Pityriasis rosea. Discrete papulosquamous lesions with larger initial patch (herald lesion). (From Callen JP, et al: Color Atlas of Dermatology. Philadelphia, WB Saunders Co, 1993.)

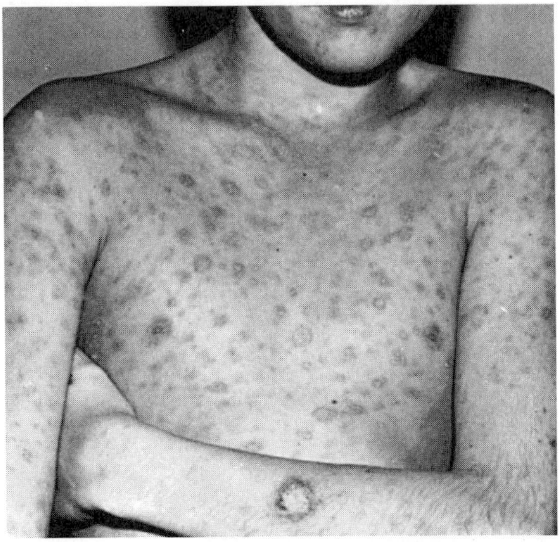

■ **Figure 29.13** Pityriasis rosea with herald patch on forearm. (From Arnold HL, Odom RB, James WB: Andrews' Diseases of the Skin, 8th ed. Philadelphia, WB Saunders Co, 1990.)

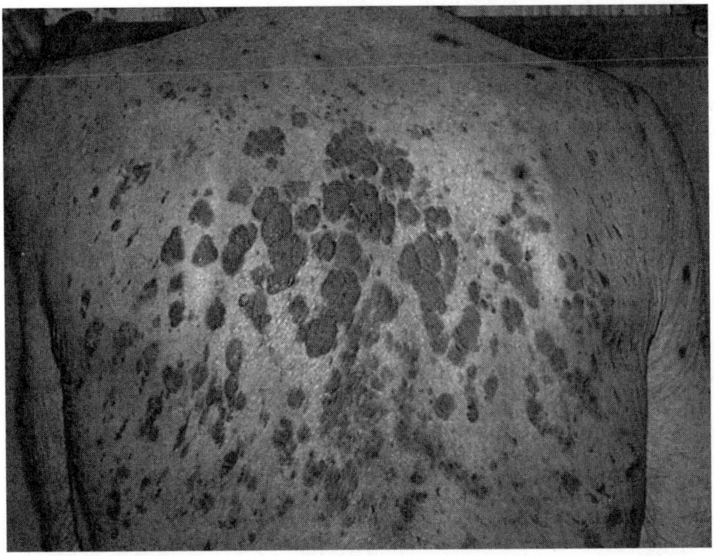

■ **Figure 29.14** Multiple seborrheic dermatoses. (From Callen JP, et al: Color Atlas of Dermatology. Philadelphia, WB Saunders Co, 1993.)

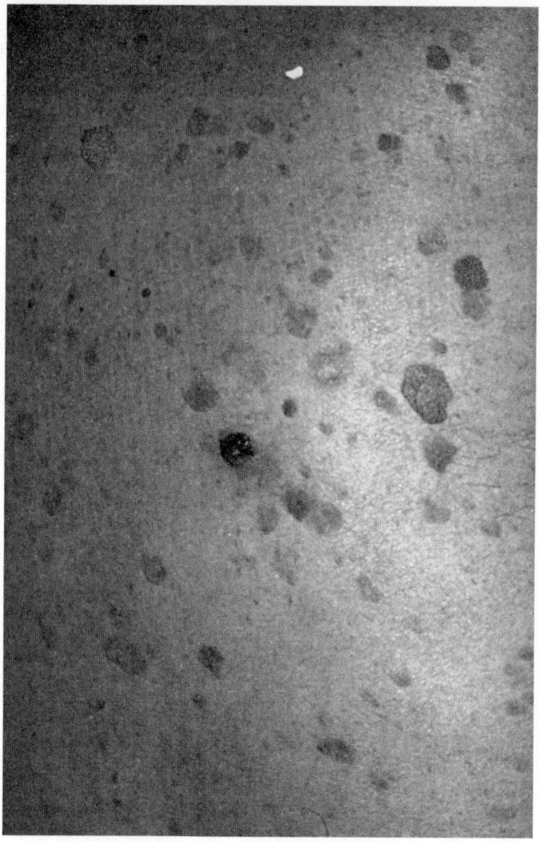

■ **Figure 29.15** Irritated seborrheic dermatoses may become lighter in color. (From Callen JP, et al: Color Atlas of Dermatology. Philadelphia, WB Saunders Co, 1993.)

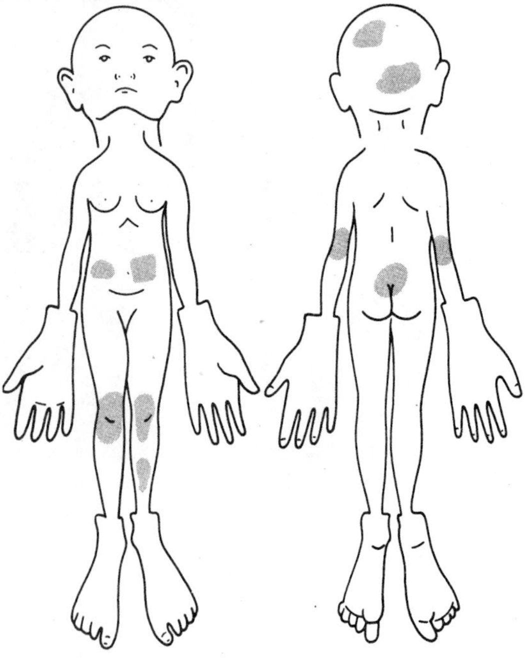

■ **Figure 29.16** Psoriasis tends to be found on extensor surfaces and areas of repeated trauma, such as the waistline. (From Lamberg SI: Common problems of the skin. *In* Barker LR, Burton JR, Zieve PD [Eds]: Principles of Ambulatory Medicine. Baltimore, Williams & Wilkins, 1982.)

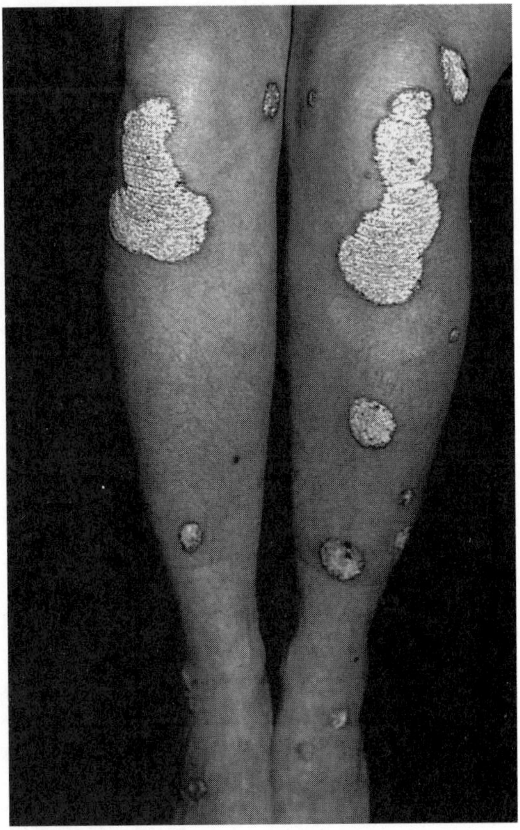

■ **Figure 29.17** Psoriasis vulgaris. (From Callen JP, et al: Color Atlas of Dermatology. Philadelphia, WB Saunders Co, 1993.)

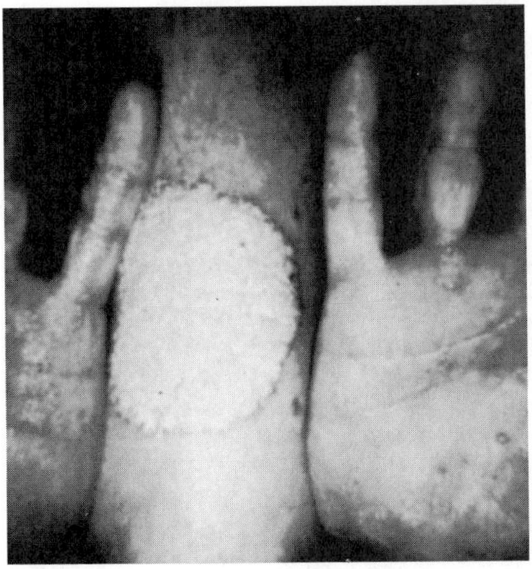

■ **Figure 29.18** Psoriasis. White scale and palm lesions. (From Welton W: Dermatology and syphilology. *In* Rakel RE, Conn HF [Eds]: Family Practice, 2nd ed. Philadelphia, WB Saunders Co, 1978.)

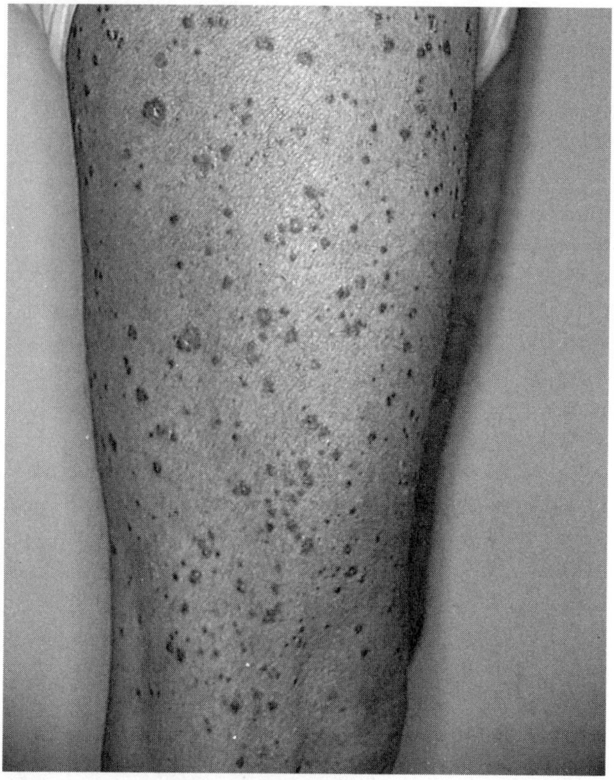

■ **Figure 29.19** Guttate psoriasis of thigh. (From Callen JP, et al: Color Atlas of Dermatology. Philadelphia, WB Saunders Co, 1993.)

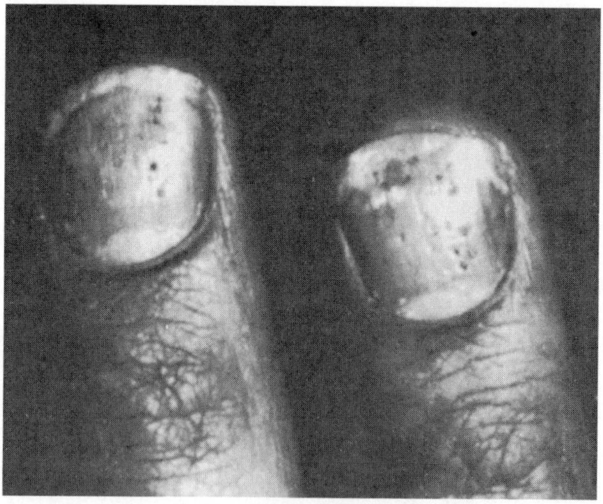

■ **Figure 29.20** Minute pits typically are seen on the surface of nails in patients with psoriasis. (From Lamberg SI: Common problems of the skin. *In* Barker LR, Burton JR, Zieve PD [Eds]: Principles of Ambulatory Medicine. Baltimore, Williams & Wilkins, 1982.)

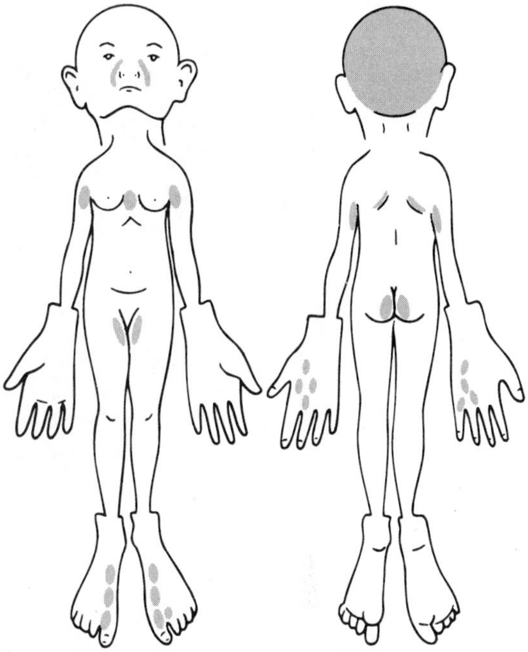

■ **Figure 29.21** Usual location of erythema and scale in seborrheic dermatitis. (From Lamberg SI: Common problems of the skin. *In* Barker LR, Binton JR, Zieve PD [Eds]: Principles of Ambulatory Medicine. Baltimore, Williams & Wilkins, 1982.)

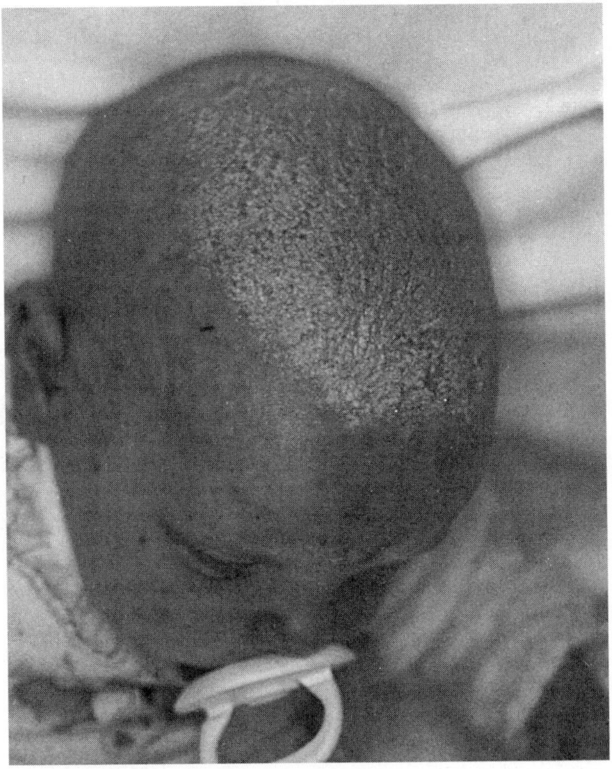

■ **Figure 29.22** Seborrheic dermatitis of scalp ("cradle cap"). (From Callen JP, et al: Color Atlas of Dermatology. Philadelphia, WB Saunders Co, 1993.)

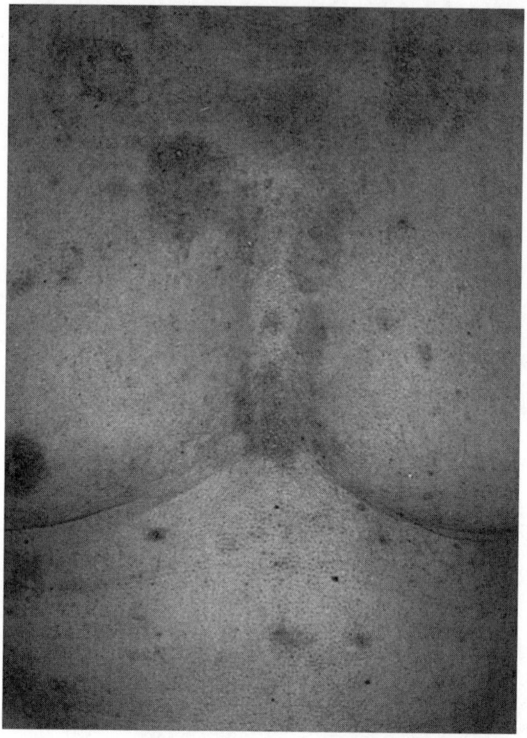

■ **Figure 29.23** Seborrheic dermatitis of chest with greasy-looking scale and erythema. (From Callen JP, et al: Color Atlas of Dermatology. Philadelphia, WB Saunders Co, 1993.)

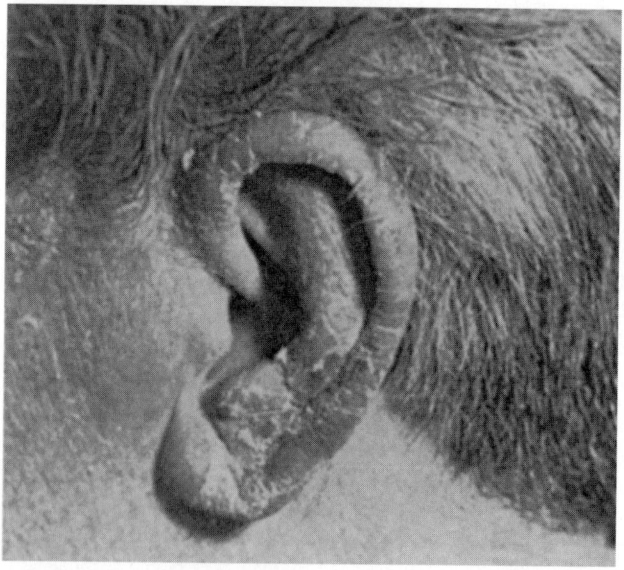

■ **Figure 29.24** Seborrheic dermatitis. Erythema and scaling on ears and scalp is typical of this condition. (From Medical Times, June 1977, p 67.)

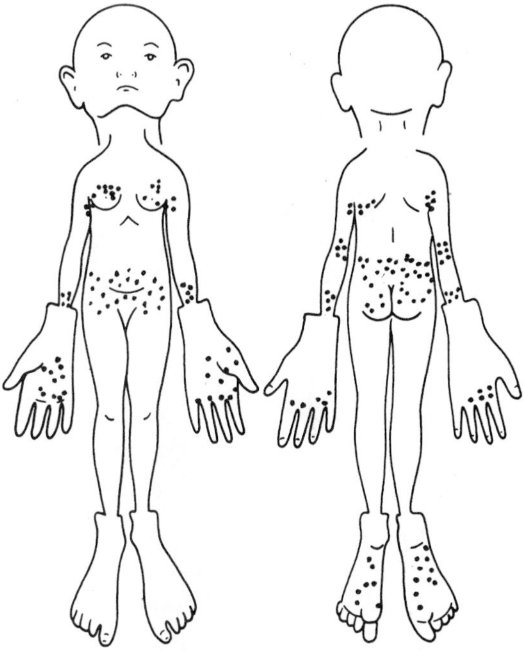

■ **Figure 29.25** Pruritic papules are most prevalent about the waist, pelvis, elbows, hands, and feet in scabies. (From Lamberg SI: Common problems of the skin. *In* Barker LR, Burton JR, Zieve PD [Eds]: Principles of Ambulatory Medicine. Baltimore, Williams & Wilkins, 1982.)

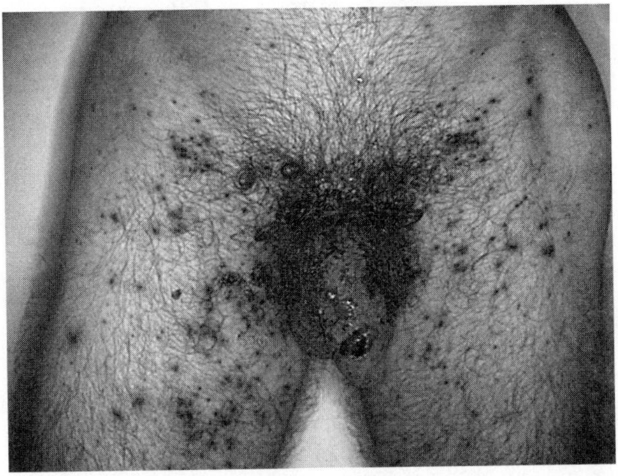

■ **Figure 29.26** Scabies of groin. (From Callen JP, et al: Color Atlas of Dermatology. Philadelphia, WB Saunders Co, 1993.)

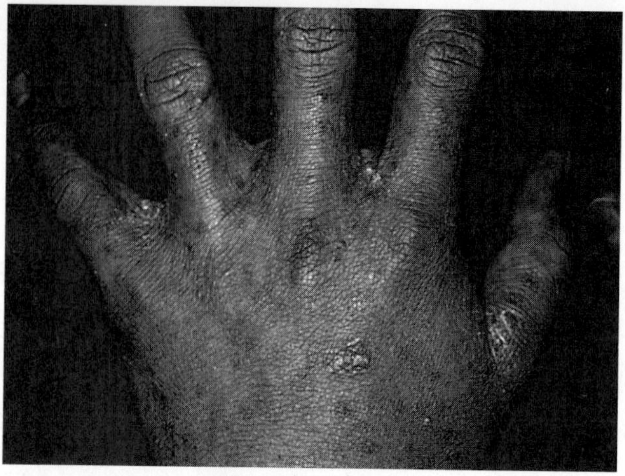

■ **Figure 29.27** Scabies of hand. (From Callen JP, et al: Color Atlas of Dermatology. Philadelphia, WB Saunders Co, 1993.)

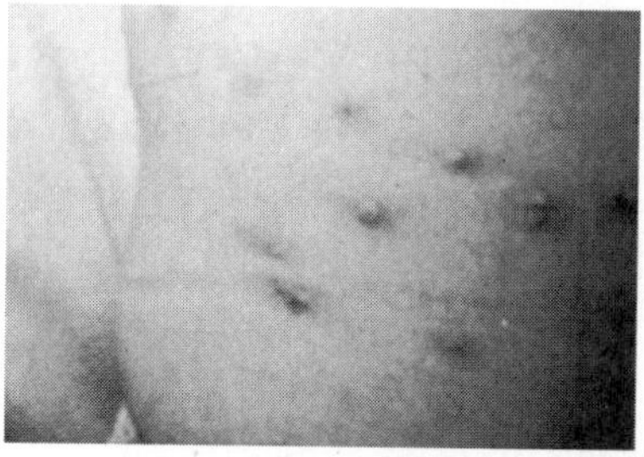

■ **Figure 29.28** Insect bites (clustered itching papules). (From Vickers HR: Problems of dermatological diagnoses. Br J Clin Pract 32:159-166, 1978.)

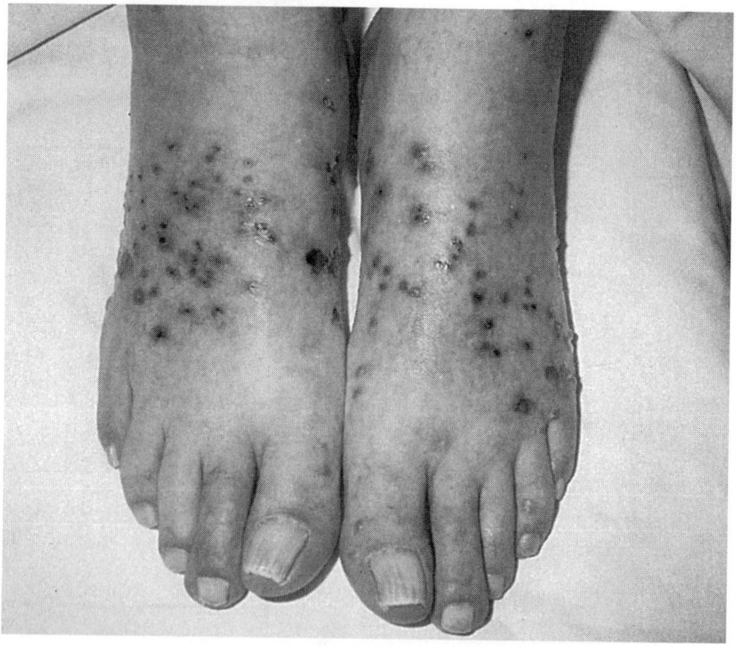

■ **Figure 29.29** Flea bites of feet. (From Callen JP, et al: Color Atlas of Dermatology. Philadelphia, WB Saunders Co, 1993.)

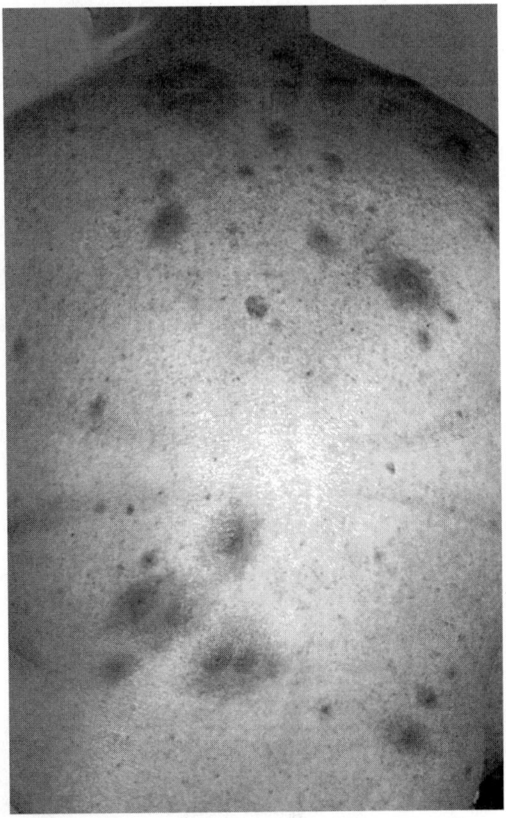

■ **Figure 29.30** Bed bug bites causing erythematous papules. (From Callen JP, et al: Color Atlas of Dermatology. Philadelphia, WB Saunders Co, 1993.)

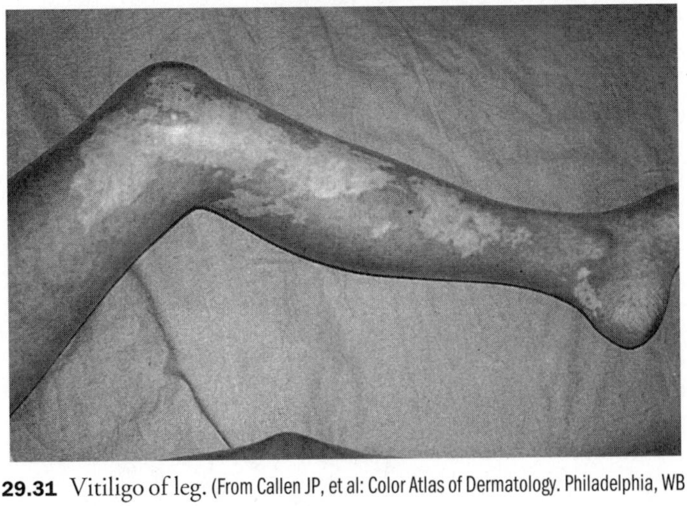

■ **Figure 29.31** Vitiligo of leg. (From Callen JP, et al: Color Atlas of Dermatology. Philadelphia, WB Saunders Co, 1993.)

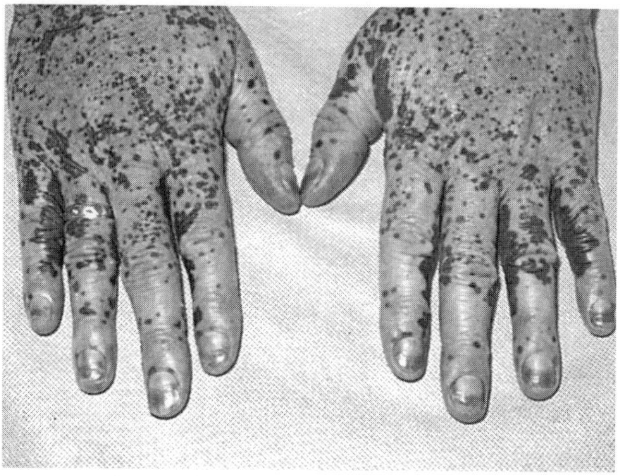

■ **Figure 29.32** Vitiligo of hands. (From Callen JP, et al: Color Atlas of Dermatology. Philadelphia, WB Saunders Co, 1993.)

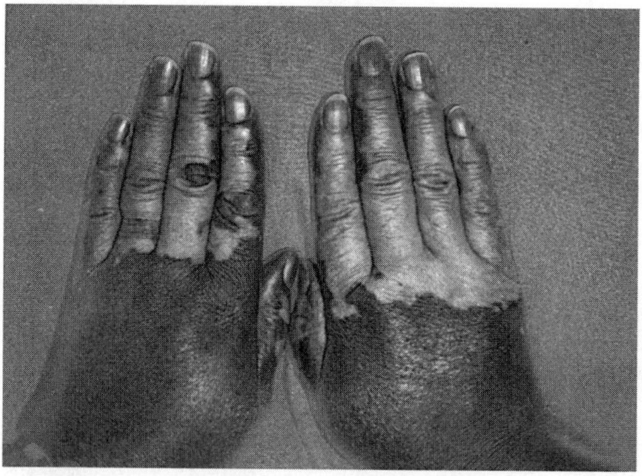

■ **Figure 29.33** Chemical (phenolic) depigmentation of hands simulating vitiligo. (From Callen JP, et al: Color Atlas of Dermatology. Philadelphia, WB Saunders Co, 1993.)

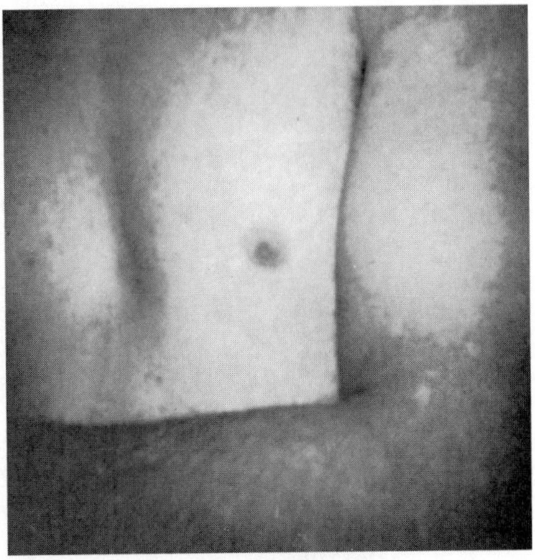

■ **Figure 29.34** Tinea versicolor of chest and arm showing varying stages of pigmentation and depigmentation. (From Welton W: Dermatology and syphilology. *In* Rakel RE, Conn HF [Eds]: Family Practice, 2nd ed. Philadelphia, WB Saunders Co, 1978.)

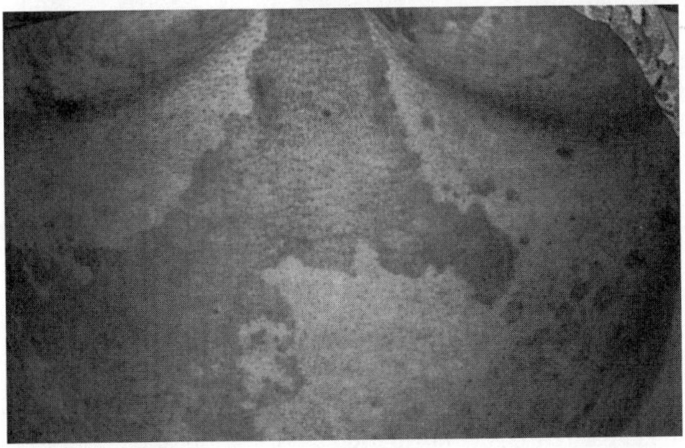

■ **Figure 29.35** Tinea versicolor of trunk. (From Callen JP, et al: Color Atlas of Dermatology. Philadelphia, WB Saunders Co, 1993.)

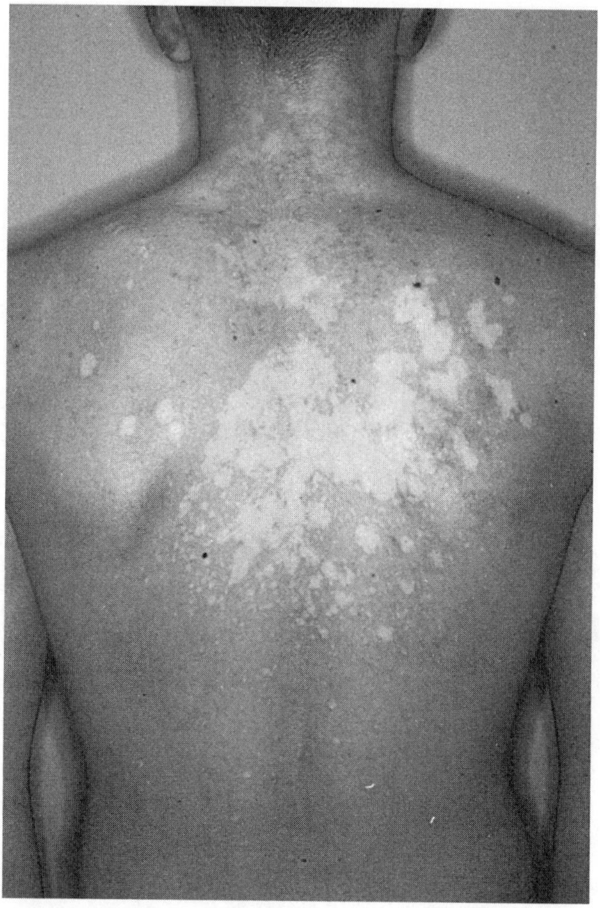

■ **Figure 29.36** Tinea versicolor showing depigmentation. (From Callen JP, et al: Color Atlas of Dermatology. Philadelphia, WB Saunders Co, 1993.)

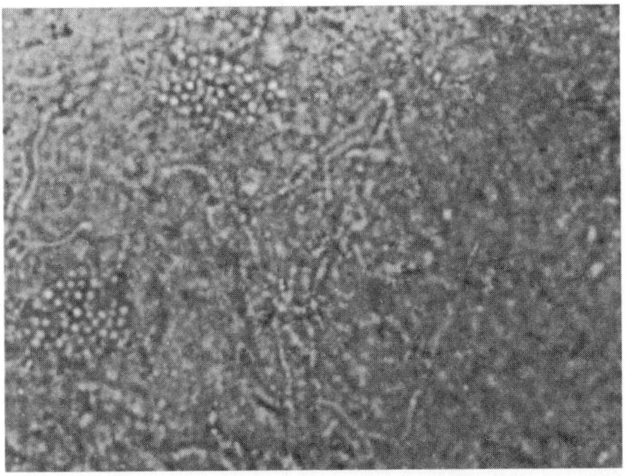

■ **Figure 29.37** Short hyphae and spores of *Malassezia furfur* seen in tinea versicolor (KOH preparation, ×400). (From Lamberg SI: Common problems of the skin. *In* Barker LR, Burton JR, Zieve PD [Eds]: Principles of Ambulatory Medicine. Baltimore, Williams & Wilkins, 1982.)

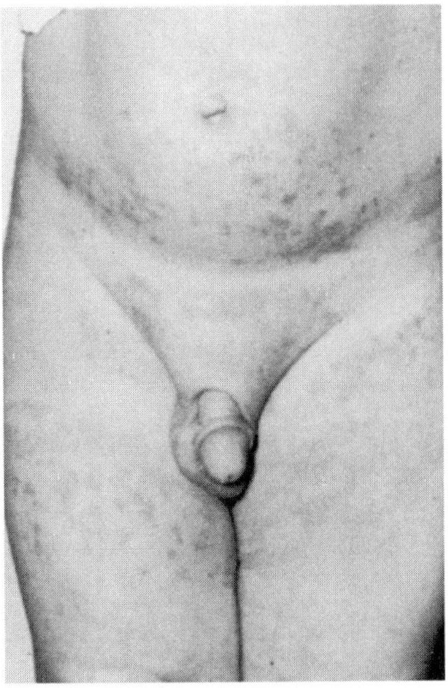

■ **Figure 29.38** Contact dermatitis caused by laundry detergent. Note sparing of the folds. (From Jacob AH: Eruptions in the diaper area. Pediatr Clin North Am 25:209, 1978.)

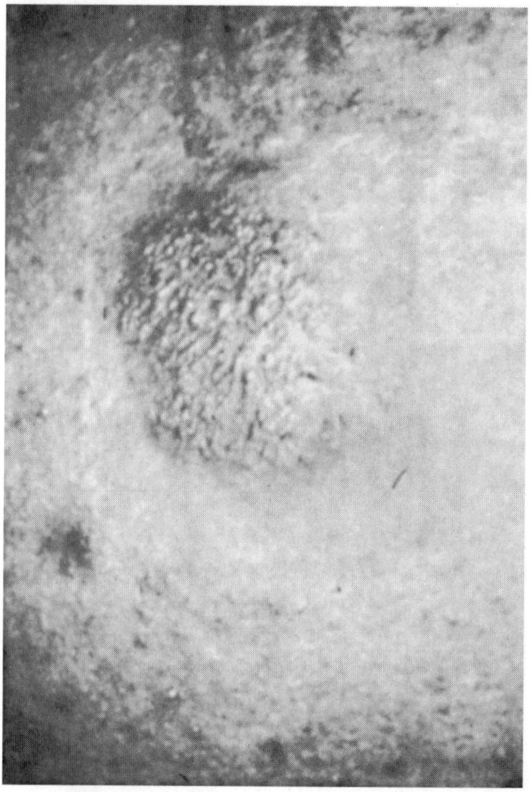

■ **Figure 29.39** Microvesicles and dermal edema in acute contact dermatitis. (From Basler RS: Contact dermatitis. Neb Med J 65:296–299, 1980.)

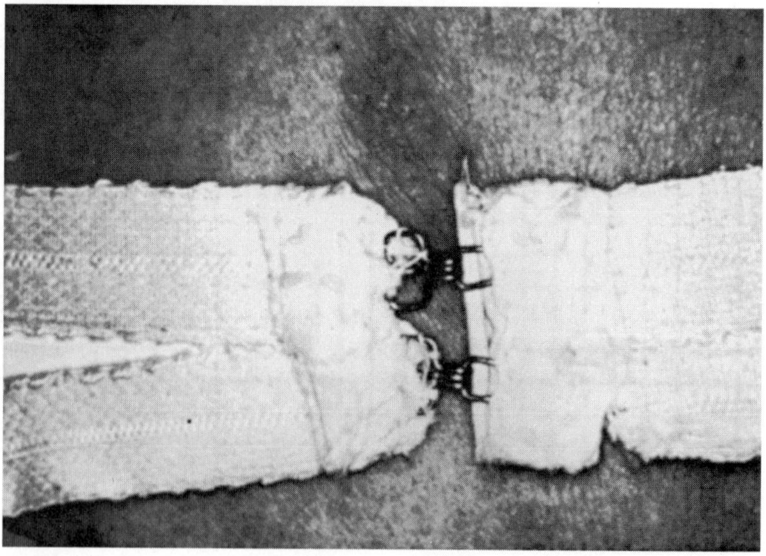

■ **Figure 29.40** Chronic contact dermatitis. (From Basler RS: Contact dermatitis. Nebr Med J 65:296–299, 1980.)

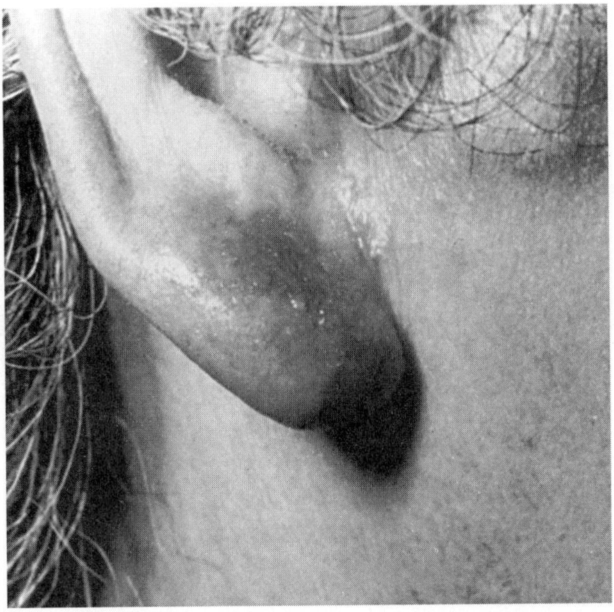

■ **Figure 29.41** Nickel dermatitis of ear lobe from earring. (From Arnold HL, Odom RB, James WB: Andrews' Diseases of the Skin, 8th ed. Philadelphia, WB Saunders Co, 1990.)

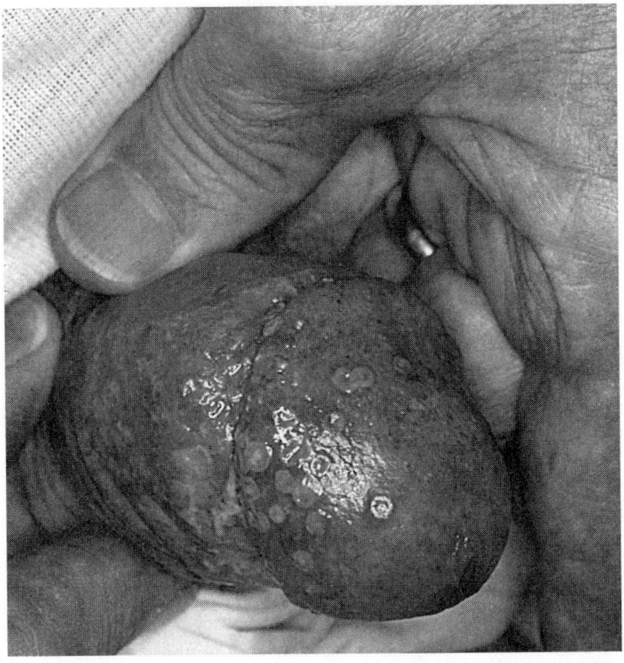

■ **Figure 29.42** Primary herpes progenitalis. (From Callen JP, et al: Color Atlas of Dermatology. Philadelphia, WB Saunders Co, 1993.)

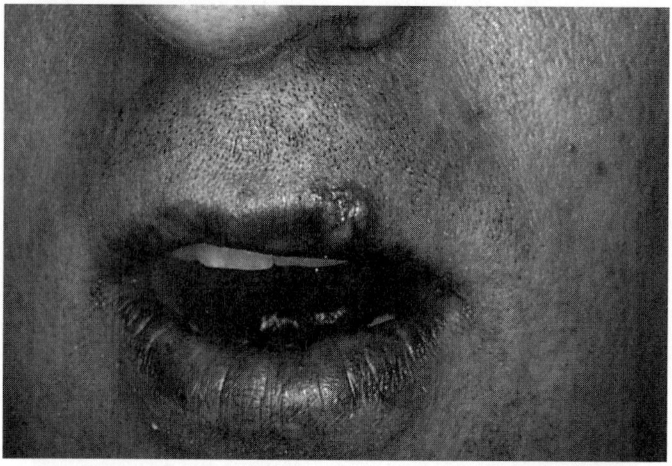

■ **Figure 29.43** Herpes simplex. (From Callen JP, et al: Color Atlas of Dermatology. Philadelphia, WB Saunders Co, 1993.)

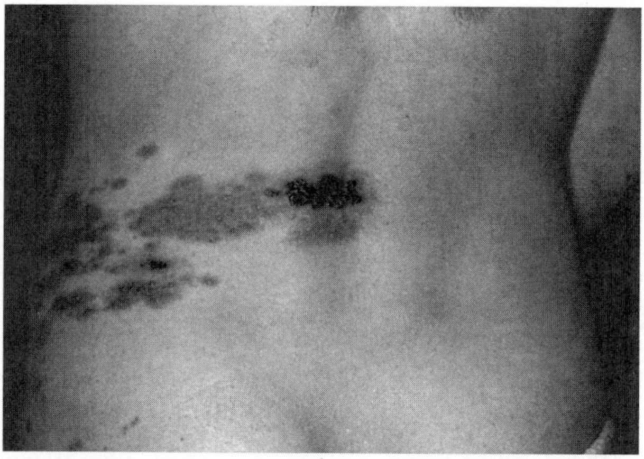

■ **Figure 29.44** Herpes zoster with dermatomal distribution. (From Callen JP, et al: Color Atlas of Dermatology. Philadelphia, WB Saunders Co, 1993.)

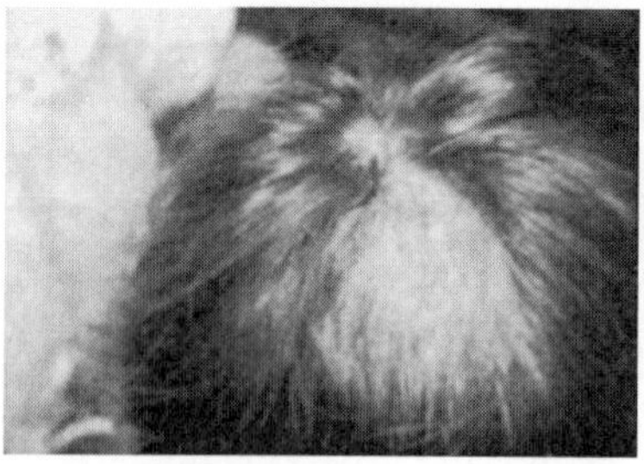

■ **Figure 29.45** Ringworm of scalp *(Trichophyton tonsurans)*. (From Vickers HR: Problems of dermatological diagnosis. Br J Clin Pract 32:159-166, 1978.)

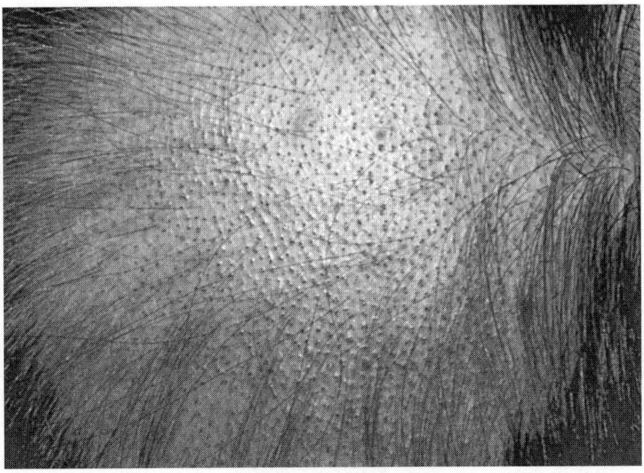

■ **Figure 29.46** Tinea capitis from *Trichophyton tonsurans* ("black dot" ringworm). (From Callen JP, et al: Color Atlas of Dermatology. Philadelphia, WB Saunders Co, 1993.)

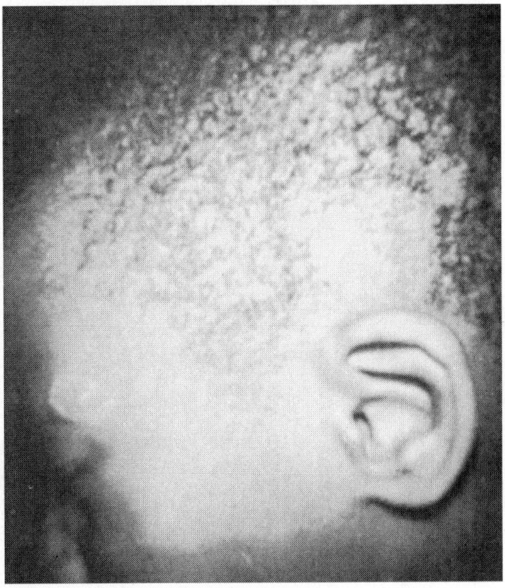

■ **Figure 29.47** Tinea capitis: round areas of broken hairs and some scale. (From Welton W: Dermatology and syphilology. *In* Rakel RE, Conn HF [Eds]: Family Practice, 2nd ed. Philadelphia, WB Saunders Co, 1978.)

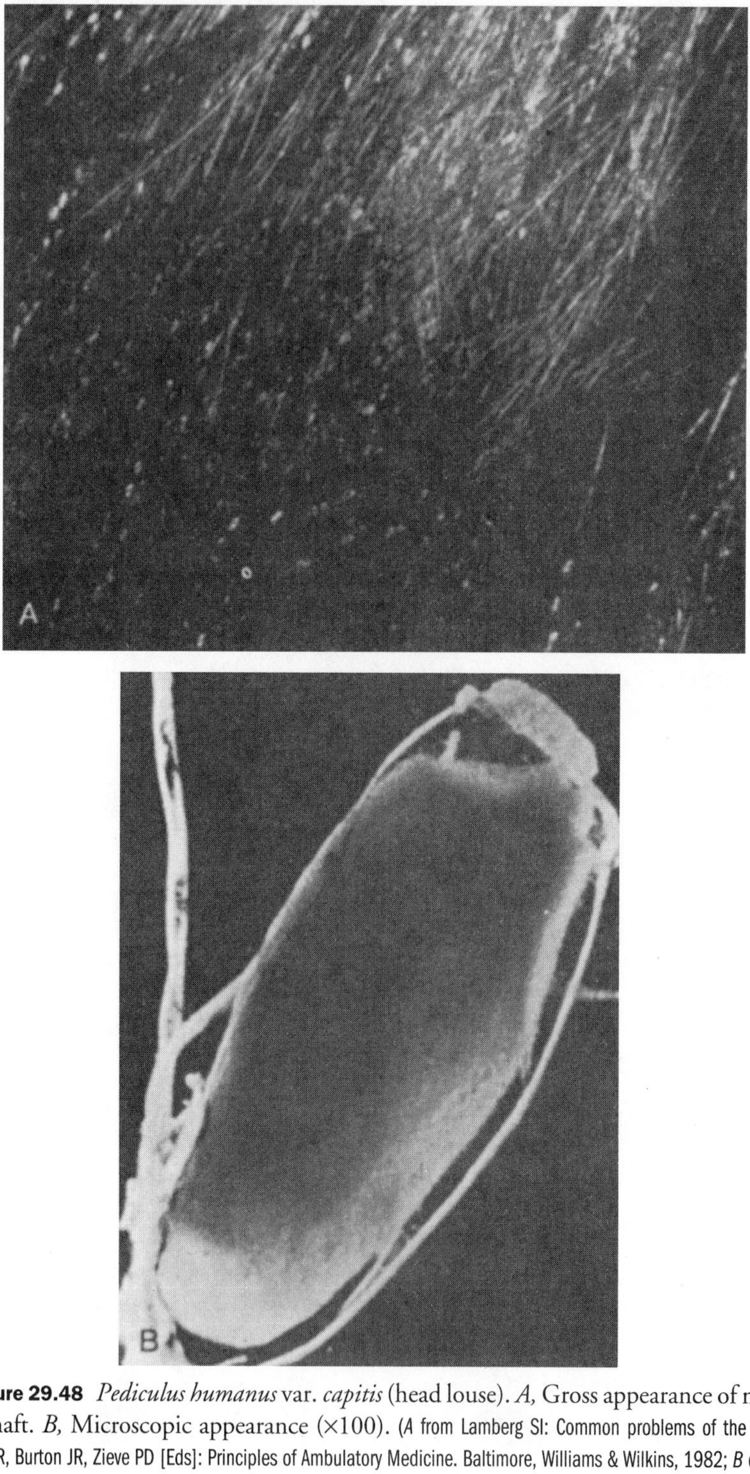

■ **Figure 29.48** *Pediculus humanus* var. *capitis* (head louse). *A,* Gross appearance of nits on hair shaft. *B,* Microscopic appearance (×100). (*A* from Lamberg SI: Common problems of the skin. *In* Barker LR, Burton JR, Zieve PD [Eds]: Principles of Ambulatory Medicine. Baltimore, Williams & Wilkins, 1982; *B* courtesy of Reed & Carnrick, Kenilworth, NJ.)

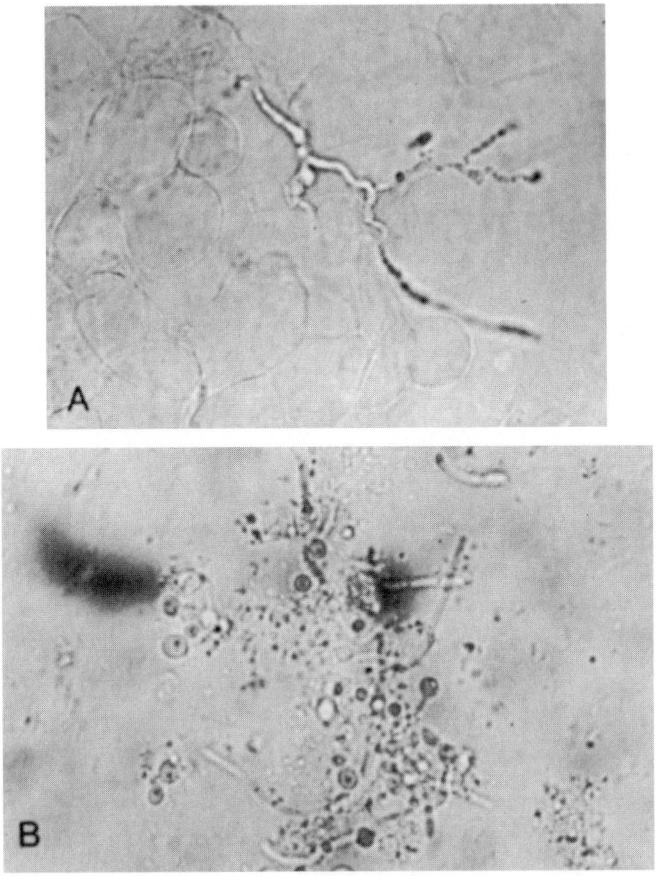

■ **Figure 29.49** *A,* Hyphae of tinea (KOH preparation, ×400). *B,* Pseudohyphae of *Candida* (KOH preparation, ×400). (*A* from Lamberg SI: Common problems of the skin. *In* Barker LR, Burton JR, Zieve PD [Eds]: Principles of Ambulatory Medicine. Baltimore, Williams & Wilkins, 1982; *B* courtesy of William G. Merz, PhD.)

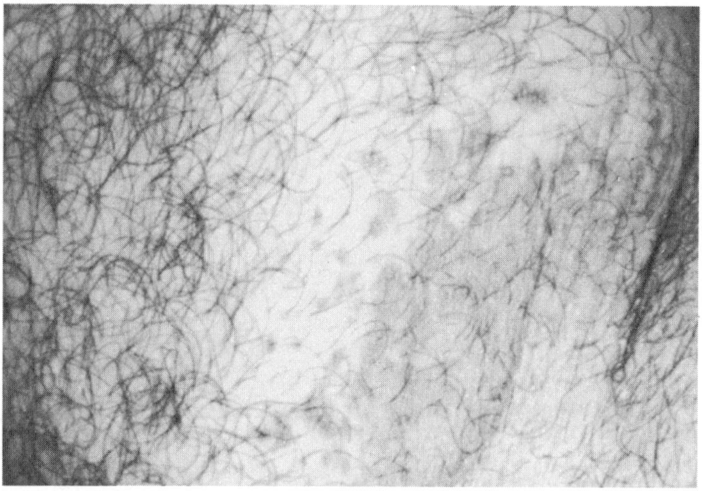

■ **Figure 29.50** Candidiasis (moniliasis). Groin with intense erythema and satellite papules and pustules. Requires blood sugar determination in adult. (From Gilbert R, Rosenthal D: Dermatology. *In* Rakel RE [Ed]: Textbook of Family Practice, 3rd ed. Philadelphia, WB Saunders Co, 1984.)

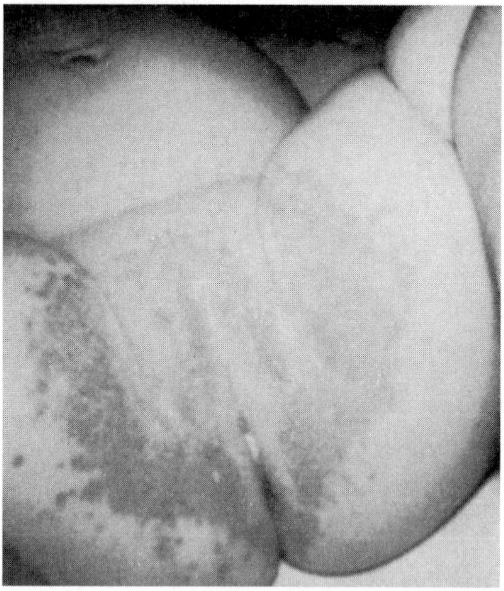

■ **Figure 29.51** Candidiasis resembling diaper rash, but papules and pustules suggest *Candida* infection. (From Welton W: Dermatology and syphilology. *In* Rakel RE, Conn HF [Eds]: Family Practice, 2nd ed. Philadelphia, WB Saunders Co, 1978.)

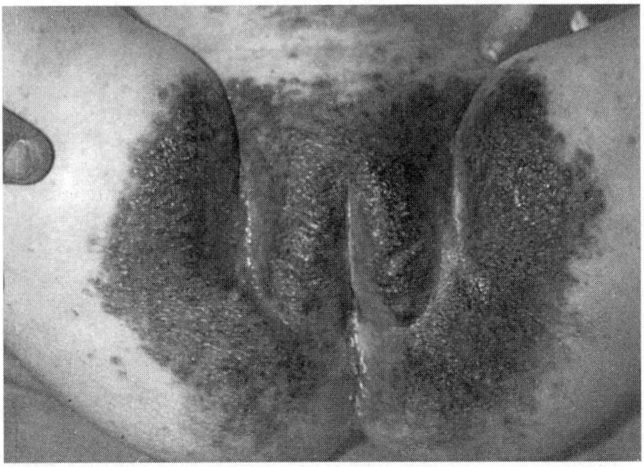

■ **Figure 29.52** Diaper rash. (From Callen JP, et al: Color Atlas of Dermatology. Philadelphia, WB Saunders Co, 1993.)

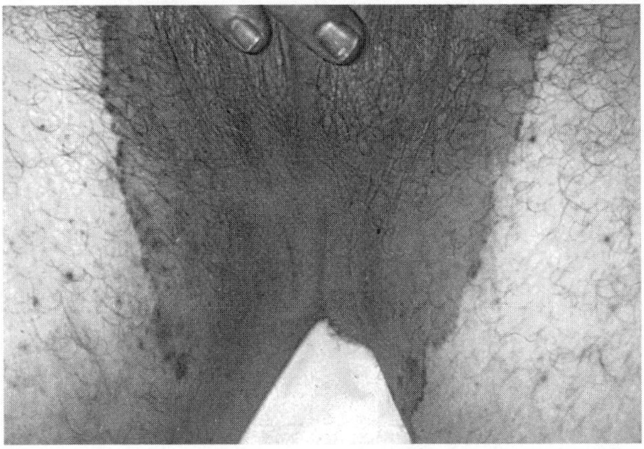

■ **Figure 29.53** Tinea cruris. (From Callen JP, et al: Color Atlas of Dermatology. Philadelphia, WB Saunders Co, 1993.)

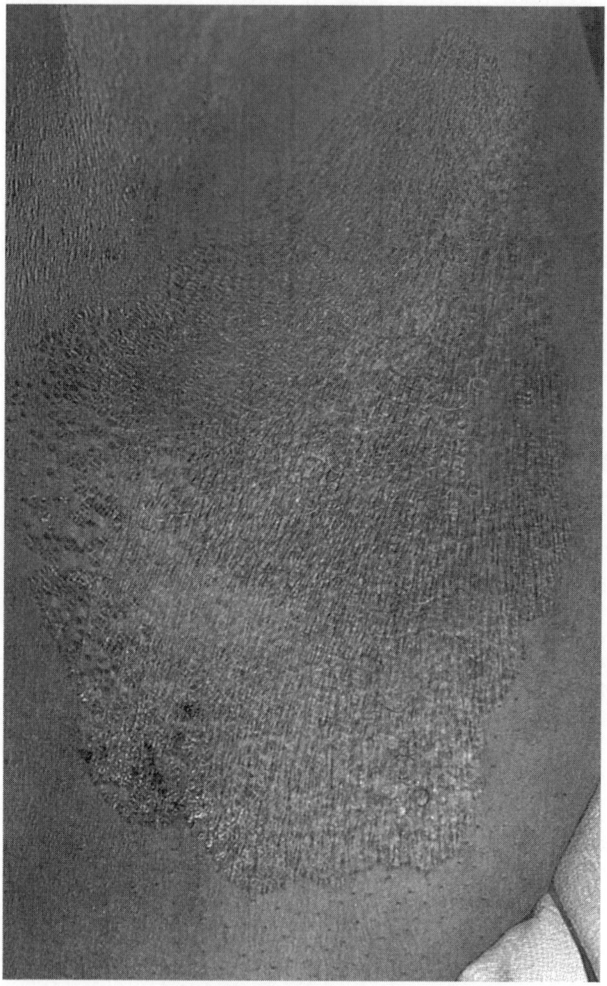

■ **Figure 29.54** Erythrasma. (From Callen JP, et al: Color Atlas of Dermatology. Philadelphia, WB Saunders Co, 1993.)

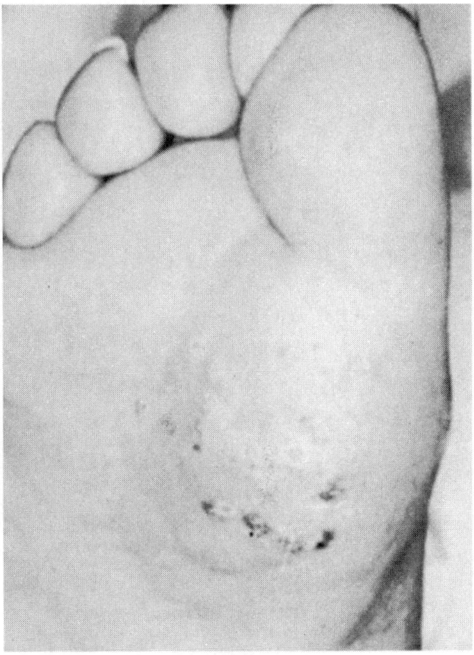

■ **Figure 29.55** Tinea pedis, macerated acute type. (From Welton W: Dermatology and syphilology. *In* Rakel RE, Conn HF [Eds]: Family Practice, 2nd ed. Philadelphia, WB Saunders Co, 1978.)

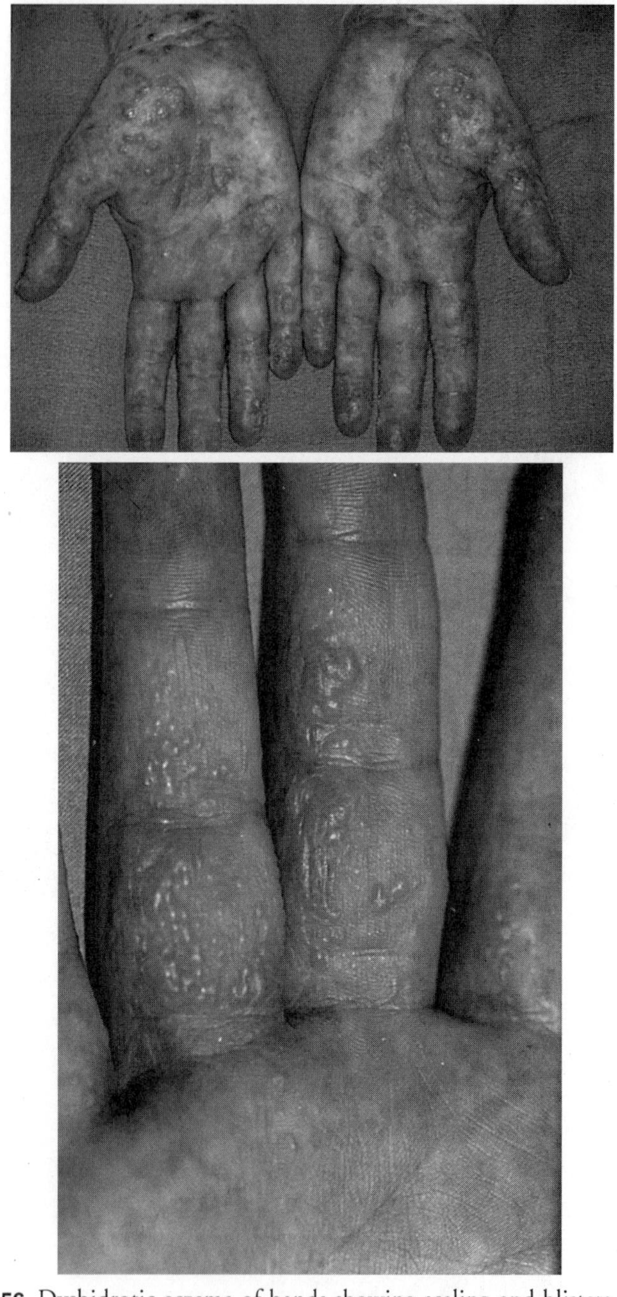

■ **Figure 29.56** Dyshidrotic eczema of hands showing scaling and blisters. (From Callen JP, et al: Color Atlas of Dermatology. Philadelphia, WB Saunders Co, 1993.)

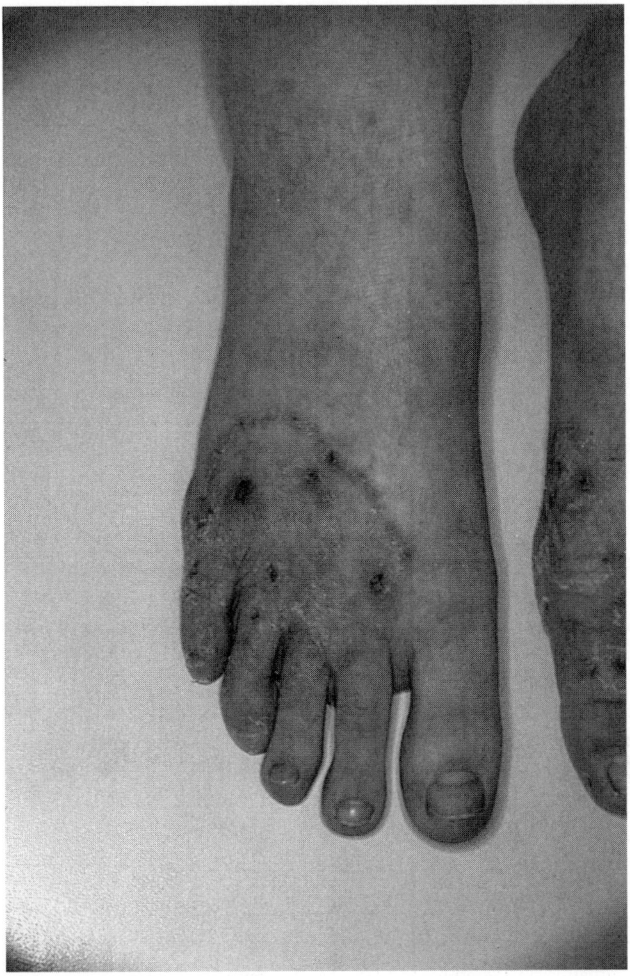

■ **Figure 29.57** Tinea pedis showing scaling, vesicles, and involvement between toes and on dorsum of foot. (From Callen JP, et al: Color Atlas of Dermatology. Philadelphia, WB Saunders Co, 1993.)

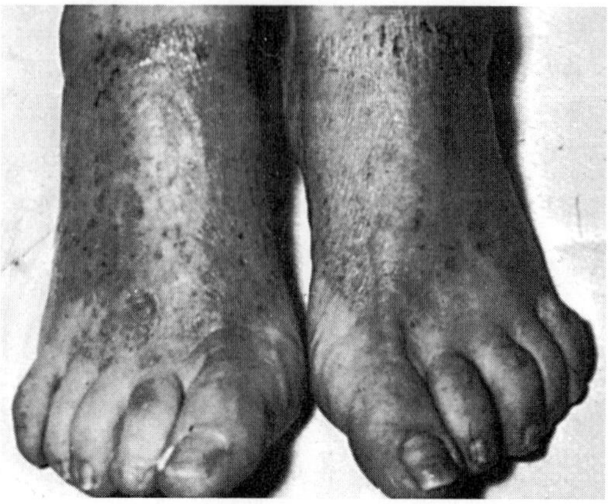

■ **Figure 29.58** Shoe dermatitis from chrome used in tanning process. (From Arnold HL, Odom RB, James WB: Andrews' Diseases of the Skin, 8th ed. Philadelphia, WB Saunders Co, 1990.)

Selected References

Arnold HL, Odom RB, James WB: Andrews' Diseases of the skin, 8th ed. Philadelphia, WB Saunders Co, 1990.

August PJ: Iatrogenic skin disease. Practitioner 224:471–478, 1980.

Bart BJ: Annular skin eruptions: not every ring on the skin is ringworm. Postgrad Med 96:37–50, 1994.

Beacham BE: Common dermatoses in the elderly. Am Fam Phys 47:1445–1450, 1993.

Ben-Amitai D, Ashkenazi S: Common bacterial skin infections in childhood. Pediatr Ann 22:225–233, 1993.

Berger TG, Obuch ML, Goldschmidt RH: Dermatologic manifestations of HIV infection. Am Fam Physician 41:1729–1743, 1990.

Callen JP, et al: Color Atlas of Dermatology. Philadelphia, WB Saunders Co, 1993.

Conklin RJ: Common cutaneous disorders in athletes. Sports Med 9:100–119, 1990.

Davidson CL: Occupational contact dermatitis of the upper extremity. Occup Med State Art Rev 9:59–74, 1994.

Feigold DS, Bachta M: Common skin diseases seen by the internist. DM 25(8):1–39, 1979.

Kirsner RS, Federman DG: Cutaneous clues to systemic disease: telltale signs enable early diagnosis. Postgrad Med 101:137–150, 1997.

Lamberg SI: Common problems of the skin. *In* Barker LR, Burton JR, Zieve PD (Eds): Principles of Ambulatory Medicine. Baltimore, Williams & Wilkins, 1982.

Martin DH, Mroczkowski TF: Dermatologic manifestations of sexually transmitted diseases other than HIV. Infect Dis Clin North Am 8:533–582, 1994.

McLauria CI: Unusual patterns of common dermatoses in blacks. Cutis 32(4):352–355, 358–360, 1983.

Prawer SE: Occupational dermatoses in primary care: a guide to recognition. Consultant 38:423–444, 1998.

Sahl WJ, Mathewson RJ: Common facial skin lesions in children. Quintessene Int 24:475–481, 1993.

Schlossberg D: Fever and rash. Infect Dis Clin North Am 10:101–110, 1996.

Scott DA: Disorders of the hair and scalp in blacks. Dermatol Clin 6:387–395, 1988.

Stevenson CJ: Occupational skin disease. Postgrad Med J 65:374–386, 1989.

Symposium on Pediatric Dermatology. Pediatr Clin North Am 25(2):189–389, 1978.

Vickers HR: Problems of dermatological diagnoses. Br J Clin Pract 32:159–166, 1978.

White JE: Skin cancer. Practitioner 224:501–503, 1980.

CHAPTER 30

Sore Throat

This chapter defines sore throat as pain in the throat at rest that often worsens with swallowing. The most common causes of sore throat without pharyngeal ulcers include *viral pharyngitis, bacterial pharyngitis* and *tonsillitis, allergic pharyngitis, pharyngitis secondary to sinusitis,* and *infectious mononucleosis.* Common causes of sore throat with pharyngeal ulceration include *herpangina, herpes simplex, fusospirochetal infection, candidiasis, herpes zoster,* and *chickenpox* (varicella). The less common primary and secondary syphilitic ulcerations are usually not painful.

Pharyngitis is a vexing problem because it is extremely prevalent and because it is difficult to establish a precise diagnosis. The annual cost of laboratory tests and medications ordered for patients with sore throats is about $300 million. Despite streptococcal and viral pharyngitis (including infectious mononucleosis) being the most common causes of sore throat, studies have shown that even with careful diagnostic techniques, a precise cause can be determined in only about 50% of patients.

Prompt diagnosis and treatment of *streptococcal pharyngitis* are essential to reducing its spread to close contacts; treatment also prevents acute rheumatic fever. Prompt antibiotic therapy also shortens the clinical course and decreases morbidity. Rapid screening tests for streptococcal antigens are useful in selected cases. For a precise diagnosis of streptococcal pharyngitis, there must be a positive culture for group A streptococci and a fourfold rise in the antistreptolysin O (ASO) titer. The carrier state exists with a positive culture without antibody response. According to one large study in which these criteria were used, most patients were found to be carriers. Because it does not rise until 1 to 6 months after an acute streptococcal infection, the ASO titer in the acute serum is of no value in the diagnosis of a current infection. This does not mean that throat cultures are of no value, but it does reinforce the need for sound clinical judgment in the diagnosis and treatment of patients with sore throats (Table 30–1).

Nature of Patient

Streptococcal pharyngitis is most prevalent in patients under age 25 years, particularly those between ages 5 and 15. Likewise, *herpangina, herpes simplex, fusospirochetal infections,* and *candidiasis* are more common in children. As a cause of pharyngitis, *infectious mononucleosis* is most prevalent in adolescents and young adults. It does occur, although less frequently, in patients over age 60. It is particularly notable that 70 percent of elderly patients with infectious mononucleosis do not develop pharyngitis, adenopathy, or splenomegaly.

TABLE 30.1 Probabilities of Streptococcal Isolation in Four Series with Different Clinical Predictors*

	PRESENT SERIES (n = 693) (%)	WALSH et al (n = 418) (%)	CRAWFORD et al (n = 472) (%)	CENTOR et al (n = 234) (%)
Tonsillar exudate	25.4	19.9	18.5	18.9
Anterior cervical adenopathy	13.8	12.6	15.3	16.5
Temperature >100°F	22.2	14.3	NR†	NR
Temperature >101°F	26.1	23.9	25.0	19.5
History of recent exposure to streptococcus	11.1	18.8	20.0	NR
No cough	15.0	14.8	14.7	19.3
No rhinorrhea	14.8	13.4	NR	11.9
"High risk" according to Walsh algorithm‡	26.4	19.0	22.7	NR

*Probabilities in all series adjusted to an assumed prevalence rate of 10%, using Bayes' theorem.

†NR = not reported.

‡"High-risk" patients are those with enlarged or tender cervical nodes *and* pharyngeal exudate *or* history of recent exposure to someone with diagnosed streptococcal infection.

From Komaroff A, et al: The prediction of streptococcal pharyngitis in adults. J Gen Intern Med 1:1–7, 1986.

Chlamydia trachomatis and *Neisseria gonorrhoeae* presenting with oropharyngeal symptoms are becoming more common as causes of pharyngitis but are often unrecognized. *Neisseria* has been cultured from the throat in 10% of patients with anogenital gonorrhea. Of those with positive cultures, most do not have pharyngeal symptoms. It is more common in people who engage in orogenital sex. Male homosexuals have a higher incidence of oropharyngeal gonorrheal infections than other groups.

Common ulcerative and vesicular pharyngeal lesions include *recurrent aphthous stomatitis, herpes zoster, herpes simplex, fusospirochetal infections,* and *candidiasis* (particularly if the patient is immunosuppressed or taking antibiotics; Table 30–2). Although rare, primary and secondary syphilitic lesions occasionally are seen in adults. They should be suspected if the lesion is not painful and the usual accompanying symptoms of upper respiratory infection (URI) are absent.

Nature of Symptoms

Marked pain in the throat (frequently associated with dysphagia), an oral temperature exceeding 100° to 101°F (37.7° to 38.3°C), and a rapid onset of symptoms suggest the probability of a *streptococcal* or *viral pharyngitis.* A low-grade temperature, gradual onset of pharyngeal symptoms, and systemic symptoms that are more persistent suggest *infectious mononucleosis.* In reality, it is difficult for the physician to determine the cause of pharyngitis on the basis of the nature of the chief complaint; predisposing factors and physical examination are frequently more useful indicators.

Associated Symptoms

Headache, nausea, vomiting, and abdominal pain may occur, especially in children.

Predisposing Factors

Herpangina, herpes simplex, and *candidiasis* are most common in immunosuppressed patients. Candidiasis also is most prevalent in diabetic patients and in those taking broad-spectrum antibiotics. Herpangina is most common in children and shows a strong seasonal propensity for summer and autumn, whereas *streptococcal pharyngitis* is most prevalent in the winter and early spring.

Physical Findings

Marked erythema and swelling of the throat (often associated with an exudative pharyngitis or tonsillitis), temperature greater than 101°F, tachycardia, and occurrence between September and April all strongly indicate *streptococcal pharyngitis.* Likewise, a history of streptococcal exposure within the family during the

TABLE 30.2 Common Infections Causing Oropharyngeal Ulceration

DISEASE	LOCATION	VESICULATION	PAIN	SIZE OF LESION (mm)	DIAGNOSTIC CRITERIA
Local herpangina	Tonsils, pillars, uvula	Yes	Yes	1–2	Characteristic clinical presentation, coxsackievirus in culture of lesion exudate, positive serologic test
Herpes simplex	Lips, gingivae, buccal mucosa, tongue	Yes	Yes	1–2	Multinuclear giant cells with ballooning degeneration in Tzanck smear of ulcer-crater exudate
Fusospirochetal infection	Gingivae, may spread diffusely	No	Yes	2–30	Characteristic legions, foul breath, anaerobic forms and spirochetes in smear of lesion exudate
Candidiasis	All parts of oropharynx	No	Yes	3–10	*Candida albicans* in Gram-stained smear and culture of scrapings
Primary syphilis	Lips, tonsils, tongue	No	No	5–15	Indurated "heaped-up" lesion, positive serologic test (periodic evaluation necessary)
Herpes zoster	Unilateral involvement of tongue, lip, buccal mucosa	Yes	Yes	2–4	Unilateral involvement, painful prodromes, giant cells in Tzanck smear of lesion exudate
Systemic hand-foot-and-mouth disease	All parts of oropharynx	Yes	Yes	1–10	Exanthem on hands and feet, coxsackievirus in culture of lesion exudate, positive serologic test
Varicella	All parts of oropharynx	Yes	No	2–4	Characteristic exanthem
Secondary syphilis	Symmetric involvement of all parts of mouth and oropharynx	No	No	2–10	Other evidence of secondary syphilis, positive serologic test, spirochetes visible on darkfield microscopy

From Brown RB, Clinton D: Vesicular and ulcerative infections of the mouth and oropharynx. Postgrad Med 67(2):107–116, 1980.

past week, prior history of acute rheumatic fever, diabetes, tender anterior cervical nodes, or a scarlatiniform rash increases the likelihood that streptococcal pharyngitis is the correct diagnosis. Streptococcal pharyngitis is rare after age 30 and is most common between ages 5 and 15.

Although many authors stress an association between tonsillopharyngeal exudate and streptococcal pharyngitis, only 50% of the patients with proven streptococcal pharyngitis have an exudate, and only 50% of all patients with a pharyngeal exudate have streptococcal pharyngitis. A nonadherent pharyngeal exudate is a sensitive but nonspecific indicator of streptococcal pharyngitis because an exudate is found in many other bacterial and viral infections. Despite this, many physicians presume a streptococcal cause if a tonsillar exudate is present and if one or more of the following signs also are demonstrated: temperature greater than 101°F, tender anterior cervical nodes, or duration of sore throat for more than 6 days, particularly with no cough (see Table 30–1). A cough militates against a strep infection.

Studies have shown that when the patient is 15 years or older, the presence of all four criteria (tonsillar exudate, tender anterior cervical adenopathy, temperature greater than 101°F, absence of cough) suggests a group A beta-hemolytic streptococcal (GABHS) infection with a probability of 50% to 60%.

The absence of fever or the presence of conjunctivitis, cough, hoarseness, coryza, anterior stomatitis, ulcerative oral lesions, viral exanthem, and diarrhea mitigates against a diagnosis of a streptococcal infection.

Viral pharyngitis is the most common cause of pharyngitis and, unlike streptococcal pharyngitis, has no particular distribution with regard to age or time of year, although it is slightly more frequent in the winter months. Patients with viral pharyngitis usually have less severe pharyngeal symptoms and more severe systemic symptoms. These patients are less likely to have an exudate or marked erythema of the pharynx. The pharynx is usually slightly injected but also may appear swollen, boggy, or pale. No exudate or follicular tonsillitis is usually present, but systemic symptoms (malaise, fever, cough, headache, fatigue) are more prominent than with streptococcal pharyngitis.

Patients with the pharyngitis of *infectious mononucleosis* may present with an exudate, although most do not. The enanthem of infectious mononucleosis (palatine petechiae) is almost diagnostic. The petechiae resemble small, red, raised grains of sand surrounded by 0.5-mm pale bases. The pharyngitis of infectious mononucleosis is almost invariably (90% of cases) accompanied by posterior cervical adenopathy. Some authors are reluctant to diagnose infectious mononucleosis in the absence of posterior cervical adenopathy.

Epiglottitis, which may occur in children but is rare in adults, is usually caused by a *Haemophilus* infection. When epiglottitis is suspected, appropriate cultures should be performed, and antibiotics should be administered promptly. *Gingivitis* is most often seen in patients with poor oral hygiene. In some cases, it can involve the entire oropharynx. The most common presentation of *ulcerative gingivitis (trench mouth)* is an acute onset of painful bloody gums, foul breath, and a grayish exudate covering the interdental papillae. Ulcerative gingivitis is a *fusospirochetal infection* and responds well to improved oral hygiene and appropriate antibiotics. Pharyngeal involvement with fusospirochetal organisms *(Vincent's angina)* may occur primarily or secondarily to a spread of fusospirochetal infection from anterior sites. In patients with this infection, sore throat is the most common complaint, and necrotic, gray, ulcerative lesions may develop about the tonsillar pillars. If the "pseudomembrane" is removed, bleeding of the undersurface usually occurs. Although in most cases involvement is initially unilateral, it often spreads and becomes bilateral.

Patients who have frequent sore throats without evidence of pharyngitis or fever may have an *allergic pharyngitis.* This is often associated with an intermittent postnasal drip that leads to minor irritation and inflammation of the posterior pharynx. Some patients with recurrent or chronic low-grade *sinusitis* may present with a sore throat induced by a postnasal drip from the affected sinuses. **When a patient complains of a sore throat that becomes worse with swallowing, and when the physical examination of the oropharynx is negative, the physician should suspect thyroiditis and palpate the thyroid for swelling or pain on palpation.** This is a common way by which the uncommon illness of thyroiditis presents.

Retropharyngeal abscess is most common in infants and young children, but it does occur infrequently in adults. The patient may have an unexplained fever, URI, loss of appetite, difficulty in swallowing, and stridor. The last sign is particularly common in children. Retropharyngeal abscess is a medical emergency and should be evaluated promptly. The study of choice is a computed tomography (CT) scan. Some investigators believe that earlier treatment with antibiotics reduces the incidence of this complication and the need for surgical intervention.

Sore throat may be the presenting complaint in children with a *peritonsillar abscess.* This complication of tonsillitis is more common in older children and adolescents. Dysphagia, odynophagia, and trismus may be associated, but the tonsil may be without significant inflammation or exudate. The tonsil is usually displaced medially.

The presence of oropharyngeal ulcerations, with or without vesiculation, is often helpful in differential diagnosis (see Table 30–2). In patients with *herpangina,* usually children, the painful ulcerations measure 1 to 2 mm and occur on the tonsils, pillars, and the uvula. The pharyngeal ulcers (2 to 30 mm) due to *fusospirochetal infections* are usually present on the gingivae, but they may spread diffusely throughout the oropharynx. These lesions are usually painful, but there is no associated vesiculation. In adults and children with *herpes simplex,* the painful ulcers measure 1 to 2 mm and can occur on the lips, gingivae, buccal mucosa, or rarely the tongue. The painful ulcerations of *herpes zoster* usually are unilateral and involve the tongue, lip, or buccal mucosa. These lesions are usually 2 to 4 mm and associated with vesiculation. In infants and adults with *candidiasis,* the ulcerations measure 3 to 11 mm and can involve any part of the oropharynx. Vesiculation does not occur with candidiasis.

Diagnostic Studies

Tests that are often helpful in the differential diagnosis of sore throat are a complete blood count (CBC) with differential, throat cultures, Gram staining, monospot test, and ASO titers. With the advent of rapid antigen detection tests (RADTs) for streptococcal antigens, the most recent recommendation is treatment if a double-swab RADT is positive. If it is negative, a throat culture should be performed and treatment begun if the culture is positive. One approach recommends culture if any one of the following is present: age less than 25 years, definite streptococcal exposure during the previous week, history of acute rheumatic fever, diabetes, known epidemic of streptococcal pharyngitis, oral temperature greater than 99.5°F, exudate, tender anterior cervical nodes, or scarlatiniform rash.

Difficulty with follow-up, a known epidemic of nephritogenic streptococcal infections, or presence of a scarlatiniform rash is an indication for both throat culture and treatment with penicillin. In addition, if there is a history of rheumatic fever or if diabetes is present, treatment with penicillin is indicated despite the clinical picture. **A patient with a temperature greater than 101°F, tonsillar exudate, tender anterior cervical nodes, and no cough probably has a streptococcal pharyngitis, and immediate treatment is justified.** A CBC with a lymphocytosis of greater than 50% or an absolute lymphocytosis of greater than 4500 lymphocytes per mm^3 with more than 10% atypical lymphocytes suggests *infectious mononucleosis.* This is confirmed by a positive monospot test. **Virtually no false-negative monospot tests exist, although some studies have shown 10% false-positive results.** Most of these characteristic hematologic and serologic abnormalities occur within 1 week from onset of symptoms in 80% of patients.

Less Common Diagnostic Considerations

Patients with *thyroiditis* may present with sore throat or dysphagia or both. In a patient complaining of a sore throat whose throat examination is negative, the thyroid gland should be palpated. If it is tender, thyroiditis should be suspected. Patients with *hypothyroidism* may complain of sore throat or hoarseness, regardless of whether a goiter is present. Some patients with seasonal *allergy* present with sore throat. Most patients have minimal pharyngeal swelling. Occasionally, a postnasal drip is seen, and other allergic symptoms usually can be elicited as well.

Patients who have swallowed a coarse *foreign body* such as a bone, rough vegetable, or piece of meat may complain of sore throat with or without dysphagia, even if they have successfully swallowed the object. If this complaint persists or is severe, the possibility that a foreign body is lodged in the posterior pharynx or proximal esophagus should be considered.

Patients with *leukemia, agranulocytosis,* or *diphtheria* may also present with sore throat.

Differential Diagnosis of Sore Throat

TYPE OF PHARYNGITIS	NATURE OF PATIENT	NATURE OF SYMPTOMS	PREDISPOSING FACTORS	PHYSICAL FINDINGS	DIAGNOSTIC STUDIES
Without pharyngeal ulcers					
Viral	All ages	Pain in throat Rapid onset Systemic symptoms		Exudate less likely than with streptococcal infections	
Infectious mononucleosis	Adolescents and young adults Uncommon in elderly	Gradual onset		Low-grade temperature Occasional exudate Enanthem Posterior cervical adenopathy Hepatosplenomegaly	Monospot test
Streptococcal pharyngitis	Patients younger than age 25, especially ages 6–12	Pain in throat Rapid onset Few systemic symptoms	Fall and winter Streptococcal infection in family Diabetes	Marked erythema and throat swelling Temperature >101°F Tender anterior cervical nodes Scarlatiniform rash Tonsillar exudate more likely than with viral infection	Culture Rapid streptococcal antigen screening Increased ASO titer
Gonococcal pharyngitis	Most common in male homosexuals and those with anogenital gonorrhea	Often no symptoms	Orogenital sex		Culture

Without pharyngeal ulcers *Continued*					
Sinusitis with postnasal drip	Adults	Mild throat soreness Symptoms often worse with recumbency		Evidence of sinusitis Postnasal drip	Sinus radiographs
Allergic pharyngitis			Seasonal allergies	No fever Intermittent postnasal drip Swollen pharynx with minimal injection	Eosinophils in nasal secretions
With pharyngeal ulcers					
Herpangina	More common in children	Painful ulcers on tonsils, pillars, or uvula	Immunosuppression Summer and autumn	Vesicles 1–2-mm ulcers	Serologic tests
Fusospirochetal infection (Vincent's angina)	Children and those with poor oral hygiene	Painful ulcers Bleeding gums Foul breath		No vesicles Ulcerative gingivitis Gray necrotic ulcers 2–30-mm ulcers Pseudomembrane	Gram stain: spirochetes
Candidiasis	Children Immunosuppressed patients Those taking antibiotics		Immunosuppression Antibiotics	3–11-mm ulcers No vesicles	KOH smear: *Candida* Culture
Herpes simplex	Most common in children	Not usually a cause of sore throat	Immunosuppression	1–2-mm painful ulcers Vesicles present on lips, gingivae, buccal mucosa, or tongue	Tzanck smear shows multinucleated giant cells

Selected References

Balciunos BA, Overholser CD: Diagnosis and management of common oral lesions. Am Fam Physician 35:206–220, 1987.

Bisno AL, et al: Diagnosis and management of group A streptococcal pharyngitis: a practice guideline. Clin Infect Dis 25:574–583, 1997.

Brown RB, Clinton D: Vesicular and ulcerative infections of the mouth and oropharynx. Postgrad Med 67(2):107–116, 1980.

Komaroff AL: A management strategy for sore throat. JAMA 239:1429–1432, 1978.

Komaroff AL, et al: The prediction of streptococcal pharyngitis in adults. J Gen Intern Med 1:1–7, 1986.

McIsaac WJ, et al: Reconsidering sore throats. Part 2. Alternative approach and practical office tool. Can Fam Physician 43:495–500, 1997.

Middleton DB: Pharyngitis. Prim Care 23:719–739, 1996.

Perkins A: An approach to diagnosing the acute sore throat. Am Fam Physician 55:131–138, 1997.

Sloan PD: Sore throats. Consultant 22(5):110–127, 1982.

Todd JK: The sore throat: pharyngitis and epiglottitis. Infect Dis Clin North Am 2:149–162, 1988.

Vukmir RB: Adult and pediatric pharyngitis: a review. J Emerg Med 10:607–616, 1992.

CHAPTER 31

Swelling of the Legs

Swelling of one or both legs is a frequent presenting complaint. Common causes include systemic edema states such as *heart failure, nephrotic syndrome, cirrhosis, acute* and *chronic thrombophlebitis, chronic venous insufficiency, cellulitis, lymphedema,* and *drugs,* as well as mechanical factors such as *dependency* and *constricting garters or pantyhose.* Although the causes are numerous and the pathophysiology complex, diagnosis is simplified by determining whether one or both legs are involved, whether onset is sudden or gradual, whether pain is present, and whether other associated symptoms exist. **Certainly the most common cause of unilateral leg edema is chronic venous insufficiency, and the most common causes of bilateral leg edema are the systemic edema states, venous insufficiency, salt-retaining drugs, dependency, and primary lymphedema.**

Nature of Patient

Primary lymphedema is an inherited defect in the lymphatic system caused by hypoplasia, aplasia, or digitation of the lymphatic vessels. In the neonate, unilateral edema of a leg is termed *congenital lymphedema* and is caused by a form of primary lymphedema. If the swelling of the leg becomes apparent around 10 years of age, it is called *lymphedema praecox.* Traumatic thrombophlebitis, cellulitis, and *compartment syndromes* also cause unilateral leg edema in children. In children, bilateral leg edema usually is caused by a *systemic illness,* such as acute glomerulonephritis, nephrotic syndrome, hypoproteinemia, and primary lymphedema.

Unilateral or bilateral edema in adolescents or older women may be caused by constricting garments such as tight jeans, pantyhose, or rarely garters. In a runner, sudden onset of painful calf swelling suggests a *ruptured gastrocnemius muscle,* whereas intermittent pain and swelling of the upper or lower leg suggest a compartment syndrome.

In obese women, the development of bilateral leg swelling that spares the feet suggests *lipedema.* Lipedema occurs exclusively in obese women and is a bilateral and symmetric deposition of fat in the lower extremities. The foot is not involved in lipedema, whereas in lymphedema the swelling starts in the most distal part of the foot; this differentiates the two conditions.

In a chronic alcoholic, bilateral edema of the leg suggests edema caused by *cirrhosis,* with or without ascites. In a diabetic patient, unilateral and occasional bilateral swelling of the legs suggests *cellulitis,* especially if it is accompanied by warmth and tenderness. Leg swelling due to *venous insufficiency* is more common in women, and frequently there is a history of varicose veins in female relatives. In patients with *heart failure* or cirrhosis, bilateral leg edema is usually a manifestation of their systemic disease. In patients with *rheumatoid arthritis,* a painful unilateral swelling of the calf may result from a ruptured Baker's cyst, sometimes referred to as *pseudophlebitis.* A localized, pretibial swelling in a patient with tachycardia, exophthalmos, or other signs or symptoms of hyperthyroidism suggests *pretibial myxedema,* which is a rare finding in hyperthyroidism.

Unilateral swelling of the lower leg may be the presenting complaint in patients with *Kaposi's sarcoma,* which is more common in acquired immunodeficiency syndrome (AIDS).

Nature of Symptoms

Unilateral swelling of the lower or upper leg suggests local mechanical or inflammatory processes. These include *lymphedema, venous insufficiency* (the most common cause of unilateral leg edema), *thrombophlebitis, cellulitis, ruptured gastrocnemius muscle, compartment syndrome, ruptured Baker's cyst,* and rarely an acquired or inherited *arteriovenous fistula.* Bilateral leg swelling is most often caused by systemic conditions, including *congestive heart failure, nephrotic syndrome, cirrhosis, acute glomerulonephritis, salt-retaining drugs, constricting garments,* or *prolonged dependency* of the legs. Less common causes of bilateral leg swelling include *idiopathic edema, lipedema, primary lymphedema,* and exposure to *extremes of temperature.*

A sudden onset of calf swelling suggests a ruptured Baker's cyst, ruptured gastrocnemius, arterial occlusion, thrombophlebitis, cellulitis, or a compartment syndrome. Chronic bilateral swelling of the legs occurs in the systemic illnesses mentioned as well as in lymphedema, lipedema, lymphatic obstruction, chronic venous insufficiency, and cellulitis, which may be secondary to bilateral venous stasis dermatitis. The gradual onset of edema that starts in the distal part of the foot and involves the dorsum of the foot and ankle suggests lymphedema. **Painless unilateral leg edema in a woman over age 40 should make the physician suspicious of a gynecologic cancer with obstruction of the lymphatics, causing secondary lymphedema.**

Associated Symptoms

If warmth, redness, moderate pain, and tenderness to palpation are associated with calf swelling, cellulitis or thrombophlebitis is probable. The absence of pain does not eliminate the diagnosis of thrombophlebitis. If pain is associated with calf swelling, thrombophlebitis, compartment syndrome, arterial thrombosis, ruptured Baker's cyst, or ruptured gastrocnemius should be suspected.

Dyspnea on exertion, orthopnea, or paroxysmal nocturnal dyspnea suggests heart failure as the cause of leg edema. If spider angioma, palmar erythema, hepatomegaly, or jaundice is present in a patient with swollen legs, cirrhosis should be suspected. Patients with nephrotic syndrome often have generalized edema and swelling of the eyelids, which is particularly noticeable after prolonged recumbency. If leg swelling is absent or minimal after recumbency but develops as the day progresses, venous insufficiency is most likely.

Precipitating and Aggravating Factors

Prolonged sitting or standing may cause swelling of the lower extremities, particularly in patients with venous insufficiency. Garments such as jeans or pantyhose tight enough to impede venous return may also cause swelling of the legs. Patients may gain weight gradually so that their thighs are fatter yet are not recognized as such by the patient. The garments that previously fit adequately now impede venous return. Elastic knee bands may be used intermittently by patients with arthritis of the knee for pain relief and tendonesis. They can impede venous return and cause lower leg swelling. The physician should inquire about their use because they may not be worn at the visit.

Trauma to a vein resulting in thrombophlebitis may cause unilateral, painful swelling of the leg. Conditions such as pregnancy and large uterine fibroids that increase intraabdominal pressure may mechanically impede venous return and cause painless unilateral or bilateral swelling of the legs.

Fluid-retaining drugs such as estrogens, oral contraceptives, nonsteroidal antiinflammatory drugs (NSAIDs), psychotropic agents (lithium, tricyclic antidepressants), and vasodilators (calcium channel blockers, nitrates, prazosin, minoxidil) can cause fluid retention with minimal to moderate painless swelling of both legs. Other drugs that may give rise to bilateral gradual leg swelling include corticosteroids, progesterone, testosterone, methyldopa, hydralazine, and diazoxide.

Ameliorating Factors

Cessation of salt-retaining and vasodilating drugs will alleviate edema if these drugs were causal. Marked weight loss alleviates some of the swelling of lipedema. Support hose alleviate the edema of venous insufficiency. Muscle activity of the lower legs alleviates the edema of dependency. Edema due to a ruptured gastrocnemius or ruptured Baker's cyst gradually subsides, as does the edema from thrombophlebitis and cellulitis. Diuretics and aldosterone blocking agents often assist in the mobilization of edema in patients with cirrhosis, nephrosis, and heart failure.

Physical Findings

Physical examination of the legs should include inspection, measurement, and palpation. The lower leg should be examined, in the erect and recumbent position, for dilated superficial veins, perforators, and multiple small, superficial veins on the foot. The patient should be examined to determine the area of the swelling, which may be in the knee, the anserine bursa, or Cooperman's fat pad, none of which causes true edema of the lower extremity. Lipedema excludes the foot and is a deposition of fat in the leg, whereas lymphedema begins at the distal area of the foot and involves the dorsum of the foot with a so-called "hump."

The character of the skin in the area of edema is also diagnostically helpful. Typically, the patient may have pitting edema with acute deep vein thrombosis, chronic venous insufficiency, and systemic edema conditions, whereas the swelling of lymphedema and lipedema is nonpitting. Thick, taut, and fibrotic skin suggests that the causative process is chronic rather than acute. Redness or lymphangitic streaks suggest a cellulitis. Ecchymoses in the dependent part of the ankle associated with midcalf pain suggest a tear of the gastrocnemius muscle. Tenderness to palpation over the vein, warmth, low-grade fever, and a positive Homans' sign suggest thrombophlebitis. Painful swelling of one calf in a patient with the stigmata of rheumatoid arthritis and popliteal cyst on the opposite side suggests pseudophlebitis, a ruptured Baker's cyst.

Physical findings of systemic illnesses associated with swelling of the legs include pulmonary rales, distended neck veins, tachycardia, gallop rhythm, cardiac enlargement, heart failure, hepatomegaly, jaundice, ascites, palmar erythema, gynecomastia, spider angiomas, cirrhosis, hypertension, periorbital edema, nephrotic syndrome, peau d'orange skin, and lymphatic obstruction.

Diagnostic Studies

Although venography is the "gold standard" for the diagnosis of deep vein thrombosis, it is not necessary or advisable in all patients. Duplex ultrasonography or, if not available, Doppler ultrasonography can be used to confirm the diagnosis of venous thrombosis when invasive or radiographic procedures are contraindicated. Magnetic resonance imaging (MRI) has also been used in pregnant women to evaluate lower leg edema, but its use in the first trimester is not recommended.

A computed tomography (CT) scan can be used to determine the distribution of edema in instances of leg swelling: venous obstruction exhibits an increased cross-sectional area of muscle tissue and edema in the muscular and interstitial compartment; obesity and lipedema exhibit increased subcutaneous fat; lymphedema exhibits increased fluid in the interstitial space with a honeycombed pattern when the condition is chronic; and popliteal cysts exhibit an extension of fluid from the joint space to between the muscle planes.

Direct and indirect lymphangiography is used to visualize lymphatics, which are dilated in instances of congenital and acquired lymphatic obstruction, although lymphangiography has been replaced by CT scanning in most cases. Occasionally, lymphoscintigraphy is helpful in the evaluation of a swollen leg.

Differential Diagnosis of Swelling of the Legs

CAUSE	NATURE OF PATIENT	NATURE OF SYMPTOMS	ASSOCIATED SYMPTOMS	PRECIPITATING AND AGGRAVATING FACTORS	AMELIORATING FACTORS	PHYSICAL FINDINGS	DIAGNOSTIC STUDIES
Systemic							
Heart failure	Hypertension, coronary artery disease	Bilateral	Dyspnea on exertion Orthopnea Paroxysmal nocturnal dyspnea	Myocardial infarction		Pulmonary rales Distended neck veins Tachycardia Cardiac enlargement Gallop	Chest radiograph Echocardiogram
Cirrhosis	Alcoholic	Bilateral	Ascites Jaundice Abdominal swelling			Hepatomegaly, jaundice, ascites, gynecomastia	Abnormal liver function tests Liver biopsy
Nephrotic syndrome	Often children	Bilateral	Polyuria Eyelid swelling			Edema of eyelids, hypertension	Albuminuria Hypercholesterolemia Serum protein Electrophoresis
Hypoproteinemia	Malnourished	Bilateral					
Venous insufficiency	Usually female	Often unilateral	Minimal on arising		Recumbency	Varicose veins	
Thrombophlebitis		Usually unilateral, sudden onset of swelling with redness and pain	Pain, warmth, redness	Trauma Immobilization Childbirth Drugs (estrogen, oral contraceptives)		Tender cord Positive Homans' sign Warmth, low-grade fever	Duplex ultrasonography Venogram Doppler ultrasonography CT scan

Table continued on following page.

Differential Diagnosis of Swelling of the Legs *Continued*

CAUSE	NATURE OF PATIENT	NATURE OF SYMPTOMS	ASSOCIATED SYMPTOMS	PRECIPITATING AND AGGRAVATING FACTORS	AMELIORATING FACTORS	PHYSICAL FINDINGS	DIAGNOSTIC STUDIES
Mechanical							
Ruptured gastrocnemius	Runners	Sudden onset	Pain			Ecchymoses of ankle	CT scan
Baker's cyst	Rheumatoid arthritis		Arthritis				Arthrogram
Constrictive garments	Usually female		Painless	Weight gain	Weight loss	Fat thighs	
Dependency	After stroke		Impaired mobility	Venous insufficiency	Muscle activity of legs		
Lymphatic							
Congenital	Neonate	Unilateral					
Secondary lymphedema	Over age 40, usually female			Pelvic cancer Radiation		Peau d'orange skin, involves foot, dorsal hump	Lymphangiography
Lipedema	Obese, female	Bilateral	Obesity	Weight gain	Weight loss	Spares foot	
Salt-retaining drugs		Bilateral		Estrogen, oral contraceptives, NSAIDs, lithium, vasodilators			

Less Common Diagnostic Considerations

Lipedema is a bilateral, symmetric deposition of fat in the lower extremities that spares the foot. Spontaneous *venous thrombosis* occurs more frequently during pregnancy, parturition, surgical trauma, severe illness, polycythemia, malignant disease, multiple myeloma, and dehydration. *Retroperitoneal fibrosis* (most often induced by the antimigraine drug methysergide) can cause obstruction of lymphatic or venous drainage. The swelling may be unilateral or bilateral.

Erythema nodosum can cause unilateral or bilateral leg swelling. *Reflex sympathetic dystrophy* can cause unilateral leg swelling, but usually a precipitating factor exists, such as trauma, venous or arterial thrombosis, or infection. Pretibial *myxedema* occurs in patients with hyperthyroidism. Thrombosis of the iliac vein and iliac vein compression by a distended bladder are other rare causes of unilateral edema of the leg.

Cyclic or *idiopathic edema* occurs mostly in obese women and is usually bilateral. These patients can develop fluid retention of several pounds in a few days.

Selected References

Merli GJ, Spandorfer J: The outpatient with unilateral leg swelling. Med Clin North Am 79:435–447, 1995.

Ruschhaupt WF: Differential diagnosis of edema of the lower extremities. Cardiovasc Clin 13:307–320, 1983.

Ruschhaupt WF, Graor RA: Evaluation of the patient with leg edema. Postgrad Med 78:132–139, 1985.

Sachs MK: The optimum use of needle aspiration in the bacteriologic diagnosis of cellulitis in adults. Arch Intern Med 150:1907–1912, 1990.

Satiani B, Rustin R, Biggers K, Bordner L: Noninvasive diagnosis of deep venous thrombosis. Am Fam Physician 44:569–574, 1991.

Vaughan BF: CT of swollen legs. Clin Radiol 41:24–30, 1990.

Wheatley DC, et al: Lymphoscintigraphy and color Doppler sonography in the assessment of leg oedema of unknown cause. Br J Radiol 69:1117–1124, 1996.

Young JR: The swollen leg: clinical significance and differential diagnosis. Cardiol Clin 9:443–456, 1991.

CHAPTER 32

Urethral Discharge and Dysuria

Dysuria denotes burning or pain associated with urination and can have several causes. Frequency, hesitancy, urgency, and strangury (slow, painful urination) are other symptoms typically associated with micturition disorders. Urinary urgency occurs as a result of *trigonal* or *posterior urethral irritation* produced by inflammation, stones, or tumor; it most often occurs with *cystitis.* Acute inflammatory processes of the bladder cause pain or urgency when only a small quantity of urine is present in the bladder.

Frequency of urination, when due to bladder problems, occurs with either a decreased bladder capacity or with pain on bladder distention. Frequency is caused most frequently by lesions of the bladder or urethra, although diseases of the nervous system involving the bladder's nerve supply (either centrally as in tabes and multiple sclerosis or peripherally as in diabetic neuropathy) may produce bladder decompensation with voiding abnormalities. Urinary frequency may also be a manifestation of overflow incontinence; this can occur with either *prostatic hypertrophy* or *neurologic bladder disorders.*

Inflammatory lesions of the prostate, bladder, and urethra are the most common cause of dysuria and frequency and include *prostatitis* in men, *urethrotrigonitis* in women, and *bladder* and *urethral infections* in men and women. Both men and women may have *chronic inflammation of the posterior urethra.* In the United States, women with symptoms of lower urinary tract infections (UTIs) account for more than 5 million office visits per year; only 50% of these women, however, have classic cystitis with urine culture bacteria concentrations greater than 10^5 organisms per milliliter. **Several studies indicate that symptomatic women with urinary bacteria counts of fewer than 10^5 organisms per milliliter (female urethral syndrome) should be considered to have an infectious cause and be treated accordingly.**

About 2 million cases of urethritis (men and women) occur annually in the United States; more than 60% of these cases are nongonorrheal. *Nongonococcal urethritis* occurs five times more frequently than gonococcal urethritis, largely because of a decline in gonococcal urethritis. *Chlamydia,* which causes nongonorrheal urethritis, is a major cause of sexually transmitted disease and infertility in the United States. Because of the frequency of complaints of dysuria and urethral discharge, the associated public health problem, and the ease of treatment, it is essential that physicians be expert in recognizing the causes of these symptoms.

Nature of Patient

In children, *meatal stenosis* may cause recurrent lower UTIs. Up to 20% of children with urinary complaints may have some degree of meatal stenosis. Dysuria and urethral discharge are uncommon in children. When these symptoms occur in young girls, they frequently are caused by a *chemical vaginitis* or a *mechanical urethritis.* When these findings are seen in young boys, they are often secondary to a mechanical urethritis, which can result from continued jarring of the perineum from bicycle riding, horseback riding, a foreign body, or masturbation. *Sexually transmitted diseases* (STDs) must be considered in cases of urethritis or vaginitis that occur in boys or girls. If discovered in young children, child abuse is usually the cause.

Bacteriuria is rare in school-age boys and occurs in only 0.1% of men. The incidence of bacteriuria increases in men at age 50 years and rises to about 1% at age 60 and 4% to 15% in later years, coinciding with the onset of prostatic disease. Women under age 18 have a 5% incidence of asymptomatic bacteriuria.

Women between ages 15 and 34 account for most who present with symptoms of UTIs. A study in Great Britain showed that 20% of women in this age group developed dysuria and frequency. Dysuria in women is most frequently caused by *cystitis, interstitial cystitis, vaginitis, female urethral syndrome,* and *mechanical irritation of the urethra.* Dysuria in men is most often caused by *urethritis, prostatitis, cystitis,* and *mechanical irritation of the urethra.* Urethral discharge, which is essentially limited to men, is usually caused by *gonorrheal* or *nongonorrheal urethritis* (*Chlamydia* or *Trichomonas*).

Nature of Symptoms

Cystitis

In women who complain of frequency, urgency, and dysuria without clinical evidence of an upper UTI, *bacterial cystitis* is usually suspected. Several studies, however, have shown that 30% to 50% of women complaining of these symptoms do not have a positive urine culture according to traditional criteria (isolation of a pathogen in concentrations greater than 10^5 bacteria per milliliter of urine in a clean-voided specimen).

Several possible reasons exist for this. First, dysuria often represents a vaginal infection rather than a UTI. When carefully questioned, women with dysuria due to cystitis usually describe an internal discomfort, whereas women with dysuria due to vaginitis usually describe a more external discomfort; their burning sensation appears to be in the vagina or the labia and is caused by urine flow over an inflamed vaginal mucosa. **All women with dysuria should be questioned about an associated vaginal discharge or irritation.**

Second, many women who present with symptoms due to bacterial cystitis (dysuria, frequency) have colony counts of fewer than 10^5 bacteria. **Various**

studies have shown that if pathogens are found in a concentration of fewer than 10^5 per milliliter in symptomatic women, there is probably a significant bacterial infection.

Third, *Chlamydia trachomatis* is frequently the causative agent. Patients who are infected with this organism have symptoms and pyuria but a negative routine urine culture. Chlamydial infections of the bladder and urethra in women are somewhat analogous to nongonorrheal urethritis in men; in both, there is pyuria but no growth on routine culture. Although rare, *urinary tract tuberculosis* also may present with pyuria and a negative routine culture.

The physician must inquire about the duration and onset of symptoms. Longer duration and gradual onset of symptoms suggest a chlamydial infection, whereas a history of hematuria and sudden onset of symptoms indicates a bacterial infection. Dysuria that is more severe at the end of the stream, particularly if associated with hematuria, suggests *cystitis;* dysuria that is worse at the beginning of the stream is a sign of *urethritis.* Patients with the *female urethral syndrome* often have dysuria, frequency, suprapubic pain, onset of symptoms over 2 to 7 days, and some pyuria. Besides having dysuria, frequency, and suprapubic pain, patients with *cystitis* demonstrate symptoms that develop quickly—pyuria, bacteriuria, and positive urine cultures (Table 32–1). Fever, nausea, back pain, and leukocytosis are not common findings in either female urethral syndrome or cystitis.

Urethritis

Urethral discharge in male patients is accepted as objective evidence of *urethritis,* but patients may have urethritis without a significant urethral discharge. **If the patient has dysuria and more than four polymorphonuclear cells per high-powered field in a urethral smear, urethritis is probable.** Nongonorrheal urethritis is defined to include inflammations in men who have negative urethral

TABLE 32.1 Clinical Features of Female Urethral Syndrome and Cystitis

CLINICAL FEATURES	FEMALE URETHRAL SYNDROME	CYSTITIS
Dysuria, frequency, suprapubic pain	+	–
Fever, nausea, back pain, other systemic signs	–	–
Duration of symptoms (days)	2-7	1-2
Leukocytosis	–	–
Urinalysis:		
Pyuria	+ or –	+
Bacteriuria	–	+
Hematuria	–	+ or –
White blood cell casts	–	–
Urine cultures	–	+
Blood cultures	–	–

From Meadows JC: The acute urethral syndrome: diagnosis, management, and prophylaxis. Contin Educ, December 1983, pp 112–120.

cultures for *Neisseria gonorrhoeae* and a urethral discharge or more than four cells per field in the urethral smear. *Chlamydia trachomatis* is the most common isolate from patients with nongonorrheal urethritis (Table 32–2). Other causative organisms may include *Mycoplasma,* group D streptococci, *Trichomonas,* and rarely *Candida albicans.*

Although a significant number of patients with nongonorrheal urethritis are asymptomatic, most have mild dysuria and a minimal or absent urethral discharge. When a discharge does appear, it is usually clear or whitish. In contrast, about 80% of patients with gonorrheal urethritis have a moderate to heavy urethral discharge that is usually purulent. Dysuria with a mucoid or mucopurulent urethral discharge usually develops 1 to 3 weeks after coitus with an infected partner.

Urethral discharges are usually observed on awakening, after a long period without urination, or after penile stripping. Other symptoms include urgency, frequency, and meatal or urethral irritation. The usual presentation of nongonorrheal urethritis is a low-grade inflammation; the symptoms of gonorrheal urethritis tend to be more acute and more severe and include a urethral discharge that is purulent, spontaneous, and greater in volume. **It is important to recognize that a patient may have gonorrheal as well as nongonorrheal urethritis at the same time.** Both may be contracted simultaneously from the same contact.

Associated Symptoms

When hematuria accompanies dysuria, *cystitis* is most probable, although the possibility of a *tumor* or *stone* should be considered. If a middle-aged woman complains of recurrent dysuria associated with bladder pain, urgency, marked frequency, and nocturia, *interstitial cystitis* is most probable. The patient obtains some relief by voiding. Urine culture is usually sterile, and pyuria is absent. The diagnosis is made by cystoscopy.

If dysuria and frequency are associated with a high fever or chills, an upper UTI such as *pyelonephritis* may be present. When frequency and dysuria are associated with backache or costovertebral angle tenderness, *pyelonephritis* or *prostatitis* should be suspected. Patients who have prostatitis often present with an unexplained backache, with or without fever. The physician should perform a gentle rectal examination on any man who complains of frequency, dysuria, and fever to determine whether the prostate is tender to palpation. Pyelonephritis should be suspected if nausea and vomiting accompany dysuria. Patients who demonstrate prostatic enlargement or experience severe pain on micturition that causes them to resist voiding have outflow obstruction. This causes bladder distention, which may also induce nausea, vomiting, or mild ileus, resulting in abdominal distention.

Frequency of urination without discomfort on voiding may be caused by a *diminished bladder capacity, overflow incontinence,* or *habit* in patients with a

TABLE 32.2 Comparison Between *Chlamydia trachomatis* and *Neisseria gonorrhoeae* as Venereal Disease Agents

SUBJECT	*C. TRACHOMATIS*	*N. GONORRHOEAE*
Organism	Obligate intracellular parasite	Gram-negative diplococcus often found within cells (as leukocytes on Gram's stain)
Transmission	Venereal	Venereal
Incubation period	8–21 days	2–6 days (can be longer, up to 10–16 days in rare cases)
Major infection	Urethritis (men); cervicitis (women)	Urethritis (men); cervicitis (women)
Local complications	Yes: epididymitis, bartholinitis, urethral syndrome, salpingitis, others	Yes: same as for *C. trachomatis,* and others, including prostatitis
Systemic complications	Possibly: arthritis, perihepatitis, peritonitis, and endocarditis reported	Well known: gonococcal septicemia, with resultant arthritis, dermatitis, endocarditis, and meningitis; perihepatitis and peritonitis also reported
Pharyngitis	Yes	Yes
Conjunctivitis	Yes	Yes
Proctitis	Cultured from the rectum	Yes: common venereal infection in homosexuals
Maternal infection with effect on neonate or infant	Well known: inclusion conjunctivitis and pneumonia	Less well established
Carrier state	Recognized, especially in women; can last for months	Recognized, especially in women; can last for months
Reservoir	Cervix (male urethra a minor role)	Cervix (male urethra a minor role)
Treatment	Tetracycline (antibiotic of choice) Erythromycin, sulfonamides, streptomycin, and trimethoprim-sulfamethoxazole also effective Regimen of 14 days often used	Procaine penicillin, ampicillin, amoxicillin, tetracycline, or spectinomycin; probenecid used; shorter treatment regimen
Treatment of sexual contacts	Yes	Yes

From Greydanus DE, McAnarney ER: *Chlamydia trachomatis:* an important sexually transmitted disease in adolescents and young adults. J Fam Pract 10:611–615, 1980.

normal bladder. It also is observed in patients who pass a large volume of urine because of diabetes, hypercalcemia, hypokalemia, congestive heart failure, loss of renal concentrating capacity, or use of diuretics. The absence of nocturia in a patient with urinary frequency suggests that the increased frequency of urination may be of psychogenic origin. Rarely, this may result from a polyp or irritative lesion in the posterior urethra that is relieved by recumbency.

Testicular pain due to an *epididymitis* suggests a chlamydial infection, since this is the most common cause of epididymitis in young men.

Precipitating and Aggravating Factors

Patients who have multiple sexual contacts are more likely to develop an STD such as *gonorrheal* or *nongonorrheal urethritis* or *cervicitis.* An abrupt alteration in the frequency of ejaculation may result in symptoms of *prostatitis.* This often occurs on the patient's return from a vacation during which the frequency of intercourse and subsequent ejaculation was increased. The use of vaginal sprays, douches, and bubble baths (particularly in children) may induce a *chemical vaginitis* that may present with dysuria. It is important for the physician to ask women who complain of dysuria whether a vaginal discharge is present because, in the absence of a recognizable discharge, *vaginitis* is an unlikely cause of dysuria.

Ameliorating Factors

Some patients with *cystitis* believe that they can alleviate their pain by avoiding urination; they actually mean that the pain is made worse with micturition, particularly at the end of urination, when the inflamed bladder walls become apposed. Some symptoms of cystitis are ameliorated by warm tub baths. Patients who complain of persistent frequency, nocturia, terminal hematuria, and suprapubic pain relieved by voiding may have *chronic interstitial cystitis,* a condition that is most common in middle-aged women.

If *N. gonorrhoeae* is the offending organism, the symptoms of urethritis occasionally abate without treatment after a few months. In contrast, the symptoms of nongonorrheal urethritis, although low grade, usually persist if not treated appropriately.

Physical Findings

The physical findings of gonorrheal urethritis in men include a spontaneous urethral discharge or one that can be elicited by penile stripping. The most common physical finding in patients with dysuria due to cystitis is suprapubic tenderness to palpation or percussion. When dysuria is caused by vaginitis, a vaginal discharge is apparent on pelvic examination.

Diagnostic Studies

In men, *urethritis* is present if a urethral smear shows more than four polymorphonuclear cells per high-power field. All urethral discharges should be examined by Gram stain and culture. A culture should be obtained for *N. gonorrhoeae* and *Chlamydia.* Urine cultures should be obtained from all patients with symptoms of cystitis. In uncomplicated cases, some physicians use only reagent test strips, including the leukocyte esterase test strips, before beginning empiric antibiotic therapy. When sterile pyuria is demonstrated on routine culture, the urine should be cultured for *Chlamydia* and tuberculosis-causing species of *Mycobacterium.*

Laboratory tests are required to distinguish gonorrheal from nongonorrheal urethritis. Because it is frequently difficult to culture *Chlamydia,* physicians often diagnose nongonorrheal urethritis by establishing the presence of urethritis and then excluding gonorrheal infection by smear and culture. *Trichomonas vaginalis* and *C. albicans* are uncommon causes of urethritis and need not be considered at the initial visit. A Gram smear or a KOH preparation may help identify patients with candidal urethritis, and a saline wet-mount should be examined if trichomonal urethritis is suspected.

The following are considered indications for urologic evaluation: an initial UTI in a child, UTI in men, UTIs in pregnant women, recurrent UTIs (three per year) in women, severe acute UTIs suggesting upper tract involvement, and painless hematuria. Patients with symptoms of chronic cystitis with no apparent cause should have cystoscopic examination to rule out tumor and interstitial cystitis.

Less Common Diagnostic Considerations

Less common causes of dysuria and urinary frequency include genital herpes simplex virus, *Trichomonas* infection, and *Candida* urethritis. Rarely, frequency is an early symptom of a bladder tumor or carcinoma in situ of the bladder. Drug-induced cystitis is not usually recognized. Nonsteroidal antiinflammatory drugs (NSAIDs), especially tiaprofenic acid, are the most common offenders, but cyclophosphamide may also cause cystitis.

Relatively uncommon causes of urethritis include infections with *Mycoplasma hominis.* Urethritis secondary to *Mycoplasma* is most common in lower socioeconomic groups and in men and women who have multiple sexual partners. *Mycoplasma genitalium* is present in 26% of men with nongonococcal urethritis who are *Chlamydia* negative.

Another uncommon cause of urethritis is *Reiter's syndrome,* which frequently begins with a urethritis after sexual contact and is followed in a few days by conjunctivitis, mucocutaneous lesions (including balanitis), and arthritis. This type of urethritis is characterized by mucopurulent discharge and dysuria, but it may be asymptomatic. Sometimes Reiter's syndrome may be initiated by a gonorrheal urethritis. In such cases, the urethritis responds to penicillin, so that the purulent discharge disappears and is replaced by the less purulent, mucoid discharge of nonspecific urethritis.

Differential Diagnosis of Urethral Discharge and Dysuria

CAUSE	NATURE OF PATIENT	NATURE OF SYMPTOMS	ASSOCIATED SYMPTOMS	PRECIPITATING AND AGGRAVATING FACTORS	AMELIORATING FACTORS	PHYSICAL FINDINGS	DIAGNOSTIC STUDIES
Cystitis	Most common in women ages 15–34	Dysuria (worse at end of flow) Urgency Frequency "Internal" discomfort Acute onset of symptoms with bacterial infection	Hematuria Nocturia Fever	Meatal stenosis may cause recurrent UTI in children Drugs (e.g., NSAIDs, cyclophosphamide)	Avoidance of urinating Warm baths	Suprapubic tenderness to palpation or percussion Fever	Urine culture positive Cystoscopy Special test for *Chlamydia* Pyuria by urinalysis or leukocyte esterase test
Interstitial cystitis	Women ages 20–50	Dysuria Marked frequency of small volume of urine	Nocturia Bladder pain Urgency	Some relief of pain with voiding		Tenderness of bladder base	Urine culture: sterile Cystoscopy: Hunner's ulcers
Female urethral syndrome		Dysuria Urgency Frequency Gradual onset of symptoms over 2–7 days	Suprapubic pain			Suprapubic pain No fever	Minimal pyuria Urine culture usually negative

Table continued on following page.

Differential Diagnosis of Urethral Discharge and Dysuria *Continued*

CAUSE	NATURE OF PATIENT	NATURE OF SYMPTOMS	ASSOCIATED SYMPTOMS	PRECIPITATING AND AGGRAVATING FACTORS	AMELIORATING FACTORS	PHYSICAL FINDINGS	DIAGNOSTIC STUDIES
Vaginitis (see Chap. 33)	Candidiasis more common in diabetic patients	Dysuria "External burning"	Vaginal itching			Vaginal discharge on pelvic examination	KOH and saline wet mounts for *Candida* and *Trichomonas* Gram stain and culture for gonococci
Chemical vaginitis	Common cause of dysuria and urethral discharge in young girls	Dysuria "External burning" Urethral discharge (minimal)		Bubble baths Vaginal sprays and douches		Vaginitis	
Prostatitis	Men over age 50	Dysuria Frequency	Backache Fever Decreased or intermittent stream	Abrupt change in frequency of ejaculation (e.g., after a vacation)		May be costovertebral tenderness Prostate tender to palpation on rectal examination	Examination and culture of prostatic secretions
Meatal stenosis	Children	Dysuria Recurrent UTI symptoms					

Urethritis							
Gonorrheal	Most common in men	Sexually transmitted Urethral discharge is moderate to large, purulent, mucoid, or mucopurulent and develops 1–3 wk after coitus with infected partner Dysuria (worse at beginning of urine flow)		Sexual contact		Urethral discharge is spontaneous or elicited by penile stripping	Gram's stain and culture of urethral smear
Nongonorrheal (chlamydial or trichomonal)	Most common in men	Sexually transmitted Symptoms usually minimal or absent Discharge (if present) is observed on awakening, thin and clear or whitish Dysuria (ranges in severity) Urgency Frequency	Meatal or urethral irritant	Multiple sexual partners		Thin, scanty, and whitish Urethral discharge appears on penile stripping	Gram's stain and culture of urethral smear Special test for *Chlamydia* Saline wet mount for *Trichomonas*
Mechanical	Most common in young boys and girls	Dysuria Minimal urethral discharge		Horseback or bike riding Masturbation Foreign body			

Selected References

Bodner DR: The urethral syndrome. Urol Clin North Am 15:699–703, 1988.

Greydanus DE, McAnarney ER: *Chlamydia trachomatis:* an important sexually transmitted disease in adolescents and young adults. J Fam Pract 10:611–615, 1980.

Kiel DP, Moshowitz MA: The urinalysis: a critical appraisal. Med Clin North Am 71:607–624, 1987.

Komaroff AL: Urinalysis and urine culture in women with dysuria. Ann Intern Med 107:212–218, 1986.

Krieger JN: Trichomoniasis in men: old and new issues. Sex Transm Dis 22:83–96, 1995.

Kurowski K: The woman with dysuria. Am Fam Physician 57:2155–2163, 1998.

Lipsky BA: Urinary tract infections in men: epidemiology, pathophysiology, diagnosis, and treatment. Ann Intern Med 110:138–150, 1989.

Martin DH, et al: *Chlamydia trachomatis* infections in men with Reiter's syndrome. Ann Intern Med 100:207–213, 1984.

Maskell R: Broadening the concept of urinary tract infection. Br J Urol 76:2–8, 1995.

McNulty A, Bodsworth N: Urethral discharge in men. Aust Fam Physician 22:157–165, 1993.

Mobley DF, Baum N: Interstitial cystitis: when urgency and frequency mean more than routine inflammation. Postgrad Med 99:201–214, 1996.

Parrott TS: Cystitis and urethritis. Pediatr Rev 10:217–222, 1989.

Richardson DA: Dysuria and urinary tract infections. Obstet Gynecol Clin North Am 17:881–887, 1990.

CHAPTER 33

Vaginal Discharge and Itching

Vaginal discharge, which may be accompanied by vulvar itching or burning, is one of the most common problems seen in the physician's office. Usually, these symptoms indicate *bacterial vaginosis* (a polymicrobial superficial infection characterized by an increase in aerobic bacteria, especially *Gardnerella,* and a decrease in lactobacilli), *candidiasis* or *moniliasis (Candida albicans),* or *trichomoniasis* (*Trichomonas* infection). Other common causes of vaginal discharge include *acute cervicitis, gonorrhea,* and *herpes genitalis.*

Many discussions of vaginitis emphasize a "typical" appearance of the discharge: cheesy, frothy, or mucoid. Appearances, however, may be misleading. **In addition, 15% to 20% of patients in one series had two coexistent infections.** Other studies of patients with vaginitis have shown that 35% had bacterial vaginosis, 25% had candidiasis, and 20% had trichomoniasis. The remaining 20% had less common types of vaginitis.

Vaginitis, in contrast to cervicitis, is an inflammatory change of the vaginal mucosa in the absence of profuse discharge from the cervix. A vaginal discharge can be produced by cervicitis without a significant vaginal infection, as can be the case with *gonorrhea. Chlamydia* also causes a mucopurulent cervicitis.

Nature of Patient

Prepubertal Patients

Prepubertal girls may develop a vaginal discharge in association with *vulvovaginitis* or an *exocervicitis.* These young girls are particularly susceptible to vulvovaginitis because of the anterior location of the vagina, the proximity of the vagina to the anus, the lack of labial fat pads, a neutral to alkaline vaginal pH, a thin atrophic vaginal wall, and occasionally poor hygiene.

Trichomonal vaginitis is rare in children and in women over age 60 but does occur in neonates of infected mothers. Conversely, *candidal (monilial) vaginitis* can occur at any age but is uncommon in prepubertal girls unless they have been receiving antibiotics. It is a common cause of vulvovaginitis in children. In prepubertal girls, vulvovaginitis is more common than vaginitis. Vulvovaginitis can be caused by bubble baths, other chemical irritants, tight nylon panties, mixed bacterial infections, and foreign bodies.

Bacterial vaginosis is uncommon in premenarchal girls. **Gonorrheal infections**

in premenarchal children are rare but do occur. In such cases, sexual abuse must be suspected. Although a girl may be asymptomatic when a gonococcal infection is present, vulvovaginitis and exocervicitis are usually present.

Adolescents

After puberty, a vaginal discharge may be caused by physiologic factors, cervicitis, or vaginitis. Although *trichomonal vaginitis* and *candidal vaginitis* may occur in adolescents, the most common cause of vaginitis with discharge in adolescent girls is *bacterial vaginosis. Candida* infection is the second most common cause of specific leukorrhea in adolescents. There is a high and increasing incidence of chlamydial and gonococcal infections among postpubertal girls. Among young mothers, the growing prevalence of *Chlamydia trachomatis* may increase the incidence of this infection among neonates and some children. It is important to question the patient about genital or urinary tract infections (UTIs) in other family members (male or female) or sexual partners (male or female).

The physician must remember that *physiologic leukorrhea* may occur in menarchal girls. This is not usually profuse or associated with itching. Although these girls may be concerned about a vaginal discharge, they may not present with it as a chief complaint. Therefore, the physician should provide reassurance concerning this and other normal changes that may occur with menarche. The discharge that occurs just before and after menarche is often thick, grayish white, and odorless and has a pH of less than 4.5. No signs of inflammation exist because this discharge is a physiologic reaction to the initial phase of cyclic estrogen production.

Adults

In adult women of reproductive age, the common causes of vaginitis are bacterial vaginosis, *Candida,* and *Trichomonas,* in decreasing order of frequency. The three most common causes of cervicitis are *C. trachomatis, Neisseria gonorrhoeae,* and herpes simplex virus. In elderly, postmenopausal women, *senile atrophic vaginitis* often causes a discharge, as do other specific forms of vaginitis.

Nature of Symptoms

Vulvovaginitis in premenarchal girls usually causes only minor discomfort, which may include perineal pruritus, burning, and a discharge that may be profuse or scanty.

The duration and type of symptoms do not consistently distinguish the common infectious causes of vaginitis. Certain symptoms and findings, however, strongly suggest the diagnosis. For instance, although an acute onset of vaginal discharge or vulvar irritation indicates that a yeast infection is the probable cause, these symptoms are often unreliable. Likewise, a curdlike discharge (resembling cottage cheese) strongly suggests a yeast vaginitis; **however, the gross appearance is less sensitive and less specific in establishing the diagnosis than microscopic examination of the vaginal discharge.** A curdlike appearance virtually eliminates the possibility of trichomonal vaginitis, which usually produces a profuse, frothy, white or grayish green, malodorous discharge. The discharge from *trichomonal vaginitis* is typically described as frothy, whereas the discharge from bacterial vaginosis is described as homogeneous.

Because itching and burning may occur with virtually all forms of vaginitis, these symptoms are not particularly helpful in differentiating the cause. It is important to differentiate vulvar pain from vulvar itching. Itching is most prominent in *candidal vaginitis* and least prominent in bacterial vaginosis. Itching and burning are uncommon with *gonococcal infections,* but a significant percentage of patients with a gonococcal infection have a combined infection. They may have gonorrhea with their itching caused by *Trichomonas* or *Candida.*

Systemic causes of vulvar itching include diabetes that predisposes to candidiasis, liver disease, polycythemia, psoriasis, seborrheic dermatitis, and medications such as penicillin, ampicillin, and sulfa drugs.

If a vaginal discharge is sticky, brown, or yellowish and occurs in an elderly woman, *atrophic vaginitis* should be suspected.

Associated Symptoms

Dysuria may be a symptom of both a vaginal infection and a UTI. **Therefore, all women who complain of dysuria should be asked about the presence of a vaginal discharge or irritation or both.** About 30% of patients who have vaginitis but no evidence of UTI complain of dysuria. Usually, these patients complain of "external" dysuria (pain felt in the inflamed vaginal labia as the urinary stream passes) rather than "internal" dysuria (felt inside the body). Internal dysuria seems to correlate with UTIs, whereas external dysuria usually corresponds to vaginal infections.

Dyspareunia usually indicates vulvar disease rather than vaginitis. When dyspareunia is associated with a purulent discharge, *acute cervicitis* should be suspected. *Trichomonal vaginitis* is often associated with gonococcal or *Bacteroides* cervicitis. *Trichomonas* and *Chlamydia* may produce a vaginitis as well as a coexisting urethritis that causes dysuria and increased frequency. If dysuria, rectal infections, or pain on walking or climbing stairs is present, *gonorrhea* should be suspected.

If there are symptoms of diabetes or ingestion of birth control pills or antibiotics, *candidal vaginitis* is probable. Refractory fungal vulvovaginitis may be secondary to undiagnosed diabetes.

Precipitating and Aggravating Factors

Oral contraceptives, antibiotics, and pregnancy predispose the patient to *candidal vaginitis.* Uncontrolled diabetes and long-term use of tetracycline for acne increase the intestinal reservoir of *Candida,* which predisposes the patient to recurrent vaginitis. *Bacterial vaginosis* is common and increasing in incidence. It is most frequently spread through venereal contacts. *Trichomonal vaginitis* is usually transmitted by sexual intercourse; in children, however, it may be spread by direct nonsexual contact. The increasing incidence of venereal diseases such as gonorrhea, bacterial vaginosis, and trichomoniasis results from sexual activity in younger adolescents, multiple partners, and failure to use protective barrier contraceptives (e.g., diaphragms, condoms).

In young children and in some adults, inappropriate genital hygiene (e.g., wiping perineal region from back to front) may increase the incidence of recurrent vaginal infections. *Chemical vaginitis* is precipitated by douches, bubble baths, and vaginal sprays. It may be aggravated by powders and panties made of synthetic fibers.

Physical Findings

Physical examination should include thorough evaluation of the genital and pelvic areas. The appearance of the labia, vulva, entire vagina, and cervix should be noted, and the vaginal discharge should be inspected. *Nonspecific vaginitis,* which occurs particularly in premenarchal girls, usually does not extend above the lower one third of the vagina.

Atrophic vaginitis can occur in premenarchal girls, as can infections due to insertion of foreign bodies into the vagina. When atrophic vaginitis occurs in postmenopausal women, there is often a sticky, brownish vaginal discharge, and the vaginal mucosa is usually thick, pale, and smooth, demonstrating loss of normal rugosal folds.

The pelvic examination should include adnexal palpation and cervical manipulation so that the physician can determine whether any masses or points of tenderness exist. Adnexal tenderness and pain on motion of the cervix ("chandelier sign") suggest *pelvic inflammatory disease,* not merely cervicitis. When these findings occur in conjunction with a vaginal discharge, a *gonococcal infection* is probable. In such cases, if smear and culture are negative for gonorrhea, *Chlamydia* should be suspected and appropriately treated.

Diagnostic Studies

Ninety percent of patients with vaginitis can be classified into one of four major clinical categories on the basis of symptomatology, vaginal pH, and wet smear findings (Table 33–1).

In patients whose only symptom of vaginitis is vaginal discharge, a Gram stain is not indicated because it is not specific. However, if a patient has a purulent discharge from the cervical os and a Gram stain that reveals more than three polymorphonuclear leukocytes per high-power field, a chlamydial or gonococcal infection is likely. Intracellular gram-negative diplococci are highly specific for a gonococcal infection. False-positive results are rare. A Gram stain is recommended

TABLE 33.1 Classification of Vaginitis

TYPE OF VAGINITIS	SYMPTOM	pH	WET SMEAR FINDINGS
Candidiasis (moniliasis)	Pruritus	<4.5	Hyphae or spores
Bacterial vaginosis	Malodorous	>4.7	"Clue" cells
Trichomoniasis	Profuse discharge	5.0–6.0	Protozoa, white blood cells
Atrophic vaginitis	Discharge	7	Parabasal cells

whenever there is purulent discharge from the cervical or urethral os. **Simultaneous chlamydial infections are present in 30% to 50% of patients with cervical gonococcal infections.**

In some populations with a high prevalence of asymptomatic gonococcal carriers, a cervical culture for *N. gonorrhoeae* on Thayer-Martin medium is considered appropriate whenever a patient has a pelvic examination. It certainly should be performed in any woman with a purulent discharge from the cervical os or urethra.

In all patients with a vaginal discharge, saline and KOH wet mounts should be examined. The saline mount should be inspected for "clue cells" (epithelial cells with bacilli adherent to their surface), which are virtually pathognomonic of *bacterial vaginosis.* The pH range of secretions in patients with bacterial vaginosis is usually greater than 4.7. A positive "whiff test" (presence of a fishy or amine odor when 10% KOH is added to a sample of the discharge) also indicates bacterial vaginosis.

The saline wet mount is the most reliable laboratory test for confirmation of the motile protozoan *Trichomonas.* It should be done as soon as possible after the specimen is obtained. The pH of the vaginal secretions in patients with *Trichomonas* infection ranges from 4.9 to 6.0.

The best test for detection of candidal vaginitis is microscopic examination of the discharge in a KOH preparation; this will show the *Candida* mycelia. The pH in patients with candidal (monilial) vaginitis is less than 4.5. Cultures, though most sensitive, should be reserved for certain circumstances because 15% to 20% will be positive in asymptomatic healthy women.

Less Common Diagnostic Considerations

Increased physiologic leukorrhea has a pH of less than 4.5, an absence of yeast and *Trichomonas,* and a culture with a preponderance of *Lactobacillus.* Dermatoses (e.g., psoriasis, seborrheic dermatitis) and infestations with parasites (e.g., amebiasis, pinworms, lice) can cause vaginal discharge in rare cases. Allergy to nylon underwear and feminine deodorants, sprays, and douches may cause a vulvovaginitis leading to vaginal discharge or itching. Vaginal and cervical neoplasms can cause a serosanguineous discharge. Poor anal and vulvar hygiene also may produce vaginal discharge and itching. Tuberculosis is a rare cause of vulvovaginitis. In

Differential Diagnosis of Vaginal Discharge and Itching

CAUSE	NATURE OF PATIENT	NATURE OF SYMPTOMS	ASSOCIATED SYMPTOMS	PRECIPITATING AND AGGRAVATING FACTORS	PHYSICAL FINDINGS	DIAGNOSTIC STUDIES
Vulvovaginitis *Candida* Chemical irritants Douches Vaginal sprays Bubble baths Bacteria Foreign bodies	Most common cause of vaginal discharge in prepubertal girls	Variable discharge (scanty to profuse) Perineal pruritus Burning	May be "internal" dysuria		Vulvovaginitis does not usually extend above lower third of vagina Thin atrophic vaginal wall	
Physiologic discharge	Menarchal girls	Discharge: thick, grayish white, odorless, but not profuse No pruritus		Beginning estrogen effect occurs just before or after menarche	No signs of inflammation	pH of discharge <4.5
Candidiasis (moniliasis)	Any age Common cause of vulvovaginitis in children Common during reproductive years	Acute onset of discharge or vulvar irritation Discharge is often curdlike (resembles cottage cheese) Pruritus prominent	May be "external" dysuria	Diabetes Antibiotics Oral contraceptives Pregnancy	Vaginitis	Saline or KOH wet mount: hyphae or spores Vaginal pH <4.5

Trichomoniasis	Common cause of vaginal discharge in women of child-bearing age Rare in children Rare in women over age 60 May occur in neonates of infected mothers	Discharge usually profuse, frothy, gray-greenish, malodorous Varying degrees of pruritus	May be associated with gonococcal or *Bacteroides* infection Urethritis may cause dysuria and frequency	Often sexually transmitted Multiple sex partners	Vaginitis Vaginal petechiae Mucosal inflammation	Vaginal pH >6.0 Saline wet mount: white blood cells and motile protozoa
Bacterial vaginosis	Most common cause of vaginitis in adolescents Common during reproductive years Rare in premenarchal girls	Discharge is malodorous but not usually frothy Pruritus not prominent	Urethritis may cause dysuria and frequency	Change in vaginal secretions at menarche Sexually transmitted Multiple sex partners	Vaginal mucosa not inflamed Adherent grayish white discharge	Saline wet mount: "clue" cells Vaginal pH >4.7 Positive "whiff test"
Gonorrhea	Increased incidence in neonates of infected mothers Rare in premenarchal girls (if present, sexual abuse must be suspected)	Itching and burning uncommon Purulent cervical discharge Pelvic pain Fever	Dysuria Rectal infection (often asymptomatic) Pain on walking or climbing stairs	Symptoms often worse near time of menstrual period Sexually transmitted	Cervicitis and cervical discharge Pain with cervical manipulation Adnexal tenderness	Intracellular gram-negative diplococci Positive culture Chlamydial infections common
Chlamydia infection			Dysuria	Sexually transmitted	Cervicitis and cervical discharge Pain with cervical manipulation	Tests for chlamydia Often coexists with cervical gonococcal infections

Table continued on following page.

Differential Diagnosis of Vaginal Discharge and Itching *Continued*

CAUSE	NATURE OF PATIENT	NATURE OF SYMPTOMS	ASSOCIATED SYMPTOMS	PRECIPITATING AND AGGRAVATING FACTORS	PHYSICAL FINDINGS	DIAGNOSTIC STUDIES
Herpes genitalis	Usually sexually active adolescents Less frequently patients over age 35 years	Pain can be excruciating Vulvar pruritus uncommon Burning Vulvar tenderness	Dyspareunia Dysuria	Secondary *Streptococcus* or *Candida* infection	Cervicitis Widespread clusters of vesicles over vulvar and perineal areas, vagina, and cervix *Herpetic lesions:* Affect vulva and adjacent areas Begin as vesicles Progress in 5–10 days to shallow, painful ulcers Ulcers last 3–10 days Recurrent Do not usually produce vaginitis	Tzanck smear
Senile atrophic vaginitis	Elderly women	Discharge is sticky, brown, or yellowish		Loss of estrogen effect	Vaginal mucosa: thin, pale, smooth (from loss of rugosal folds)	Vaginal pH 7.0 Parabasal cells

premenarchal girls, particularly young children, coliform bacterial infections may produce vaginitis. This is usually a low-grade, somewhat chronic infection and may be associated with pinworm infestation or insertion of a foreign body into the vagina. Retained tampons and other foreign objects occasionally may be found in adults.

Herpes genitalis is a relatively uncommon cause of vaginal discharge (although a common cause of cervicitis), but it is increasing in frequency. It is most common in adolescents and appears less frequently in patients over age 35. Herpetic lesions, which can be excruciating, affect not only the vulva but also adjacent areas (thighs, buttocks, vagina, and cervix). The lesions begin as vesicles that progress in 5 to 10 days to shallow, exquisitely painful ulcerations with a clear, watery discharge. The ulcers last for 3 to 10 days and are prone to secondary infections, especially *Streptococcus* and *Candida.*

Unfortunately, genital herpes is often recurrent; some patients experience repeated flare-ups for many years. The presenting symptoms may include pain, vulvar pruritus, burning, and frequently extreme vulvar tenderness that makes intercourse unbearable. Micturition also may be excruciating. Examination reveals widespread clusters of vesicles that may involve the vulvar and perineal areas as well as the vagina and cervix. The physician must remember that herpes does not usually produce vaginitis, although it may infect the vagina and cervix. A Tzanck smear from the base of the vesicle is a simple, definitive diagnostic test.

Rarely, what appears to be a clear, gelatinous vaginal discharge in infants may be due to leakage of absorbent jelly material from the new generation of diapers that contain this chemical substance to increase the absorptive capacity.

Selected References

Biswas MK: Bacterial vaginosis. Clin Obstet Gynecol 36:166–176, 1993.

Carr PL, Felsenstein D, Friedman RH: Evaluation and management of vaginitis. J Gen Intern Med 13:335–346, 1998.

Eschenbach DA, Hillier SL: Advances in diagnostic testing for vaginitis and cervicitis. J Reprod Med 34(8 suppl):555–564, 1989.

Farrington PF: Pediatric vulvovaginitis. Clin Obstet Gynecol 40:135–140, 1997.

Fox KK, Behets FM-T: Vaginal discharge: how to pinpoint the cause. Postgrad Med 98:87–104, 1995.

Hammill HA: Unusual causes of vaginitis (excluding trichomonas, bacterial vaginosis and *Candida albicans*). Obstet Gynecol Clin North Am 16:337–345, 1989.

Majeroni BA: Bacterial vaginosis: an update. Am Fam Physician 57:1285–1289, 1998.

Schneider GT: Vaginal infections: how to identify and treat them. Postgrad Med 73:255–262, 1983.

Sobel JD: Vaginal infections in adult women. Med Clin North Am 74:1573–1603, 1990.

Woodruff JD: Vulvar disease: a spectrum of clinical pictures. Postgrad Med 73:232–245, 1983.

CHAPTER 34

Vision Problems

Patients may think that discomfort in the eyes or noticeable redness is serious. **Visual symptoms, however, are always more serious than nonvisual ones.** Blurred vision is the most common visual complaint, but it is often the most difficult visual symptom to evaluate. Other common vision problems include diplopia, "floaters," "stars," or light flashes, and visual blurring associated with pain or eye soreness. A correct diagnosis requires knowing the patient's age and deciding whether symptoms are unilateral or bilateral, whether onset is sudden or gradual, and whether symptoms are constant or intermittent. The prevalence of severe visual impairment is increased in elderly patients. **In all instances, visual acuity must be determined by using a Snellen chart.**

The most common causes of visual symptoms include *refractive errors, contraction of the vitreous, migraine, acute angle-closure glaucoma, cataracts, dry eyes, drug side effects,* and *transient ischemic attacks* (TIAs).

Nature of Patient

In young patients the most common cause of visual blurring is *refractive error.* The two most frequent refractive errors are *myopia* (nearsightedness) in teenagers and *presbyopia* (loss of accommodation) in patients about age 40 when glasses become necessary for reading. Scintillating scotomas, another common visual problem in adolescents and adults, are experienced by patients with *migraine* as a prodrome to their headache. Some patients note only the scintillating scotoma but do not develop a headache, a condition known as *ophthalmic migraine,* also called "migraine sans migraine."

The remainder of the common visual symptoms listed in the introduction generally occur in older adults. *Cataracts, glaucoma,* "floaters," light flashes, *senile macular degeneration, TIA, drug side effects,* and *dry eyes* occur almost exclusively in elderly patients. Older women often develop dry eyes, which may result in visual blurring sometimes associated with a sense of grittiness and warmth in the eyes. In elderly patients a sudden onset of painless unilateral blurred vision often associated with a relative central scotoma and visual distortion suggests *senile macular degeneration,* the most common cause of blindness after age 55.

Two neuroophthalmologic vascular emergencies occur in elderly patients: temporal arteritis and third nerve palsy. *Temporal arteritis* presents as a transient (in some cases progressive) unilateral visual loss often associated with visual field defects. Temporal arteritis is twice as common in elderly women as in elderly men. Patients with *third nerve palsy* present with a sudden onset of diplopia with pain around the eye or diffusely in the head. Since approximately 20% of these elderly patients have an aneurysm causing the third nerve palsy, their cases must be investigated promptly.

Nature of Symptoms

The physician must inquire whether the blurred vision (1) is equal or unequal in each eye, (2) is unilateral or bilateral, (3) is constant or intermittent, (4) is present for near or distant vision or both, (5) had a sudden or gradual onset, and (6) has improved or worsened since it was first noted. Monocular blurring, particularly of sudden onset, is more likely to be serious and of ocular origin. If the blurring is binocular and has occurred gradually over months in an otherwise healthy individual, a *refractive error* is most likely.

In an elderly patient, when primarily distant vision is blurred, the cause is most often *cataracts,* but if near vision mainly is affected, a *retinal circulatory disturbance* or *macular degeneration* should be suspected. Monocular blurring of sudden origin (days or weeks) is generally not a refractive error. In some patients, monocular blurring due to a refractive error may be longstanding but only recently noted.

Episodic blurring is virtually never caused by a refractive error. In older adults it can result from *glaucoma, multiple sclerosis* (MS), or *TIAs.* Brief episodes of blurred vision or loss of vision, usually monocular but occasionally binocular, are typically caused by transient impairment of retinal circulation resulting from *atherosclerotic emboli* from the carotid circulation or heart, *carotid insufficiency,* or *vertebrobasilar insufficiency.* Patients with the latter condition may have transient diplopia, blurring accompanied by dizziness, or both. Episodic blurring due to carotid insufficiency is often referred to as *amaurosis fugax.* Since 11% of these patients develop permanent visual loss, they should be investigated promptly.

Several types of visual auras are experienced by patients with *migraine. Scotomas* are areas of indistinct or totally obscured vision. A *negative* scotoma is a circumscribed, obscured region in the visual field that appears translucent or as a dark or shimmering area. Negative scotomas most often begin in the central region of the visual field and then expand across the visual field, sometimes encompassing part of the right or left field. Homonymous hemianopsia may be present, or the vision may be totally obscured. Vision may also be obscured by *positive* scotomas, which are often described as bright, shimmering, shooting, or scintillating lights. These also occur initially in the center of the visual field, then expand to fill the entire visual field.

When transient blurring (with associated pain and redness) occurs unilaterally in older patients, *acute angle-closure glaucoma* should be suspected. The sudden loss of central vision in one eye and ocular pain without redness suggest *optic neuritis.* Fifty percent of patients with optic neuritis eventually develop *MS.* Optic neuritis preceding MS is virtually always unilateral, and the blurring may last several days. Ischemic neuropathy, often due to *giant cell arteritis,* usually presents with variable blurring and superior or inferior field defects. Visual loss is usually permanent.

Patients often confuse *diplopia* (double vision) with *blurred vision.* Patients with diplopia see two separate objects either side by side or one above the other. Most diplopia in adults is caused by paralysis or weakness in one or more of the extraocular muscles. This paralysis may be caused by *trauma, cerebrovascular lesions, MS, thyroid disease, myasthenia gravis,* or *brain tumors.* Diplopia due to *strabismus* is most common in children and leads to eyes that fail to coordinate. Patients may have intermittent exotropia or esotropia. Young children with these symptoms usually suppress one image and therefore do not complain of double vision. Diplopia due to strabismus is more common in adults when the angle of their squint changes.

Diplopia may be monocular or binocular as well as constant or intermittent. Patients with *monocular* diplopia experience double vision with one eye occluded. It is most often the result of *lens opacities.* A slightly *dislocated lens* associated with *trauma* or *Marfan's syndrome* is a rare cause of monocular diplopia. Monocular diplopia in an otherwise healthy individual should suggest the possibility of *hysteria.*

Constant *binocular* diplopia may be caused by *head trauma* or pathology involving the extraocular muscles or their cranial nerves. If total third nerve palsy exists and the pupil is involved, an *aneurysm* is probable.

After blurring, the next most common visual complaints are spots floating in the visual field and light flashes. Floaters and flashes are caused by *contraction of the vitreous* and occur in middle-aged and older patients. *Light flashes* are usually noted in the temporal field, particularly when the patient is in the dark or in poorly illuminated areas. Flashes are caused by the vitreous shrinking away from the retina and thus stimulating it. *Vitreous floaters* are produced when the vitreous pulls away from the retina, thus detaching particles suspended in the vitreous. Patients describe these as black spots in the visual field when they look at a bright background such as the sky or a light-colored wall. Neither light flashes nor vitreous floaters are serious, but they should be investigated by an ophthalmologist because they may signal *retinal detachment.* Likewise, if a peripheral field defect occurs after the patient experiences light flashes and a shower of floaters, *retinal detachment* should be suspected, and the patient should be examined by an ophthalmologist.

Halos around lights are a common symptom in patients with *acute angle-closure glaucoma.* The rapid development of a relative central scotoma associated with visual distortion is often caused by *senile macular degeneration.*

Associated Symptoms

If blurred vision or diplopia occurs intermittently and is associated with dizziness, *TIAs* involving the vertebrobasilar system must be suspected. When an older patient complains of difficulty in driving at night because of glare from headlights or difficulty with daytime driving in bright sunlight, *cataracts* may be present. If blurred vision is associated with halos around lights, pain in the eye, and headache, *glaucoma* is most probable, particularly in elderly patients. With *acute narrow-angle glaucoma* the eye often is red and nausea and vomiting occur. When intermittent or progressive monocular blurring occurs in an elderly patient and is associated with a nocturnal headache, *temporal arteritis* should be suspected, particularly if there is tenderness to palpation over the temporal artery. Elderly patients who are visually impaired often have an associated restriction of mobility.

When visual disturbances are associated with pain in the eye, iritis and acute glaucoma must also be considered. Pain in the eye without visual symptoms or redness suggests a neurologic etiology such as *trigeminal neuralgia.* Since most serious causes of red eye do not affect both eyes at once, monocular redness is more a portent of serious disease than is binocular redness. When a red eye is associated with pain in the eye, *iritis, glaucoma, periorbital cellulitis,* and *corneal abrasion* must be considered. Photophobia and a red eye suggests iritis, *keratopathy,* or glaucoma. A sudden onset of blurred vision in both eyes can be precipitated by sudden changes in the blood sugar, such as occurs in diabetic patients. Although a sudden onset of blurred vision in both eyes can occur with established diabetes, it also could be the initial symptom of *diabetes mellitus.*

Precipitating and Aggravating Factors

Many drugs, including anticholinergic, antihypertensive, and psychotropic agents, can cause blurred vision by interfering with *accommodation.* The chronic administration of corticosteroids or phenothiazines predisposes to *cataract* formation, which causes visual blurring. Antihistamines that decrease tear formation as well as hot, dry environments may aggravate the condition of patients with dry eyes. Visual hallucinations and *metamorphopsia* can be caused by *hallucinogenic agents.* Patients with *digitalis toxicity* may report yellow vision or complain that everything seems to be covered with snow. Drugs, particularly those that dilate the pupil, may precipitate *acute angle-closure glaucoma* and its associated symptoms of pain, redness, and blurred vision.

Amaurosis fugax can be caused by a decrease in blood pressure from drugs, arrhythmias, or decreased cardiac output, or by emboli from diseased carotid arteries. Chocolate, red wine, or vasodilator medications may precipitate the visual auras of migraine with or without a headache. Decreased illumination may aggravate the impaired vision associated with *cataracts.*

Ameliorating Factors

Improvement of visual acuity by looking through a pinhole indicates that retinal function is good and that the visual problem is caused by a *refractive error.* If diplopia is improved by occluding one eye, the cause may be paralysis or weakness of the extraocular muscles. This weakness may in turn be caused by *neuropathy,*

MS, thyroid disease, myasthenia gravis, diabetes, trauma, or an intracerebral process such as a *tumor* or an *aneurysm.* If increasing illumination improves vision, a cataract is probable. If the patient notes that dimming lights or looking beside the object improves vision, *macular degeneration* should be suspected.

Physical Findings

It is essential to evaluate visual acuity by using a Snellen chart. If visual acuity is decreased, the test should be repeated with the patient looking through a pinhole made in a paper card. If this improves visual acuity, a *refractive error* is present. The conjunctivae should be examined for redness, which would suggest an inflammatory or allergic process as well as glaucoma. *Acute glaucoma* may cause corneal edema or corneal haziness.

The patient should be tested for a *relative afferent pupillary defect* (RAPD). This test is performed by having the patient look into the distance and then shining a light into one eye, thus eliciting pupillary constriction in that eye and consensual constriction in the other eye. The light is then quickly moved in front of the other pupil, which normally should constrict further. If this additional constriction does not occur and the pupil dilates instead, RAPD is present. This test must be repeated several times. The presence of RAPD requires further investigation by an ophthalmologist. If RAPD is absent, as it should be, unilateral *optic nerve disease* or widespread *retinal damage* is unlikely. For example, RAPD is absent in *macular degeneration* and *cataracts* but is present with *chronic glaucoma, retinal detachment,* and *optic neuritis.* The size and shape of the pupil should also be evaluated. In *acute glaucoma* the pupil is vertically oval.

When the eye is not inflamed and no RAPD exists, *cataracts, vitreous opacities,* and *macular degeneration* are possible. If a white eye (absence of red eye) and RAPD are present, *chronic glaucoma* should be suspected. In addition, chronic glaucoma should be considered with excessive deepening of the optic disc and narrowing of the peripheral field. If chronic glaucoma is suspected, peripheral fields should be checked because patients may have advanced narrowing of their visual fields without being aware of it. Tonometry may be diagnostic.

When *senile macular degeneration* is present, funduscopic examination may reveal *drusen* (discrete, round yellow spots of retinal pigment in the region of the macula). Neovascularization and other signs of *diabetic retinopathy* may also be seen. Schirmer's test may reveal decreased tear production in patients with *dry eyes.*

Diagnostic Studies

Tests to rule out systemic disease include complete blood count (CBC); thyroid studies to rule out *hyperthyroidism,* which may give rise to certain oculomotor palsies); and determination of blood sugar and glycosylated hemoglobin to diagnose *diabetes,* which may give rise to *refractive errors, diabetic retinopathy,* and rarely *oculomotor palsies.*

Differential Diagnosis of Vision Problems

CONDITION	NATURE OF PATIENT	NATURE OF SYMPTOMS	ASSOCIATED SYMPTOMS	PRECIPITATING AND AGGRAVATING FACTORS	AMELIORATING FACTORS	PHYSICAL FINDINGS	DIAGNOSTIC STUDIES
Refractive errors Myopia Presbyopia	Teenagers Older than 40 years	Blurred vision: bilateral, gradual onset	Glasses needed for reading		Looking through pinhole improves visual acuity		**Determination of visual acuity using Snellen chart in *all* patients**
Cataracts	Older adults	Blurred vision, especially distant vision		Poor illumination	Increased illumination	Lenticular opacification RAPD absent	
Senile macular degeneration	Older adults	Blurred vision, especially near vision Unilateral at first Painless	Central scotomata Visual distortion Often blindness		Dark environment Looking next to object	RAPD absent Drusen near macula	
Glaucoma Acute angle closure	Older adults	Usually monocular blurring, which is often episodic	Ocular pain and redness Halos around lights Nausea and vomiting	Dark environment Drugs that dilate pupils		Red eye, corneal edema, or haziness RAPD present Pupil vertically oval	Tonometry
Chronic						White eye RAPD present Deep optic disc Narrowing of peripheral visual fields	Tonometry

Table continued on following page.

Differential Diagnosis of Vision Problems *Continued*

CONDITION	NATURE OF PATIENT	NATURE OF SYMPTOMS	ASSOCIATED SYMPTOMS	PRECIPITATING AND AGGRAVATING FACTORS	AMELIORATING FACTORS	PHYSICAL FINDINGS	DIAGNOSTIC STUDIES
Dry eyes	Usually older women	Bilateral visual blurring	Pain, soreness, gritty feeling in eyes	Antihistamines Hot and dry environment		Decreased tear formation	Schirmer's test
Transient ischemic attacks	Older adults	Episodic monocular visual blurring and/or diplopia	Dizziness			Decreased carotid pulsation or bruit	Carotid Doppler studies
Drug side effects	All ages but more common in older adults as they take more medications	Bilateral visual blurring Dry eyes	Dry mouth	Anticholinergics Antihypertensives Psychotropic drugs		Impaired accommodation Pupils may be dilated	
Contraction of vitreous	Middle-aged and older adults	Floaters and/or light flashes Usually unilateral and of sudden onset		Floaters usually seen when looking at bright background Light flashes usually noted when in dark environment		RAPD absent Vitreous opacities	
Migraine	All ages Often a family history of bad headaches	Scotomata, often scintillating and as prodrome to headache	Headache (sometimes absent) Nausea, vomiting	Stress Vasodilator drugs Certain foods Menstruation			

An erythrocyte sedimentation rate (ESR) and temporal artery biopsy should be performed if *temporal arteritis* is suspected.

Less Common Diagnostic Considerations

Brain tumors and *aneurysms* may cause central vision defects as well as oculomotor palsies. Certain drugs have toxic effects on various parts of the eye, thus impairing vision, whereas other drugs such as anticholinergics and psychotropic drugs may impair accommodation. *Central* and *branch retinal artery occlusions* are persistent equivalents of *amaurosis fugax*. Acute and painless loss of vision most often result from *carotid atherosclerosis*, in which pieces of the atheromatous plaques migrate to the retinal arteries. These conditions are much more common in elderly hypertensive patients with hyperlipidemia and prior myocardial infarction.

Giant cell arteritis, which usually affects the temporal artery, can also affect the vertebrobasilar system, giving rise to diplopia and dizziness. Rarely, *cavernous sinus syndromes* and *third nerve palsies* are caused by aneurysms. Both aneurysms and ischemic conditions can cause *oculomotor nerve palsy*.

Selected References

Bajart AM: Common eye problems in the older woman. Women Health 10:85–93, 1985.

Barton JJ, Corbett J: Neuro-ophthalmologic emergencies in the elderly. Clin Geriatr Med 7:525–548, 1991.

Belmont W: Some common visual symptoms: what they mean and what to do about them. Occup Health Nurs 29:21–24, 1981.

Bryant WM: Common toxic effects of systemic drugs on the eye. Occup Health Nurs 29:15–17, 1981.

Gardiner PA: ABC of ophthalmology: evaluating common signs and symptoms. Br Med J 1:389–393, 1979.

Gregor ZJ: Blurred vision. Br J Hosp Med 33:105–109, 1985.

Hara JH: The red eye: diagnosis and treatment. Am Fam Physician 54:2423–2430, 1996.

Kaufman DM, Solomon S: Migraine visual auras: a medical update for the psychiatrist. Gen Hosp Psychiatry 14:162–170, 1992.

Maino JH: Visual deficits and mobility: evaluation and management. Clin Geriatr Med 12:803–823, 1996.

Trudo EW, Stark WJ: Cataracts. Postgrad Med 103:114–126, 1998.

CHAPTER 35

Voiding Disorders and Incontinence

Voiding disorders and incontinence are common disorders of micturition that present to the physician. They occur more frequently in elderly persons; currently, about 15% of Americans are over age 65.

Voiding dysfunction is the rule rather than the exception in elderly men. Signs and symptoms of *benign prostatic hypertrophy* have been found in about 70% of elderly patients. **Incontinence is so frequent in women that many patients consider it normal.** Decreased bladder capacity and involuntary bladder contractions have been found in as many as 20% of continent elderly persons. About 10% to 20% of community-dwelling elderly patients have *urinary incontinence* severe enough to be considered a social or health problem. Large-scale studies have reported that one third of people over age 60 occasionally experience an involuntary loss of urine. An even larger percentage of hospitalized and institutionalized elderly patients are troubled with incontinence.

Childhood enuresis (bed-wetting), whether primary or secondary, should be considered a symptom rather than a specific diagnosis. Most cases represent *primary enuresis,* a maturational delay that occasionally is familial. Secondary enuresis occurs when a child who has been continent develops enuresis. *Secondary enuresis* may result from emotional stress (e.g., birth of a sibling, beginning school) or urinary tract infection (UTI). In these children, bacteriuria may cause uninhibited bladder contractions. Most children with nocturnal or daytime incontinence (99%) do not have an anatomic abnormality but rather a disturbance in urodynamics, such as bladder instability.

Nature of Patient

Enuresis is common until about ages 4 to 5 years. **Most children with voiding disturbances do not have anatomic or neurologic disease causing their enuresis.**

Voiding dysfunction is common in elderly men. The amount of prostatic enlargement does not necessarily correlate with the symptoms of *prostatism.* Some young men without prostatic enlargement on rectal examination have symptoms of prostatism, the so-called trapped prostate.

Incontinence is more common in women than in men. It occurs more frequently in multiparous and menopausal women and in confused patients and those with limited mobility. Age-related changes in bladder function include decreased capacity, increased residual urine, increased involuntary bladder contractions (detrusor muscle instability), and increased nocturnal urine production. **Incontinence has been reported in 26% of women during their reproductive years, but in the postmenopausal years the incidence is 30% to 40%.**

Nature of Symptoms

The symptoms of *prostatism* can be divided into two categories: obstructive symptoms (e.g., weak stream, abdominal straining, hesitancy, intermittency of stream, incomplete emptying, terminal dribbling) and irritative symptoms (e.g., frequency, nocturia, urgency). Some patients have symptoms of prostatic enlargement and also have symptoms related to unstable detrusor muscle contractions. The symptoms of *benign prostatic hypertrophy* often wax and wane spontaneously probably because of changes in dynamic factors, which include bladder tone, bladder neck obstruction, and tone in the prostate and prostatic capsule.

An abrupt onset of symptoms of stress or urge *incontinence* suggests *infection.* The gradual onset of symptoms of stress incontinence, particularly after menopause or oophorectomy, suggests *estrogen deficiency.* When the amount of urine leakage is small to moderate and coincides with increased abdominal pressure, stress incontinence is probable. Large amounts of urine and incontinence associated with the sensation of a full bladder suggest detrusor muscle instability. A precipitous loss of large quantities of urine unrelated to increased abdominal pressure suggests involuntary detrusor contractions, as does incontinence associated with an extreme desire to void because of pain, inflammation, or a sense of impending micturition. Moderate dripping suggests a partially incompetent outlet, overflow, or congenital or acquired anomalies. A bladder diary over a few days, noting leakage frequency, voiding intervals, activity or sensation with leakage, and amount and type of fluid intake, is often helpful in determining the cause of incontinence.

In children the symptoms of functional voiding disorders include increased or decreased frequency of urination, urgency, dysuria, nocturnal enuresis, daytime wetting after toilet training is completed, fever, abdominal pain, perineal pain, constipation, and encopresis. The severity and presence of symptoms vary so much that children with the same voiding disorder frequently have different symptoms. The most common symptoms are increased frequency and urgency. *Dysuria* may be caused by bladder dysfunction without infection, although *UTI* should always be suspected.

Associated Symptoms

Microscopic or gross hematuria, from rupture of blood vessels coursing over an enlarged prostate, often occurs in patients with *prostatic hypertrophy.* Cystoscopy or intravenous pyelography is indicated to rule out a stone or cancer. *Infection, neurologic disease,* and *bladder carcinoma* may produce hematuria and other symptoms similar to those of benign prostatic hypertrophy. In addition, gradual obstruction from prostatic enlargement or carcinoma may lead to a large, distended bladder with overflow incontinence. Urinary retention is more common when symptoms of prostatism develop in less than 3 months or when secondary to drugs. Urinary retention is less common when symptoms develop gradually. Recurrent *cystitis* occurs more frequently in patients with persistent residual urine due to an atonic bladder, cystocele, prostatic hypertrophy, or diabetes mellitus.

Table 35–1 shows some of the factors that help in differentiating unstable bladder contractions from stress incontinence. Nocturia is rare in stress incontinence but occurs frequently with detrusor instability. Urgency and frequency occasionally occur in patients with stress incontinence but are the rule in patients with detrusor instability. Voluntary inhibition of incontinence is frequently present in patients with stress incontinence but is less probable in patients with detrusor muscle instability.

Precipitating and Aggravating Factors

Stress incontinence may be precipitated or aggravated by coughing, lifting, exercising, and position change. Incontinence caused by detrusor muscle instability may be precipitated or aggravated by the urge to void, a full bladder, or position change. Detrusor muscle instability is aggravated by bladder wall inflammation and estrogen deficiency.

Drugs that may precipitate or aggravate stress incontinence include methyldopa, prazosin, phenothiazines, diazepam, caffeine, and diuretics. Drugs that may precipitate urinary retention include alpha-adrenergic agents, calcium channel blockers, anticholinergics, androgens, and sympathomimetic agents such as ephedrine and pseudoephedrine. Psychotropic and sedative agents may diminish alertness and facilitate or precipitate urinary incontinence. Some autonomic agents precipitate incontinence, whereas others precipitate urinary retention.

TABLE 35.1 Comparison of Presenting Symptoms in Patients with Genuine Stress Incontinence and Detrusor Instability

SYMPTOMS	GENUINE STRESS INCONTINENCE	DETRUSOR INSTABILITY
Precipitating factor	Cough, lifting, exercise, position change	Preceding urge, position change
Timing of leakage	Immediate	Delayed
Amount of leakage	Small → large	Large
Voluntary inhibition	Frequently	Possibly
Urgency, frequency	Occasionally	Yes
Nocturia	Rarely	Yes
Spontaneous remission	No	Occasionally

From Horbach NS: Problems in the clinical diagnosis of stress incontinence. J Reprod Med 35:751-756, 1990.

Ameliorating Factors

The symptoms of *prostatism* may spontaneously diminish without appreciable change in the size of the prostate. The symptoms and degree of obstruction vary over time despite the absence of change in prostatic size. Cessation of drugs that aggravate urinary retention or incontinence alleviates symptoms. Discontinuing or reducing the intake of fluids, caffeine, and alcohol may also alleviate symptoms of *incontinence.* Systemic and local estrogens often improve the symptoms of stress incontinence, although they may not have been administered for that reason. Antibiotics may improve *cystitis,* and thereby reduce detrusor instability. Improvement in mental status or mobility of the patient often ameliorates the symptoms of incontinence.

Physical Findings

Examination of patients with voiding disorders or incontinence must include assessment of their mental and neurologic status, mobility, and general health. Prostatic enlargement may be detected by rectal examination, although symptoms of bladder outlet obstruction may occur without prostatic enlargement being appreciated. In these patients, trapped prostate or median bar obstruction may be detected only by cystoscopic examination. It may be helpful to observe voiding.

Neurologic examination may provide clues to sensory or motor dysfunction of the bladder, which is under the control of the second to fourth sacral nerves (S2, S3, S4). Flexion and extension of the ankle, knee, and hip against resistance, as well as assessment of rectal sphincter tone, should be performed to assess whether S2–S4 are intact.

Pelvic examination should be performed to assess the patient's estrogen status and presence of a cystocele. The urethra, trigone, and vaginal area are all estrogen dependent. A large, distended bladder may be detected on physical examination, although more sophisticated tests are needed to assess the amount of residual urine. The typical patient with urge incontinence has a postvoid residual of less than 150 ml, whereas residual of greater than 500 ml suggests overflow incontinence.

Diagnostic Studies

Patients with voiding disturbances or incontinence may have increased residual urine. Postvoid residual urine can be assessed by abdominal ultrasonography using serial, noninvasive measurements. Likewise, residual can be determined by catheterization, transabdominal ultrasonography, and postvoid films taken after intravenous pyelography. The Q-tip test provides information on the mobility of the urethrovesical junction in the evaluation of stress incontinence. It is positive if the Q-tip inserted in the urethra moves 30 degrees or more from the horizontal with coughing or straining. Incontinent patients should have a urinalysis to rule

Differential Diagnosis of Voiding Problems and Incontinence

CONDITION	NATURE OF PATIENT	NATURE OF SYMPTOMS	ASSOCIATED SYMPTOMS	PRECIPITATING AND AGGRAVATING FACTORS	AMELIORATING FACTORS	PHYSICAL FINDINGS	DIAGNOSTIC STUDIES
Benign prostatic hypertrophy	Common in older men	Nocturia Dribbling Hesitancy Decreased force of stream Incomplete emptying	Hematuria	Prostatitis Residual urine Alcohol Anticholinergics Decongestants Sympathomimetics Antidepressants	Occasional spontaneous remission of symptoms	Enlarged prostate Distended bladder	Ultrasound for prostate size and residual volume Intravenous urography Cystoscopy Urinalysis Creatinine level
Stress incontinence	Multiparous and menopausal women Postprostatectomy men	Small-quantity incontinence with cough, sneezing, laughing, and running	Recurrent cystitis	Cystitis Laughing Coughing Upper respiratory infections		Weakness or laxity of pelvic floor or urethral sphincter Atrophic vagina in elderly women	Urinalysis Residual volume Creatinine level
Urge incontinence (unstable detrusor contractions)	Elderly men more than women Poststroke Dementia	Uncontrolled urge to void Large-quantity incontinence	Unable to delay voiding long enough to reach toilet	Cystitis Urethritis Bladder calculi Alcohol Diuretics			Cystometry Urodynamics Uroflowmetry Videourodynamics

Overflow incontinence	Multiple sclerosis Severe benign prostatic hypertrophy Atonic bladder Diabetic neuropathy Tabes dorsalis	Small-quantity incontinence, nearly continuous dribbling		Medications, including anticholinergics and sympathomimetics Prostatitis in patients with prostatic hypertrophy		Distended bladder Anatomic bladder obstruction from benign prostatic hypertrophy or stricture Spinal cord disease Diabetic neuropathy	
Functional incontinence	Impaired mobility or mental status Dementia	Can void normally with assistance		Deterioration in mental or physical status	Toilet training	Severe mental or physical disability preventing normal toilet habits Normal lower urinary tract function	
Enuresis	Children older than age 5, generally not significant if <4½ yr	Bed-wetting while sleeping	Very sound sleep	Emotional stress Urinary tract infections	Usually spontaneous improvement after age 5	Usually normal	Urinalysis and culture Urodynamics Ultrasound for hydroureteronephrosis or residual urine (rarely)

out infection or hematuria. The stress test, in which the patient (with a full bladder) coughs in both the erect and the recumbent position, is also useful.

Cystoscopy allows visualization of the bladder wall and determination of the degree of urethral obstruction. Trabeculation of the bladder wall suggests chronic obstruction. Urodynamic studies assess urine flow and force of the stream. Cystometry measures filling pressures and detrusor tone to evaluate bladder function. Videourodynamics combines video of voiding with the simultaneous measurement of intravesicular, perivesicular, and rectal pressure. Transrectal prostatic ultrasonography can be used to determine prostate size and presence of prostatic nodules. It can be used to guide prostatic biopsies. Prostate-specific antigen (PSA) is helpful in screening for prostatic cancer.

Less Common Diagnostic Considerations

Dysfunctional voiding with *vesicoureteral reflux* may occur in young children.

Multiple sclerosis, spinal cord disease, tumors, trauma, syphilis, and diabetic neuropathy can all cause voiding disorders as well as incontinence, usually overflow incontinence. Urethral stricture, dyssynergic bladder neck contracture, prostate cancer, chronic prostatitis, and bladder cancer may cause symptoms similar to those of benign prostatic hypertrophy. Urethrovaginal prolapse or prolapse of a large cystocele may cause urethral obstruction.

Nocturnal polyuria syndrome, more common in elderly patients, causes an increased volume of urine and increased frequency of micturition at night.

Selected References

Bowen LW: Voiding dysfunction. Obstet Gynecol Clin North Am 16:869–882, 1989.

Busby-Whithead J, Johnson TM: Urinary incontinence. Clin Geriatr Med 14:285–295, 1998.

Bushman W: Evaluation and treatment of urinary incontinence in the adult. Compr Ther 20:224–231, 1994.

Casale AJ: Functional voiding disorders of childhood. J Ky Med Assoc 91:185–191, 1993.

Christensen MM, Bruskewitz RC: Clinical manifestations of benign prostatic hyperplasia and indications for therapeutic interaction. Urol Clin North Am 17:509–516, 1990.

Horbach NS: Problems in the clinical diagnosis of stress incontinence. J Reprod Med 35:751–757, 1990.

Jolleys J: Urinary incontinence. Practitioner 237:630–633, 1993.

Knapp PM: Identifying and treating urinary incontinence. Postgrad Med 103:279–294, 1998.

Koff SA: Evaluation and management of voiding disorders in children. Urol Clin North Am 15:769–775, 1988.

Krissovich MT, Safran R: Urinary incontinence in adults. Prim Care 1:361–381, 1997.

Kupansuu E: Patient history in the diagnosis of urinary incontinence and determining the quality of life. Acta Obstet Gynecol Scand Suppl 166:15–18, 1997.

McLorie FA, Husmann DA: Incontinence and enuresis. Pediatr Clin North Am 34:1159–1174, 1987.

Ouslander JG, Bruskewitz R: Disorders of micturition in the aging patient. Adv Intern Med 34:165–190, 1989.

Pannill FC: Urinary incontinence for the primary care physician. Conn Med 57:299–308, 1993.

Parulkar BG, Barrett DM: Urinary incontinence in adults. Surg Clin North Am 68:945–963, 1988.
Ruff CC, Reaves EL: Diagnosing urinary incontinence in adults. Nurse Pract 14:8–18, 1989.
Saxton HM: Urodynamics: the appropriate modality for the investigation of frequency, urgency, incontinence and voiding difficulties. Radiology 175:307–316, 1990.
Smith RA, Wake R, Soloway MS: Benign prostatic hyperplasia. Postgrad Med 83:79–85, 1988.
Weiss BD: Nonpharmacologic treatment of urinary incontinence. Am Fam Physician 44:579–586, 1991.

CHAPTER 36

Weight Gain and Weight Loss

Weight Gain

The most common cause of weight gain is *increased caloric intake,* regardless of what the patient states. Recent studies have investigated causes of obesity other than excessive caloric intake. Rather than defining obesity simply as excessive weight for height and build (greater than 30 kg/m^2), it is better to define it as an abnormally high deposition of fat. This is best measured with calipers and body mass index (BMI).

Weight gain due to *fluid retention* occurs in patients with the nephrotic syndrome, congestive heart failure (CHF), or cirrhosis with ascites; these patients have clear signs of edema. *Hypothyroidism* can lead to decreased metabolic needs and to weight gain, but for significant weight gain to occur, hypothyroidism must be pronounced, and it is usually clinically apparent. A *low resting metabolic rate* contributes to obesity in some individuals. *Physiologic weight gain* occurs as a result of pregnancy and premenstrual fluid retention. Commonly prescribed *drugs* (e.g., steroids, antidepressants) can cause weight gain by promoting salt and water retention or by stimulating appetite.

Nature of Patient

Although the most common type of obesity in children is exogenous, this diagnosis requires that endocrine and genetic causes of obesity be considered. Children with *exogenous obesity* often show accelerated or at least normal linear growth and may reach puberty early. **Most children with endogenous obesity are short for their age and have other associated abnormalities. All obese children with short stature should be evaluated promptly and carefully.** Obesity in adolescents correlates directly with the amount of time spent watching television.

Patients who are obese have no distinguishing characteristics other than excessive weight. Although fat people are said to be "jolly," they may experience *depression,* which can be either the result of their being overweight or the cause of their overeating. Some patients with mild depression due to seasonal affective disorder have a carbohydrate craving. Their mood improves after carbohydrate ingestion.

Familial obesity probably represents an acquired propensity to overeat; various family members are short and obese. Their obesity tends to be proximal but can have a generalized distribution.

Weight increase in patients with *edema syndromes* (e.g., cirrhosis, nephrosis, CHF) usually is accompanied by symptoms that suggest a deteriorating clinical status.

Nature of Symptoms

Patients may present complaining of weight gain, uncontrollable appetite, inability to diet, or too-tight garments. The weight gain associated with fluid retention in the *premenstrual period* usually is described as bloating and often is accompanied by breast tenderness, breast swelling, or finger swelling. Some patients with *hypothyroidism* comment that their skin seems puffy or that they are unable to lose weight on diets that previously resulted in weight loss.

Associated Symptoms and Ameliorating Factors

Sudden, marked changes in weight that occur over 1 to 2 days usually are related to changes in fluid balance. Changes may range from a few pounds gained because of premenstrual edema or salt-retaining drugs to many pounds added as the result of cyclic edema. The weight gain of *premenstrual edema* usually dissipates after menstruation. Patients usually can alleviate fluid retention that occurs with *cyclic edema* by maintaining a recumbent posture for 48 to 72 hours. The weight gain caused by *salt-retaining drugs* is not continuously progressive; it levels off after a weight increase of several pounds.

When weight gain is progressive and the patient appears to be obese without evidence of edema, it is reasonably certain that the patient's weight gain is caused by *overeating.* Some patients with profound obesity complain of fatigue, which may result from *obstructive sleep apnea.*

Precipitating and Aggravating Factors

Weight gain results from ingestion of more calories than are metabolized. Thus, although weight gain usually is related to increased caloric intake, it also can be produced by reduction of either physical activity or metabolic rate. These weight changes occur gradually.

Although most people eat less when they are tense or upset, 15% to 25% respond to stress with increased caloric intake, or *reactive hyperphagia.* These patients often are overweight. They eat excessively when they are depressed or anxious and likewise celebrate good times with elaborate meals.

Drug ingestion is an important factor in weight gain. *Steroids, nonsteroidal antiinflammatory drugs* (NSAIDs), *phenylbutazone,* and *lithium* may cause fluid retention and produce a weight gain of several pounds. *Oral contraceptives* increase weight by causing fluid retention, increasing appetite, and creating an anabolic effect. *Psychotropic agents* (e.g., tricyclic antidepressants, some phenothiazines) may produce a carbohydrate craving in patients taking these drugs. In addition, when antidepressant drugs alleviate the anorexia of depression, a pronounced weight gain may occur. *Propranolol* may cause weight gain through its induction of hypoglycemia. Smoking cessation may contribute to weight gain equivalent to approximately 200 to 300 kilocalories per day.

Physical Findings

In obese patients, adipose tissue usually is generally distributed but occasionally is proximally concentrated in the extremities. Proximal obesity associated with a "buffalo hump," hirsutism, hypertension, or diabetes suggests *Cushing's disease.* Marked weight gain due to *edema* usually is associated with pitting edema of the legs, ascites, gallop rhythm, or, in the nephrotic syndrome, swelling of the eyelids and facial edema.

The physical findings of *hypothyroidism* may include somewhat coarse, dry skin; coarse hair; loss of the outer third of the eyebrows; a low, hoarse voice; an enlarged thyroid; and "hung-up" ankle jerks (delayed contraction and relaxation phase of deep tendon reflexes). The hung-up ankle jerk is often more readily detected when the patient kneels on a bed, chair, or examining table with the feet extended over the edge. Tapping the Achilles tendon with a reflex hammer may show a prompt contraction phase but a more readily perceived slowed relaxation phase.

Diagnostic Studies

Although hypothyroidism is an uncommon cause of obesity, it is readily diagnosed by thyroid function tests.

Less Common Diagnostic Considerations

Endogenous causes of obesity are rare but usually can be diagnosed by other associated findings. Several causes are associated with short stature. *Pseudohypoparathyroidism* is characterized by short stature, short metacarpals, hypocalcemia, and occasionally mental retardation. The *Prader-Willi syndrome* is characterized by short stature, mental retardation, and hypogenitalism. *Laurence-Moon-Biedl syndrome* is characterized by short stature, mental retardation, hypogonadism, and retinal pigmentation.

Other rare causes of obesity that are not particularly associated with short stature include *Cushing's syndrome* and *insulinomas.* Patients with insulinomas invariably have symptoms of hypoglycemia. Patients with hypothalamic tumors may present with obesity, but other findings usually are suggestive of an intracranial tumor. Cyclic edema is more common in women than in men. Postencephalitic obesity, tumors of the third ventricle, obesity that develops after cerebral trauma, and certain brain tumors (e.g., chromophobe adenomas, craniopharyngiomas) are other rare causes of hyperphagia.

Weight Loss

Unexplained weight loss of greater than 5% within 6 to 12 months suggests underlying pathology. It is important to differentiate *anorexia* (loss of the desire to

Text continued on page 409.

Differential Diagnosis of Weight Gain

CAUSE	NATURE OF PATIENT	NATURE OF SYMPTOMS	ASSOCIATED SYMPTOMS	PRECIPITATING AND AGGRAVATING FACTORS	AMELIORATING FACTORS	PHYSICAL FINDINGS
Physiologic factors Pregnancy	Females of reproductive age	Amenorrhea				Enlarged uterus
Premenstrual fluid retention	Menstruating females	Premenstrual weight gain	Breast tenderness Swelling Finger swelling	End of menstrual cycle	End of menstruation	Swelling of extremities Tender, swollen breasts
Excessive caloric intake (Most common cause of weight gain)	Patients who overeat	Gradual, progressive weight increase	Children: normal linear growth, may reach puberty early Adults: depression or psychological dependency on food	Increased stress (reactive hyperphagia) Environmental inducement	Decreased caloric intake Increased caloric needs	No evidence of edema Obesity generally distributed (may have proximal concentration)
Drugs	Users of Steroids NSAIDs Phenylbutazone Lithium Antipsychotics Antidepressants Propranolol Oral contraceptives				Cessation of drug	

Table continued on following page.

Differential Diagnosis of Weight Gain *Continued*

CAUSE	NATURE OF PATIENT	NATURE OF SYMPTOMS	ASSOCIATED SYMPTOMS	PRECIPITATING AND AGGRAVATING FACTORS	AMELIORATING FACTORS	PHYSICAL FINDINGS
Edema syndromes						
Nephrotic syndrome Congestive heart failure Cirrhosis (with ascites)		Weight increase may be sudden and rapid (over 24–48 hours)	Edema Signs of deteriorating clinical status Signs of primary condition			Depends on primary disease Edema (may be pitting in legs) Periorbital edema Gallop rhythm Ascites
Metabolic causes						
Hypothyroidlism		Patient unable to lose weight on previously successful plan	Constipation Intolerance of cold weather Skin is puffy, coarse, and dry			Enlarged thyroid "Hung-up" ankle jerk Coarse hair Loss of outer third of eyebrows Low, hoarse voice
Cushing's disease		Proximal obesity	Diabetes Proximal obesity			"Buffalo hump" Hirsutism Hypertension

Differential Diagnosis of Weight Loss

CAUSE	NATURE OF PATIENT	NATURE OF SYMPTOMS	ASSOCIATED SYMPTOMS	PRECIPITATING AND AGGRAVATING FACTORS	AMELIORATING FACTORS	PHYSICAL FINDINGS
Aging	Elderly people	Anorexia	Occasional dyspepsia	Poverty Depression Drugs Inadequate caloric intake	Increased caloric intake	Decreased lean body mass
Depression	All ages, especially elderly people	Dysphoria Anorexia	Insomnia Fatigue Decreased libido Sleep disorders	Loss of any type	Antidepressants Improved social situation	Depressed affect
Systemic diseases, especially cardiopulmonary, infectious, metabolic		Those of underlying disease	Dyspnea Edema Fatigue Fever	Deterioration of underlying disease		Those of underlying disease

Table continued on following page.

Differential Diagnosis of Weight Loss *Continued*

CAUSE	NATURE OF PATIENT	NATURE OF SYMPTOMS	ASSOCIATED SYMPTOMS	PRECIPITATING AND AGGRAVATING FACTORS	AMELIORATING FACTORS	PHYSICAL FINDINGS
Medications	Users of:			Drug administration Increased dosage	Cessation of drug	
	Sedatives		Drowsiness			
	Antidepressants		Dry mouth			
	Clonidine		Drowsiness			
	Diuretics		Cramps			
	NSAIDs		Indigestion			
	Theophylline		Nausea			
	Digoxin		Nausea			
	ACE inhibitors		Distortion of taste			
	Antibiotics					
	Thyroid supplements		Nervousness			
	Levodopa					
	Chemotherapeutic agents		Nausea and vomiting			
Cancer		Anorexia	Those of the cancer			Those of underlying disease
AIDS	More common in young men		Recurrent infections			Adenopathy

ACE, Angiotensin-converting enzyme.

eat) from true weight loss, although true weight loss results from anorexia when caloric intake is substantially reduced. Involuntary weight loss is caused most frequently by cancer, depression, gastrointestinal (GI) *disorders, dysphagia,* and *social factors.*

Significant weight loss may occur in patients with anorexia secondary to psychological, cardiac, pulmonary, hepatic, renal, and metabolic diseases as well as drug ingestion. *Drugs* may decrease appetite by causing nausea, vomiting, abdominal discomfort, and delayed gastric emptying or through central nervous system effects. Weight loss is often the presenting symptom in patients with cancer (most common cause of unexplained weight loss) and chronic infectious processes. Weight loss with anorexia occurs often in patients with *depression, anxiety, anorexia nervosa,* and *GI disorders,* including malabsorption, regional enteritis, granulomatous colitis, ulcerative colitis, chronic liver disease, and carcinoma of the stomach and pancreas.

Weight loss may occur with a normal appetite and adequate intake in patients with *diabetes mellitus, acquired immunodeficiency syndrome* (AIDS), *hyperthyroidism,* and *decreased intestinal absorption* (e.g., sprue, short bowel syndrome, parasitic infestation, inflammatory bowel disease). In their zest to decrease fatness, athletes may develop food aversion and experience weight loss.

Anorexia and weight loss occur frequently in elderly people. The many causes range from loose dentures and poverty to drug ingestion, metabolic disease, and cancer cachexia. Robbins (1989) described the "nine d's" of weight loss in elderly patients: dentition, dysgeusia, dysphagia, diarrhea, disease (chronic), depression, dementia, dysfunction, and drugs. The most common causes are *psychiatric diseases, cancer, drugs,* and *benign upper GI disease.*

Selected References

Alemany M: The etiologic basis for the classification of obesity. Prog Food Nutr Sci 13:45–66, 1989.

Fernstrom MH: Drugs that cause weight gain. Obes Res 3(suppl 4):435S–439S, 1995.

Gazewood JD, Mehr DR: Diagnosis and management of weight loss in the elderly. J Fam Pract 47:19–24, 1998.

Kalucy RS: Drug induced weight gain. Drugs 19:278–288, 1980.

Morley JE, Silver AJ, Miller DK, Rubenstein LZ: The anorexia of the elderly. Ann NY Acad Sci 575:50–59, 1989.

Olsen-Noll CG, Bosworth MF: Anorexia and weight loss in the elderly: causes range from loose dentures to debilitating illness. Postgrad Med 85:140–144, 1989.

Reife CM: Involuntary weight loss. Med Clin North Am 79:299–313, 1995.

Richmond DA, Blyer EM, Linscheid TR: The obese child. Am Fam Physician 28:129–134, 1983.

Robbins LJ: Evaluation of weight loss in the elderly. Geriatrics 44:31–34, 37, 1989.

Willard MD: Obesity: types and treatment. Am Fam Physician 43:2099–2108, 1991.

Wurtman JJ: Disorders of food intake: excessive carbohydrate snack intake among a class of obese people. Ann NY Acad Sci 499:197–202, 1987.

Index

Page numbers in *italics* refer to illustrations; page numbers followed by t refer to tables.

C

F

J

N

Q

R

S

T